1989

The International Handbook of Health-Care Systems

The International Handbook of Health-Care Systems

EDITED BY

Richard B. Saltman

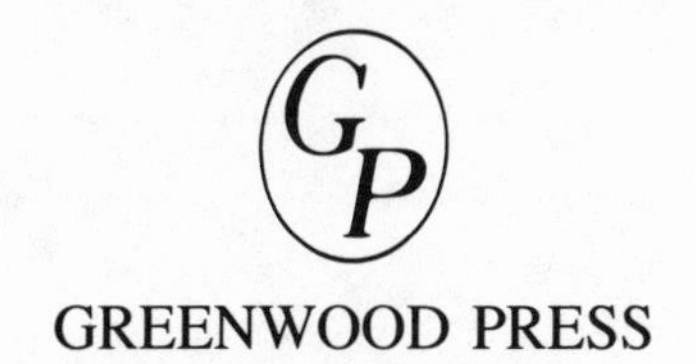

GREENWOOD PRESS

New York
Westport, Connecticut
London

Library of Congress Cataloging-in-Publication Data

The International handbook of health-care systems.

Bibliography: p.
Includes index.
1. Medical care. 2. Social medicine. 3. Medical policy. 4. World health. I. Saltman, Richard B.
RA393.I58 1988 362.1 87-17797
ISBN 0-313-24111-2 (lib. bdg. : alk. paper)

British Library Cataloguing in Publication Data is available.

Library of Congress Catalog Card Number: 87-17797
ISBN: 0-313-24111-2

First published in 1988

Greenwood Press, Inc.
88 Post Road West, Westport, Connecticut 06881

Printed in the United States of America

The paper used in this book complies with the Permanent Paper Standard issued by the National Information Standards Organization (Z39.48–1984).

10 9 8 7 6 5 4 3 2 1

CONTENTS

ACKNOWLEDGMENTS

This volume would not have been possible without the enthusiasm and support of the contributing authors. Their willingness to undertake a difficult and time-consuming assignment at the behest of a distant editor is very much appreciated.

Additionally, numerous friends and colleagues assisted in the process of identifying potential contributors. Among others I am indebted to David Bell, Philip Berman, Jan Blanpain, Richard Cash, Harvey Fineberg, Al Henn, Dieter Koch-Weser, Lennart Köhler, Michael Reich, and Per-Gunnar Svensson.

Support for editing the manuscript was provided by a curriculum development grant from the Pew Memorial Foundation to the Department of Health Policy and Management of the Harvard School of Public Health, by the Division of Public Health at the University of Massachusetts at Amherst, and by the Swedish Center for Working Life in Stockholm. Special thanks for sophisticated typing skills is due Mulberry Studios in Cambridge, Massachusetts, and to Edith Dundon and Rosemary Larrow of the University of Massachusetts.

Above all, thanks are due to my wife Denise and to our children Julian and Annika, who bore the pressure of this extended project with such good cheer.

This volume is dedicated to my father and mother.

The International Handbook of Health-Care Systems

INTRODUCTION

Richard B. Saltman

The field of comparative health systems covers a wide range of subjects and issues. Topics range from broad policy questions of system design to narrow administrative issues of local service delivery, cutting across global subsets of developed as well as developing, capitalist as well as socialist, and heterogeneous as well as homogeneous societies. Aspects of these and related subjects can be approached from a variety of social science perspectives, among them sociology, anthropology, political science, and economics, as well as a multitude of their derivatives including organization theory, management theory, and planning theory. Given this diversity of subject and approach, it is not surprising that, as a coherent area of academic activity, comparative health systems studies have developed somewhat unevenly.

Over the last decade or so, however, there appears to have been growing interest in such studies, especially among national health planners and policy-makers. These two groups, faced with a series of recent crises in national health system organization and management, are particularly interested in comparative studies that generate readily transferable administrative mechanisms with which to resolve pressing health care problems. This pattern of selective interest has been evident during the early 1980s in concerns about cost containment and financial efficiency, topics which have dominated the most recent round of comparative studies.

While this narrow, topical approach is understandable, it suffers from a number of inherent—if not always obvious—complications. A health-care system, like any form of social organization, reflects the historical, cultural, and political as well as the economic context within which it develops. Proper evaluation of a particular delivery or administrative mechanism involves a wide variety of observations about the character and mores of the population, the historical process by which the nation and the health-care system have evolved, the past and present political culture, the present governmental structure, and the central components of the national economy, as well as a list of subsidiary intra-health-system factors, such as the source of financing, the structure of medical education, the strength of personnel unions and professional associations, and the epidemiological and demographic profile of the population. Given this degree of complexity, it can be difficult to simply transplant something that works in one health-care system in one society even into an apparently similar health system and society. An example is the entirely mixed results that ensued from the 1970 Danish decision to adopt a basically Swedish model of country council administration for health-care delivery—a model which, as the chapter on Sweden in this volume indicates, has proven to be flexible and quite successful in the Swedish context.

As the 1980s unfold, there appears to be a reconsideration among health policymakers concerning comparative health systems studies. Although still unevenly distributed among different groups and countries, there has been a noticeable increase in interest in, and support for, collaborative cross-national activities seeking to compare systems rather than simply mechanisms of health-care delivery. A diverse set of studies is under way, following in the tracks of such intensive case studies as those of Deborah Stone (1981) and Robert Evans (1984). One senses a greater recognition by some health authorities of the importance and value that rigorous in-depth studies can bring to national health policy formulation.

Taken in broader historical perspective, this shift toward a more comprehensive approach follows the increasing internationalization of western economies generally. The integrated global character of various manufacturing and service sectors, supported by computer-driven communication systems, has engendered a relatively sophisticated multinational approach to many areas of economic and public policy analysis. Given this increasingly internationalized context, it is not surprising that policy analysts and scholars have begun to ask persistently comparative questions about the health-care sector as well.

The interest in rigorous health system comparisons has been fed by the apparent similarity, at least in implication, of the health-care dilemmas faced by various countries at roughly equivalent stages of economic and political development. Most developed western nations, for example, now find themselves struggling with questions of system rationalization and managerial efficiency rather than earlier issues like equal access and planned growth. Further, they increasingly confront the hegemonic aspirations of economists in health policy formulation precisely as they faced the equally narrow yet unlimited aspirations of health planners two decades ago.

Developed and developing countries are also struggling to develop mechanisms by which to pursue the World Health Organization's goal of "Health for All by the Year 2000." This worldwide strategy, as formulated in the Declaration of Alma-Ata of 1978, calls for the dramatic expansion of primary and preventive care, to be funded in good part by an equivalent contraction in the resources consumed by the high-technology hospital sector of the delivery system. Although the aggregate total and/ or budgetary percentage for health-related activities differs dramatically between developed and developing countries—a well-known observation illustrated yet again by the figures presented in this volume—both groups of nations are still searching for practical concrete processes by which to transfer successfully the necessary resources to the primary care and preventive sectors of their health-care systems.

One can point to a variety of additional policy issues that cut across national health system lines: How best to channel the diffusion of increasingly intensive high-technology machines and procedures, including the growing number of organ transplantation options; how best to resolve difficult intersectoral issues associated with the problem of social inequity in the distribution of existing health system resources; and, for developed countries, how best to respond to the growing number of what the Swedes term "the old-old"—those over 85—who will consume greater amounts of intensive curative, rehabilitative, and custodial resources. These questions all invite exploration by well-designed, well-conducted comparative health systems studies.

Beyond similarities in the *nature* of the present health-care dilemmas, however, there are also substantial differences in the *approaches* used by different countries in addressing these issues. A particularly rewarding aspect of comparative health systems studies is their ability to identify and contextualize multiple possible solutions to what appear to be equivalent problems. Properly conducted, comparative studies hold the possibility of testing culture-bound assumptions against the different practices in other societies and nations.

In this arena, too, one can point to numerous issues that now pique the analytic and administrative imaginations of national health policymakers. How is it, for example, that, among developed countries with roughly equivalent standards of living, some lose barely half as many babies during the first year of life as others? If Finland and Sweden had infant mortality rates of 6.6 and 6.4 per 1000 live births, respectively, in 1985, why did the United States have a rate of 10.9 and the United Kingdom 11.2 during the same year? One could ask a similar question of developing countries, where differences in infant mortality range along a substantially wider continuum.

A second issue concerns the relationship, again among developed countries, of the total percentage of gross domestic product expended on health care in comparison to the overall health status of the population. How is it that the countries that expend only 6.5 percent of the total gross domestic product (GDP) on health care (Finland and Great Britain) have essentially equivalent morbidity and mortality experiences as the countries that expend 10 percent or more (the Federal Republic of Germany and the United States)? Lessons in this area, when derived from analyses of developed countries, might well be applicable in developing countries as well.

One fruitful area of comparison concerns the structure of administrative systems in the health-care sector. A substantial effort has been made in a number of publicly operated health-care systems to decentralize administrative responsibility to the regional or subregional level. Service delivery in countries like Sweden and Spain, for example, has been placed under the control of regionally elected officials, whereas in the United Kingdom direct administrative duties are exercised at the district level. In pluralist systems like that of the United States and Australia, the emphasis on decentralization has been pursued via a different policy, that of developing market-based competition among relatively unregulated private health-care providers. In these instances, the pressures have been to move away from strict national control over the delivery of care, yet it remains unclear whether the selected mechanism (decentralization or privatization) can accomplish the desired national health policy goals. Privatization and market competition, in the health sector as elsewhere, tend toward vertical and horizontal monopolies that recentralize power into private, often multinational companies. Decentralization within publicly run systems runs the risk that local administrators will no longer abide by national policy guidelines—for example, to favor primary and preventive over in-patient hospital care in the resource allocation process. There is thus no certainty that either strategic approach to administrative decentralization will succeed—an uncertainty that presents a rich opportunity for comparative study.

A further set of similarities and divergences can be observed with regard to health-care financing systems. Although the rapidity of change in this sector has not (yet) matched that seen in administrative systems, the extent of variation is considerable and, from a health systems analysis perspective, intriguing. In some respects, each country appears almost to have taken its own specific approach in this area. The alternatives range from 100-percent public funding from general revenues at the national level (United Kingdom, Hungary, Poland, Soviet Union), to majority public funding but from county-level taxes mixed with national general revenue (Sweden), to a quasipublic system based predominantly on mandatory employer and employee contributions (Spain, West Germany, East Germany), to a mixed public-private system in which the public sector fills in the financing gaps from the predominantly private and voluntary (usually employee based) insurance system (USA). Once again, this diversity of alternative arrangements, and the different consequences for such economically sensitive issues as managerial efficiency, system productivity, capital reinvestment as well as broader social issues like equal access to services, provides a natural arena for comparative study and research. Moreover, the inherent cultural, political, and social complexity of such comparisons promises to provide an important check on the more solipsistic assumptions of economists working within the confines of any individual nation or society.

This volume is intended to provide baseline information for starting to think about these and similar comparative issues. To facilitate this process, contributing authors were asked not only to include a "snapshot" of their health system's current level of development, but also to detail the set of dynamic forces that drive the system's health-care decision-making processes, and which will determine its path in the future. This latter goal requires a historical and analytic perspective that has too often been lacking in health system profiles, but that is essential to a clear picture of a health delivery system's likely evolution over the long term. In the profiles written for this volume, contributors were asked to highlight unique historical, cultural, social, political, and ideological factors that help explain the particular structure that presently exists and the probable future structure as the system continues to develop. This process of critical analysis is especially important in a volume that encompasses profiles from western capitalist, eastern socialist, and developing third-world countries alike. However tautological it may appear, it is worth restating that the validity of cross-national comparisons is contingent on an appropriate understanding of the broader societal context within which each compared health-care system sits.

Contributors also were asked to provide available data on the country's response to the World Health Organization's "Health for All" strategy. While these activities are more prominent within some health systems than others, the importance of primary-care-related activities to the future development of most health-care systems, coupled with the difficulty many countries now confront in achieving primary-care-related goals, makes primary care a valuable lens through which to observe the current state of development within different delivery systems.

The profiles in this volume are not themselves comparative in character. Such an approach would have involved commissioning a series of multicountry regional essays which, by their very nature, would be of less potential utility to the reader. The methodology of this volume, which presents a series of single-country essays, provides an intensive case-study perspective that is, in the long run, more penetrating and informative. The selected approach establishes a base from which a reader can make a wide variety of different types of informed comparisons. For instance, while it is instructive to compare the health status of the Spanish population with that of other European countries, one might also find it valuable to compare the structure of Colombia's health insurance with that of its former colonial master, Spain.

It should be noted that no attempt was made to impose a rigid intellectual straightjacket on the volume's contributors. Reflecting, in part, the different structure and societal context of particular health systems and, in part, differences in their professional training, the authors have structured their national profiles along a variety of paths. Although this occasionally makes superficial comparisons more difficult, it promotes the deeper forms of comparison that are most rewarding.

It is unfortunate but true that reliable statistics for health status and also financial indices can be very difficult to obtain. In developing countries like Saudi Arabia and Mozambique, for example, certain key health statistics, like infant mortality rates, can only be estimated. Even in developed countries, some health statistics are not available—for example, the recent mortality figures from the Soviet Union have been released only on an aggregate national basis and only for certain selected years. The financial data from developed countries also can be difficult to assemble; for instance, the complex intermingling of the Spanish health-care system with the national social security structure makes precise health expenditure figures hard to isolate.

A more difficult problem is the different definitions commonly used to compile health and financial statistics in different countries. How a particular country chooses to define a "live birth," for example, can vary considerably. The issue of sorting out financial data raises a similar set of difficulties. In this regard, it should be noted that expenditure figures and percentages given in the profiles are those generated inside the country itself unless otherwise stated. Readers requiring comparative economic figures utilizing precisely the same method of calculation are advised to seek out the adjusted figures provided by such international agencies as the World Bank (World Bank, 1986) or the Organization for Economic and Community Development (1985).

In summary, perhaps the single most important aspect of comparative health-care studies is its relatively undeveloped status as an academic area of research. This status suggests the tremendous potential such studies hold for informing future policy-making activities at the national level, as well as signaling, on a methodological level, the considerable difficulties in conducting high-quality cross-national research. In this context, it does not take great foresight to predict that the future of comparative health system studies should be particularly bright over the next several decades. The 21 country profiles that make up this volume are intended to be a contribution to the development of this field of study.

References

Evans, Robert G. 1984. *Strained Mercy: The Economics of Canadian Health Care*. Toronto: Butterworths.

Organization for Economic and Community Development. *Measuring Health Care 1960–1983: Expenditure, Costs, and Performance*. Paris: Organization for Economic and Community Development.

Stone, Deborah. 1980. *The Limits of Professional Power: National Health Care in the Federal Republic of Germany*. Chicago: University of Chicago Press.

World Bank. 1986. *World Development Report, 1985*. New York and London: Oxford University Press.

World Health Organization. 1978. *Primary Health Care: Report of the International Conference on Primary Health Care, Alma Ata, USSR, 6–12 September 1978*. Geneva: WHO.

ARGENTINA

Andrés A. Santas and
Abraam Sonis

Introduction

Argentina occupies the southern-most part of South America (south cone). It is shaped like an isosceles triangle with its base in the north and its apex pointing south. Climate is subtropical in the north, mild in the center, and cool or cold in the south.

Population is now 30,000,000 (1980 census: 28,000,000)—81 percent urban and 19 percent rural, practically from European origin. Most of the population is settled in the humid pampa region, along the La Plata River (Rio de la Plata). Some one-third of the country's population (10,000,000) lives in the Buenos Aires metropolitan area. It is not only the most important political center, but also the economic, industrial, cultural, and social one.

Health Status Statistics

Argentina has had a traditionally low birth rate, lower than the rest of Latin America, except Uruguay. In some measure, immigration has compensated for the low rate: from Europe until the 1950s and afterwards from neighboring South American countries (Bolivia, Paraguay, Uruguay, and Chile). Nevertheless, the birth rate slowly began to increase during the 1970s, a trend maintained up to the present. In 1981, it stood at 23.7 per 1,000 population. As overall mortality has decreased, the rate of population growth has risen to 2 percent per year. The fertility rate increased from 86.5 per 1,000 in 1970 to 103.5 per 1,000 in 1977; in 1980, it was 98.4 per 1000. It is higher in women who have only partial or no elementary school education. Eight percent of the population is 65 years of age or older; in Buenos Aires city, the figure is 15 percent (1980). Some 30 percent of the population is fifteen years of age or younger.

Overall mortality rate was 8.4 per 1,000 in 1981. Infant mortality descended from 63 per 1,000 live births in 1970 to 33.6 per 1,000 in 1981. It is now estimated at around 32 per 1,000. The goal set by the Health for All (H.F.A.) by the Year 2000 program in Argentina is 30 per 1,000. The lowest rate is in Buenos Aires city and Tierra del Fuego in the south (17.7 per 1,000 in 1981). The northern provinces (west and east) have the highest rates (between 43 to 48 per 1,000). The most frequent contributions to infant mortality are perinatal deaths (46.4 percent) and deaths due to congenital malformations (11.8 percent). The percentage of women dying as a consequence of delivery is 0.7 percent. Hospital deliveries now make up 91 percent of the total. In the group of children between one and four years of age, the death rate is 1.4 per 1,000; the lowest rates are in Tierra del Fuego (0.3) and Buenos Aires city (0.6). The main causes of death in this group are accidents along with respiratory and gastrointestinal infections; in children between four and fifteen years old, the major factors are accidents (33.5 percent) and malignant tumors (4.3 percent).

In the population as a whole, the main causes of death are as follows:

1. Heart diseases (29 percent)
2. Malignant tumors (17.3 percent)
3. Cerebrovascular episodes (10 percent)
4. Accidents in males (6.3 percent) (females 3.4 percent) and arteriosclerosis in females (6.1 percent)
5. Diseases originating around birth (4.4 percent, the same for males and females).

In the group between 15 and 49 years of age, the main death causes are accidents in males (22 percent) and malignant tumors in females (23.1 percent); heart diseases are the second cause in both (19.9 percent and 16.1 percent respectively). Between 50 and 64 years old, the main causes are heart diseases in men and malignant tumors in women; the second causes of death are just the reverse. In those over 65, the main causes of death are the same in males and females in this sequence: heart diseases, malignant tumors, cerebrovascular accidents, arteriosclerosis, pneumonia, and influenza. According to the 1980 census, life expectancy at birth is 69.4 years; it is higher for women (72.9 years) than for men (66.1 years).

Vaccination is compulsory for children (diphtheria, measles, tetanus, whooping cough, polio, and T.B.K.) and for pregnant women. Perinatal tetanus has almost disappeared. Coverage varies between 70 percent and 85 percent according to different vaccines.

There is an estimated housing deficit of from 1 to 2 million new houses. For 18.5 percent of the population, more than three people currently live in the same room. This condition ranges from 5.1 percent in Buenos Aires city to 42.3 percent in Formosa (northeastern province).

Centralized water supply reaches 60 percent of the population; the rest has accessibility to potable water. Only in a few villages in desert areas must water be transported in trucks or by railroad; the same applies to some periurban transitory slums (''villas miserias'').

Around 45 percent of the population has centralized sewage. In Buenos Aires city, the figure is 100 percent; the lowest percentage is in Misiones (northeastern province) with only 3 percent. In nine provinces (northeastern and northwestern), it varies from 10 percent to 20 percent.

Historical Overview

From colonial times up to 1940, Argentina's history followed the pattern of many occidental countries: (1) public hospitals and philanthropic charity institutions, and (2) private health care for affluent people. The first was based on the free-of-charge public hospitals; the second was provided in doctors' offices and private small hospitals (called ''sanatoriums'').

With the influx of 5,000,000 immigrants between 1870 and 1930, ''community hospitals'' appeared as an intermediary link between charity and private health care. They were organized in the main cities following mutual aid principles and were designed to serve immigrants coming from different European countries. Over time, they became large, powerful, open institutions which are now important providers of high-quality services.

In 1949 the Federal Ministry of Health was established (a pattern also followed in the provinces). There followed a rapid expansion of the public sector. In less than ten years, the number of public hospital beds increased from 60,000 to 120,000; also, many preventive medicine programs were organized.

At the same time, for political reasons, the government favored the organization of Social Security units (''orbas sociales'') similar to Bismark's corporate approach: Each group of employees (including those working in different governmental areas) established its own organization led and administered by its trade unions or guilds. Financial resources were obtained through compulsory contribution (salary percentage) from employees and employers. The same pattern was followed in numerous public service enterprises which had been state owned (railroads, telephone, and light and power).

Thus in Argentina, social security is not a centralized organization as it is in most Latin American countries. Today, the social security sector covers 75 percent of the population including rural workers and all retired people over 65 years of age. The dominant principle was (and is) to allow low-income groups to have access to the same level of health care as the affluent. This philosophy understands Social Security to provide a supplemental income; however, it produced a massive redirection of financial resources into the private sector. This trend was reinforced by the 1970 law that defines the system and later (after 1976) by the general economic policy applied. Support for public hospitals diminished, and private health insurance grew. The private sector was further favored by the elimination (under some conditions) of custom taxes on the importance of high-technology equipment.

Since late 1983, the new constitutional government has engaged in organizing a national health insurance system, an old goal of all sectors. The current objective is to generate adequate coordination and utilization of existing structures and facilities, and to set up pluralistic, rational, efficient, and equitable delivery services.

Current Health System Structure

The present health-care system in Argentina is a complex, if not chaotic, organization. Health care is provided by three sectors: (1) public, with three subsectors: federal, provincial, and municipal; (2) Social Security; and (3) private, both profit and nonprofit. They are independent with regard to planning, organization, and management; however, they are linked, if only minimally, at the operational level.

Public Sector

The base of the government sector is the public hospital, which has an acknowledged tradition of quality health care, mainly as a consequence of the capability and prestige of its professional personnel. Many doctors were (and are) world-known leaders of medical or surgical groups (''schools''). The development of Argentine medicine is closely related to the public hospital, where postgraduates and graduates (Argentine and Latin American) are educated and trained. Until the early 1970s, modern technological equipment was almost exclusively introduced to Argentina through these public units.

Public hospitals operate 63 percent of the country's hospital beds (1980). They are open and provide free-of-charge health care to patients without insurance coverage, to those incompletely covered by Social Security, and also to some middle-class patients attracted by the reputation of certain doctors or institutions. They also take care of chronic patients (mental, handicapped, tubercular) and old people without coverage when their families cannot afford or are unwilling, to look after them.

Since most public hospitals belong to provincial or municipal governments, their characteristics, efficiency, and performance are far from homogeneous. As a rule, however, over the last ten to fifteen years, they have decayed as a consequence of low budgets, inadequate salaries and capital investments, rigid administrative regulations, and poor management. Nevertheless, these public hospitals still appeal to a large group of patients, something that makes them an outstanding base for a national health-care system.

Some attempts have been made to introduce organizational and managerial changes, in particular seeking to create a better relation with Social Security and the private sector. This was the case for certain ''community hospitals'' established in the 1960s in some rural areas or small cities. However, lack of continuity due to political changes, as well as the opposition of organized medicine, prevented them from growing or even led to their disappearance. This and other attempts have provided useful experiences for future changes.

The Social Security Sector

The Social Security system in Argentina is fragmented into nearly 400 units ("obras sociales") of different size, power, and characteristics. Additional complicating factors are these units' different political links (to trade unions, to federal, provincial, or municipal governments, and to state-owned or private corporations), different target populations (metropolitan, urban, or rural), and dissimilarities among regional and local economies. Overall, the Social Security sector owns only 5 percent of the country's hospital beds. It has thus become a third-party payer for services overwhelmingly provided by the private sector.

As already mentioned, financial resources are obtained through compulsory contributions. The 1970 law established a National Institute of Social Security to standardize, coordinate, and supervise the social security health-care system. This institute's main tasks were to supervise and act as an economic regulatory body between financially powerful as against weak organizations in an attempt to ensure more egalitarian delivery of services and to fix the price of hospital services and doctors' fees. Following its purely formal beginning, the institute has been placed since 1983 under the Federal Ministry of Health and Social Affairs in order to improve the likelihood that it will carry out its broad legal mandate.

Fee-for-service payment is the general approach in Buenos Aires city, although some organizations employ doctors on fixed salaries or on a capitated basis. In the provinces, however, all Social Security units, directly or through a common agency, sign global contracts with local medical federations (guilds) to employ physicians on a capitation basis, and these local federations then pay their member doctors on a fee-for-service arrangement. These nonprofit medical organizations ensure accessibility for Social Security patients to all practising doctors in the province.

Social Security now covers 75 percent of the population (the figures doubled between 1970 and 1980), but an important number of beneficiaries do not use its services because of inadequate accessibility, time-consuming bureaucratic requirements, established or irregular compensatory payments, and an unsatisfactory service level. A very low percentage turn to private practice, but most Social Security beneficiaries use free-of-charge public hospitals. In this way, the public hospitals effectively subsidize Social Security. This happens with only some acute patients, but it is the rule for the chronically ill.

Lack of reliable information makes it difficult to determine the total annual expenditures of Social Security and the structure. An appraisal based on partial studies estimates a yearly expenditure of more than 2.5 billion U.S. dollars. A rather reliable 1978 study showed that the Social Security cost structure was as follows:

Drugs	35 percent
Hospital services	25 percent
Doctors' fees	20 percent
Ambulatory diagnostic or therapeutic procedures	13 percent
Odontology services	7 percent

Social Security's strong and continuous development has been (and is) the most important element in the continued growth of the private sector in Argentina. In particular, Social-Security-generated support has enabled the private sector to acquire complex and sophisticated equipment that from ten to fifteen years ago was found almost exclusively in the public sector, in large urban and university hospitals. As a consequence, the private health sector has become attractive to capital investors as in any other industrial or commercial area. The economic crisis that emerged in the middle of 1982 began to reverse this trend, however. Higher costs, unemployment, lower salaries, and inefficient administration and management clearly demonstrated the intrinsic weaknesses of the private sector and led to a financial crisis for Social Security. Undoubtedly, Social Security must undergo a major change in the future.

Private Sector

The private sector contains several kinds of providers with different interests and working approaches. First are the small and middle-size clinics (called "sanatoriums"), which, established at the beginning of the twentieth century, remain widespread over the entire country, particularly in provincial centers. Typically, they are owned by the professional groups that established them in order to have a common working place. Second are the large private hospitals, providers of high technological and specialized care, which are usually located in metropolitan areas. Ownership of these generally is in the hands of private stockholders. Third are the large private nonprofit hospitals established at the end of the last century to care for immigrants on a mutual aid basis. Gradually, these have become open institutions with high standards of service. They are now, of course, financially dependent on Social Security and private health insurance (as is the entire private sector).

Fourth, Argentina has a substantial private health insurance (prepaid health care) sector. These highly lucrative enterprises have varying owners (stockholders, insurance corporations, large hospitals) and they have increased to more than 100 in number over the last ten years. These enterprises serve individuals or whole corporations and even some social security units, mainly providing care for acute patients less than 65 years of age. Policies vary from one company to another, and even inside the same company. Some have closed lists of doctors and hospitals; others allow free choice of physician with subsequent reimbursement up to previously established amounts. Ambulatory services are provided in doctors' offices. Some companies cover periodical checkups or ambulatory mental health services.

Reliable information on the number of people covered, the services actually utilized, and their cost is not available. Many middle- and upper-income subscribers pay for compulsory Social Security coverage but, not satisfied by the levels or quality of services, also carry private health insurance.

Fifth and last, there are private physicians who provide office-based services. These services are paid directly by patients, or through Social Security or private paid health insurance. Widely spread all over the country, they constitute the real source of primary care for most of the population, with doctors acting as family physicians or specialists.

Except in Buenos Aires city, doctors are grouped in regional or provincial medical federations (guilds). These federations represent the physicians in dealings with the government, Social Security, or private health insurance, and they act to defend physicians' rights, privileges, and fees. Clearly, any attempt to rationalize health services or to introduce a system of national health insurance will have to accommodate this private physician network since it is the backbone of the delivery system.

Argentina has 150,000 hospital beds (5 per 1,000 inhabitants) in 3,200 hospitals and clinics. Forty-two percent of the hospitals and clinics belong to the public sector with 63 percent of the total beds. The private sector owns 54.5 percent of these institutions with 32 percent of the beds. This means that large hospitals are government property: 87 percent of those with more than 200 beds are state owned. The Social Security system owns only 5.4 percent of the hospital beds. These recent data (1984) show an important shift: In 1965, 76 percent of the beds were in the public sector and only 20.6 percent were in the private one. Private sector hospitals are more efficient than public sector institutions, but it should be noted that private sector patients are almost exclusively acute middle-income patients. Public hospitals, conversely, also must care for patients with scarce resources and for the chronically ill. Thus, global comparisons of managerial efficiency are not helpful.

In the last ten to fifteen years, high-technology equipment has become concentrated in the private sector. In 1979, the private sector owned 56 percent of the extracorporeal circulation machines, 67 percent of the CAT scanners, and 65 percent of the intensive-care beds. This trend has been favored by exemptions from custom taxes for equipment that Argentine industry only partially produces.

The only requirement was that it be used 25 percent of the working hours by public hospitals. This obligation has proved difficult to implement and even more difficult to evaluate. In the public sector, equipment maintenance has created problems owing to lack of budget and qualified personnel, bureaucratic rigidity, and, in some cases, lack of interest in creating public competition with the private sector where the same personnel also work and even earn their main income. Due to all these factors, a high percentage of public sector equipment is frequently out of order.

Health System Financing

Argentina invests between 7 and 8 percent of its gross national product in health care. The public sector share is 23 percent, Social Security is 38 percent, and the private sector provides 39 percent of that total. The public, Social Security, and private sectors are each legally and administratively independent; however, they are interrelated at the operational level.

The public sector is dependent on federal, provincial, or municipal budgets. Health care receives approximately from 2 to 3 percent of total federal and from 5 to 15 percent (with a mean of 10 percent) of total provincial expenditures. Buenos Aires city, however, allocates 20 percent of its budget for health, mainly to support sixteen tertiary hospitals. Financial resources from provincial and municipal budgets represent 70 percent of the total amount of public sector funds allocated to the health-care system.

In spite of their recent deterioration, public hospitals still provide care of a large number of patients, including many with Social Security coverage. In the last decade, attempts have been made to charge for the cost of services provided. These efforts were abandoned since they would affect primarily low-income patients. The notion of poverty certificates was morally and socially depressing, and hospital administrators were ill-prepared to successfully implement such an approach. Nevertheless, a small number of public hospitals currently have special arrangements with some Social Security organizations.

Social Security's financial resources are provided by compulsory contributions (salary percentages) of employees and employers (including the federal government for state-owned corporations). There are also general public contributions (established by law) for certain working groups: Customer fees in some companies include a percentage for employees' Social Security (insurance and banking) or are lower for these employees (light and power, telephone, natural gas, railroads, airlines).

Social Security's payments are established in a National Nomenclator (Nomenclador Nacional) with fees and hospital reimbursement schedules fixed by the National Institute of Social Security. The present fee system favors high-technology-based medicine, and thus promotes overuse of intensive capital equipment and subspecialists, to the detriment of primary health care. This reimbursement approach has been heavily criticized by professional federations, scientific associations, university leaders, public health people, social security organizations, and provincial and municipal health authorities. However, vested interests and the population's preferences as shaped by media propaganda have blocked corrective measures.

The private sector provides care for Social Security patients and those with voluntary insurance; these are the principal, if not the only, source of its financial resources.

Current Issues

There is a severe lack of coordination among the three main health delivery sectors in Argentina. Each sector pursues its own objectives in isolation and in accordance with its own particular regulations and requirements. Moreover, within each sector, there are substantial differences as well. The public sector alone is divided into three uncoordinated subsectors: federal, provincial, and municipal. Multiplicity and diversity of Social Security components and those of the private sector (hospitals and clinics) add to the confusion. It is not surprising, therefore, to find that the population feels a generalized disappointment with the present system.

The existence of multiple sectors and subsectors is not, of course, a problem in itself. For cultural and historical reasons, Argentinians will not accept a uniform rigid health-care system; however, they would accept a pluralistic unified, and coordinated delivery system.

Beyond lack of coordination, current problems include lack of evaluation, overlapping services, over and under utilization, resource waste, inefficiency, and considerable public confusion as to how to utilize services appropriately. There are, additionally, several important personnel issues. Doctors must work simultaneously in different sectors, running from place to place. Public hospital physicians receive very low salaries, and consequently they work only mornings in the hospital, subsequently seeing Social Security and, if possible, private patients in their offices during the afternoons. There is also a large surplus of physicians—some 1 per 400 population. This situation leads to reduced physician working capacity, lower quality of care, and poor professional morale. The lack of qualified nurses and technicians also is a long-standing problem. There is only one nurse for every three doctors; most are "auxiliary" or nonregistered nurses. This shortage is caused by low salaries and poor social status.

Combined, these factors make it very difficult to organize a properly structured referral-based delivery system. Some provinces do, however, have well-planned public sectors that work satisfactorily. They provide an example of continuous leadership with clear ideas and objectives, as well as sound management and methodology.

A second important example is that of the National Institute of Retired People and Pensioners, which is responsible for the health care for 3,000,000 people, most over 65 years of age. It has organized a primary care program in doctors' offices; providers can be freely chosen by its subscribers. When necessary, referral is made to a group of connected public or private hospitals. It is a good example of intersectorial coordination and reliable health care.

The Future

The present severe crisis of Argentina's health-care organizations is recognized by governmental authorities, by leaders of different sectors, by health professionals, and by the population as a whole. In the last twenty years, many attempts have been made to solve it. Lack of understanding, vested interests, and jealous leaders have led, however, to failure.

A uniform and coordinated system that is pluralistic, participative, rational, efficient, and equitable is badly needed. To achieve this goal, every sector must understand that voluntary compromise of some of its interests and prerogatives is necessary for the benefit of all.

The public sector must reorganize its hospitals giving them administrative and financial autonomy, improving management, modernizing facilities to make them functional and comfortable, purchasing up-to-date equipment, maintaining facilities, and evaluating the quality of doctors' work and costs. Social Security must be transformed into a uniform and organic system, to ensure efficient and equitable services through consistent and parallel agreements with public and private providers. The private sector must fully participate in coordinating services and investments with the public sector and Social Security, according to regional characteristics, resources, and requirements. Finally, firm and active participation and support by professional associations is fundamental, since physicians and members of allied professions are responsible for the quality of services. In retrospect, they have always shown their interest in having a well-organized health-care system that could satisfy people's needs as well as their own expectations.

In September 1984, the Federal Ministry of Health and Social Affairs introduced a working paper proposing basic principles to plan "National Health Insurance." It suggested an integrated and coordinated system with voluntary participation of the private sector. It would be administered by a joint commission of employers and employees, under state guidance. Each sector would keep its legal individuality; primary care would be a basic objective; and all providers would have the same rights and duties, thus forming a net of services for the whole of the population. Administrative decentralization at the provincial level would be emphasized. Working norms, fares, and fees would be established at the federal level by a steering committee with representatives of all sectors. Special preventive medicine programs would receive financial support.

This working paper was studied and discussed by all groups working in the health field, and everybody agreed that this plan or one similar to it could resolve Argentina's health-care difficulties. Finally, in 1985 it was proposed as a law to the congress of the country and until now is in discussion.

References

Instituto Nacional de Estadisticas y Censos (INDEC). 1984. *La pobreza en la Argentina*. Buenos Aires.

Kohn, R., and K. L. White. 1976. *Health Care: An International Study*. London: Oxford University Press.

Kurian, G. T. 1982. *Encyclopedia of the Third World*, rev. ed. Vol. 1. New York: Facts on File, Inc.

Medicina y Sociedad. 1985. *Caracteristicas de la Organizacion de la atencion medica en la Argentina*. Buenos Aires.

Ministerio de Salud y Accion Social—P.A.H.O/W.H.O. 1985 *Argentina, Descripcion de su situacion de salud*. Buenos Aires.

Ministerio de Salud y Accion Social—Argentina. 1984. *Bases para una legislacion sobre Seguro Nacional de Salud*. Buenos Aires.

Ministerio de Salud y Accion Social, Argentina Direccion de Estadisticas de Salud. 1984. *Recursos humanos en operacion en los establecimientos asistenciales*. Serie 4; N 8. Buenos Aires.

Ministerio de Salud Publica y Medio Ambiente, Argentina. 1982. *Encuesta de Utilizacion de Servicios y Gastos en Atencion Medica*. Buenos Aires.

Neri, Aldo. 1982. *Salud y Política Social*. Buenos Aires: Ed. Hachette.

Weil, E. et al. 1974. *Area Handbook for Argentina*. Washington, D.C.: U.S. Government Printing Office.

Wilkie, J. W., and A. Perkal, eds. 1986. *Statistical Abstract of Latin America*. Vol. 24. Los Angeles: Latin American Center Publications.

AUSTRALIA

John G. Youngman

Introduction

Australia is an island in which 40 percent of the landmass is located north of the Tropic of Capricorn. It can best be described as a land rich in natural resources, with a multicultural society that lives an urbanized life style: 70 percent of the population lives in the major cities, most of which are situated on the coastline.

First settled by the British in 1788, Australia has a population approaching 16 million persons of whom less than 1 percent are indigenous Australian aborigines. A net immigration increase of 0.47 percent (most of whom came from Europe and Indochina) and the natural population increase of 0.85 percent resulted in an overall population gain of 1.32 percent in 1983. This is representative of gains in population during recent years.

The Commonwealth of Australia was created in 1901 by an act of the British Parliament, which formalized the federation of the six sovereign states that had developed since colonization. The Commonwealth Government (hereafter known as the Australian Government) has its powers defined in the Australian Constitution. Some of these powers are exclusive (at the time of federation, the states vested certain powers such as defense and foreign affairs to the commonwealth) while others are shared with the states, with the provision that commonwealth law always overrides state law if inconsistencies in law exist in areas where the constitution is applicable. Powers not defined in the constitution remain as state powers. The definition of the powers of the commonwealth and the states has important ramifications for health-care delivery and financing in Australia.

Both the commonwealth and the states have elected legislatures in which the majority representative political party forms the government. A third tier of government, the local authority, is well developed within Australia. The function of the local authority is determined by the state government, with the main emphasis on community services such as roads, water, waste disposal, town planning, and immunization programs.

Health Statistics

Health indicators for the latest available year (1983) demonstrate that the health status of the Australian population (excluding the aborigine population) is comparable with that found in most other developed countries. The crude death rate for the country was 7.6 per 1,000 population (aborigines are estimated at 10.1 per 1,000), and the infant mortality rate was 10.3 per 1,000 non-aborigine births (aborigines are estimated at 30.8 per 1,000). Life expectancy at birth was 72.1 years for males and 78.7 years for females; life expectancy at age 65 was 13.7 years for males and 17.9 years for females. The cause of death statistics reflect many of the standard problems of industrialized nations, in particular the prominence of diseases of the circulatory system and malignant neoplasms (Table 1).

Historical Overview

In the late eighteenth century, a convict settlement was established in Australia to ease the overcrowding in English prisons. Medical services were provided by doctors accompanying these early settlers. Public health measures were similar to those already accepted in England. As the population of the colonies increased, socioeconomic classes could be identified, and the lower classes were seen as needing attention if poverty was not to become a major problem. Charitable societies were formed to provide shelter and medical care for the indigent and the sick who could not afford the cost of private medical care. Physicians provided their services to these societies on an honorary basis. These societies were the forerunners of the present public hospital system which was, at a later stage, funded and managed by the state governments.

At the same time, a group of citizens, who could not afford private fees but who did not fit the criteria of those utilizing the public system, encouraged the development of Friendly Societies. These relied on their members' paying a fixed regular fee and, in return, they received medical care. The doctors were remunerated through a capitation arrangement.

Following federation in 1901, the states retained the responsibility for public health and the Australian government the responsibility for quarantine. The role of government at this time was one of nonintervention in health services if possible. During the early part of this century, Friendly Societies were expanding and, with an excess number of doctors, could dictate terms to the physicians. The British Medical Association, which perceived a threat to the autonomy of the medical profession, intervened with the result that capitation disappeared and fee-for-service medicine was introduced. This resulted in increased fees to

Table 1
Deaths by Cause, 1980 to 1984

Cause of death	Number					Deaths per 100 000 mean population				
	1980	1981	1982	1983	1984(a)	1980	1981	1982	1983	1984
Diseases of the circulatory system	55 767	56 045	57 686	54 661	54 289	379.5	375.4	380.2	355.5	349.0
Ischaemic heart disease	*30 728*	*31 433*	*32 345*	*31 388*	*30 951*	*209.1*	*210.5*	*213.2*	*204.1*	*199.0*
Other heart/hypertensive disease	*7 501*	*7 065*	*7 438*	*6 958*	*6 985*	*51.0*	*47.3*	*49.0*	*45.2*	*44.9*
Cerebrovascular disease	*13 723*	*13 706*	*13 977*	*12 652*	*12 660*	*93.4*	*91.8*	*92.1*	*82.3*	*81.4*
Atherosclerosis	*1 774*	*1 724*	*1 653*	*1 463*	*1 469*	*12.1*	*11.5*	*10.9*	*9.5*	*9.4*
Other	*2 041*	*2 117*	*2 273*	*2 200*	*2 224*	*13.9*	*14.2*	*15.1*	*14.3*	*14.3*
Malignant neoplasms	23 333	23 812	24 914	25 587	25 820	158.8	159.5	164.2	166.4	166.0
Digestive organs and peritoneum	*7 191*	*7 273*	*7 553*	*7 832*	*7 683*	*48.9*	*48.7*	*49.8*	*50.9*	*49.4*
Lung	*4 997*	*5 074*	*5 337*	*5 405*	*5 391*	*34.0*	*34.0*	*35.2*	*35.1*	*34.7*
Other	*11 145*	*11 465*	*12 024*	*12 350*	*12 746*	*75.8*	*76.8*	*79.2*	*80.3*	*81.9*
Diseases of the respiratory system	7 429	7 335	8 910	7 776	7 802	50.6	49.1	58.7	50.6	50.2
Bronchitis, emphysema and asthma	*2 257*	*2 123*	*2 359*	*2 094*	*2 148*	*15.4*	*14.2*	*15.5*	*13.6*	*13.8*
Pneumonia	*1 766*	*1 727*	*2 137*	*1 677*	*1 623*	*12.0*	*11.6*	*14.1*	*10.9*	*10.4*
Influenza	*133*	*40*	*332*	*126*	*79*	*0.9*	*0.3*	*2.2*	*0.8*	*0.5*
Other	*3 273*	*3 445*	*4 082*	*3 879*	*3 952*	*22.3*	*23.1*	*26.9*	*25.2*	*25.4*
Motor vehicle accidents	3 555	3 373	3 458	2 919	2 785	24.2	22.6	22.8	19.0	17.9
All other accidents	2 698	2 493	2 719	2 592	2 391	18.4	16.7	17.9	16.9	15.4
Diabetes mellitus	1 634	1 717	1 609	1 692	1 838	11.1	11.5	10.6	11.0	11.8
Diseases of the genito-urinary system	1 649	1 598	1 717	1 711	1 715	11.2	10.7	11.3	11.1	11.0
Suicide and self-inflicted injuries	1 607	1 672	1 777	1 726	1 712	10.9	11.2	11.7	11.2	11.0
Chronic liver disease and cirrhosis	1 231	1 214	1 258	1 162	1 112	8.4	8.1	8.3	7.6	7.1
Congenital anomalies	909	937	1 052	982	882	6.2	6.3	6.9	6.4	5.7
Perinatal conditions	1 076	956	1 006	915	823	7.3	6.4	6.6	6.0	5.3
Alcohol dependence syndrome	177	141	135	141	153	1.2	0.9	0.9	0.9	1.0
Tuberculosis	65	81	63	54	58	0.4	0.5	0.4	0.4	0.4
Intestinal infectious diseases	78	84	70	40	41	0.5	0.6	0.5	0.3	0.3
All other causes	7 487	7 545	8 397	8 126	8 493	51.0	50.5	55.3	52.8	54.6
All causes	108 695	109 003	114 771	110 084	109 914	739.7	730.1	756.3	715.9	706.6

Source: Australian Bureau of Statistics, *Commonwealth Department of Health Annual Report 1985–86* (Canberra: Australian Government Publishing Service, 1986).

join the Friendly Societies and consequently their membership decreased. The public hospital system had to support these additional patients.

These events stimulated a government-led discussion of a national health insurance scheme. The arguments for and against such a scheme continue today. What did transpire was the development of a public salaries system within the public hospitals and a private fee-for-service system. The hospital component of the private sector was supported by the development of insurance schemes operated by nonprofit health insurance organizations.

By the end of World War II, all political movements, as well as organized medicine, saw a need for a more systematic service structure; however, the two major political parties proposed contrasting policies. The scheme proposed by the Conservatives would incorporate a system of payment to doctors by capitation for the health care of low-income earners, while most of the population would join a contributory scheme based on a freedom of choice of doctor, with payment based on a fee-for-service system. The Labour Party believed that health services should be available to all at no cost, with funding being provided through a national insurance scheme. This would also result in some redistribution of wealth. Organized medicine continued to support only a voluntary fee-for-service system. The Labour Government introduced legislation to implement a pharmaceutical scheme designed to provide medications at no charge to the patient. Organized medicine successfully challenged the concept of the legislation because of its inconsistency with the Australian Constitution.

In 1946, the most significant legislation in the health field was introduced into the Australian Parliament. The Constitution Alteration (Social Services) Act of 1946 empowered the commonwealth to make laws with respect to: "the provision of maternity allowances, widow's pensions, child endowment, unemployment, pharmaceutical, sickness and hospital benefits, medical and dental services (but not so as to authorize any form of civil conscription), benefits to students and family allowances." This constitutional amendment empowered the Australian Government to enact legislation on the forementioned matters. Even though legislation could not address the actual delivery of health care, it did affect the financing, and, through this avenue, the Australian Government has introduced measures which dictate the style of health-care delivery.

During the 1970s and 1980s, there were numerous changes to the funding of the health delivery system through variations in health benefits paid by the Australian Government and nonprofit voluntary health insurance organizations. In the early 1970s, a Liberal Government continued to support the concept of private medicine funded through a nonprofit health insurance industry. The government subsidized these health insurance funds and established rules in which the maximum amount payable by a patient for any one procedure was A$5. This was adopted in conjunction with the acceptance of "the most common fee" principle, i.e., a standard set of fees approved by government for insurance reimbursement purposes and accepted by the medical profession. These policies did not reduce the continuing escalation of national health expenditures.

In 1972, a Labour Government was elected with the issues of equity and access to health care a major election issue. This mandate resulted in the introduction of a national health insurance scheme known as Medibank, which upgraded the status of the primary care physician through educational grants for training purposes and the provision of increased community support services. It also involved activity in the areas of aboriginal health, school dental services, nursing homes, and psychiatric services.

Funding of the national health insurance scheme was obtained through direct government grants with no contribution from the population. Doctors were encouraged to bill the government directly and were reimbursed 85 percent of the agreed scheduled fee. Disputes occurred between the government and the medical profession because of fee levels, and, between 1973 and 1975, significant fee increases occurred following investigation by an independent arbitrator.

In the hospital sector, the Australian Government met 50 percent of the operating costs of hospitals and provided large financial grants to the states for new capital expenditures. Prior to this scheme, the states were entirely financially responsible for public hospital operating costs.

In 1975, the national government changed. Health costs had risen to 7.7 percent of the gross national product, and a 2.5-percent income tax levy was imposed to help cover the cost of the Medibank system. However, the government allowed this to be waived if the individual enrolled in a private health insurance scheme. In 1978, the insurance levy was abolished, and the government agreed to fund all medical fees to the extent of 40 percent for those members of the community who were insured. Disadvantaged and aged citizens had all fees reimbursed by the government. Another change in government occurred in 1982, and the Labour Government again had a mandate to introduce a national health insurance scheme.

The dominant force in the health system since the 1930s has been organized medicine, in the form of the British Medical Association until 1962, at which time the Australian Medical Association was formed. This group has been supported by entrenched conservative forces in government for most of this period. The Australian Medical Association has pursued the ideology of professional autonomy for its members, symbolized by private medicine delivered through fee-for-service payments funded by voluntary health insurance mechanisms. It has been aided by the lack of government alternatives relating to funding service delivery.

Health System Structure

Role of National Government

The Australian Government has the responsibility for formulating national health policy. The Commonwealth Department of Health implements the policies of the Australian Government through the regulation of health insurance; the provision of financial grants to the states; and the provision of financial benefits related to nursing homes, domiciliary nursing care, home nursing, assistance for patients living in isolated areas of the continent, pharmaceuticals, and aids for the disabled.

The direct provision of health services is a state responsibility with the national role in the health delivery function related only to quarantine and occupational health. National government support is essential for organizations such as the Royal Flying Doctor Service, the Red Cross, and the National Heart Foundation if these groups are to continue to fulfill a useful role.

The forementioned 1946 Constitutional Amendment enabled the national government to develop a national health care system through the provision of medical and hospital benefits. The present Australian health scheme, "Medicare," is the culmination of policies developed by the Australian Labour Party Government elected in 1982.

Medicare was introduced in 1984 following the enactment in 1983 of the Health Legislation Amendment Act the purpose of which was to: (a) amend the National Health Act of 1953 and the Health Insurance Act of 1973 to establish a health insurance scheme; (b) enter into arrangements with the states for the provision of public hospital services without charge to eligible Australians; and (c) amend the Health Insurance Commission Act of 1973 to authorize the commission to plan and operate that scheme relating to the payments of Medicare medical benefits.

Medicare was described as a self-funding national health insurance providing free medical and hospital care for all Australians. The self-funding aspect was not realistic since only one-third of the cost of the scheme was derived from a 1-percent personal income tax levy (raised to 1.25 percent in December 1986); the remaining funds were provided from consolidated revenue. It has been suggested that, by 1990, a levy of 7 percent would be necessary to cover the total annual cost.

The act provided for subsidies to be paid by the Australian Government to private hospitals, which were categorized according to the level of services provided. The enacting legislation enabled doctors to bill the government directly and, in doing this, the doctors accepted the 85 percent reimbursement as total settlement for the service rendered. This practice, known as "bulk billing," is strongly opposed by most organized medical associations except in the cases of the elderly and the indigent. The objection is based on the concept that the procedure leads to overservicing by the doctor and to excessive utilization of medical services by the patient, because the patient is unaware of the costs of the services being delivered and billed by the doctor. However, the government strongly supports the concept.

The scheduled fee, to which the 85 percent relates, is derived by a government-appointed independent arbitrator following representation by all interested groups including both government and organized medicine. This fee is the basis of the Medicare reimbursement system for clinical services. The scheduled fees acceptance is not universal, as many members of the medical profession and their representative societies believe the individual practitioners have a right to set their own fees. Within the defined fee structure, there are also differentials between specialist and family physicians for the same procedure. This aggravates previously stated opposition and divides the profession itself.

Medicare functions by reimbursing 85 percent of all medical fees (with a maximum of A$20 being payable by the patient for any one service, or A$150 being the maximum payable by a patient for medical costs in one year), and provides for block financial grants to be allocated to the states to enable them to provide a free public hospital system. The gap of 15 percent between the scheduled fee and the 85 percent Medicare reimbursement is paid by the patient if the doctor bills the patient rather than the government. The gap is seen as a deterrent against excessive use of health services by the patient. However, this argument is suspect when the scheme allows direct billing of the government to occur without any patient contribution. Patients were prohibited from purchasing supplementary insurance for the gap. Recently, the government has yielded to pressure from the medical profession and has allowed gap insurance for hospital services.

If a citizen prefers private medical and hospital treatment, Medicare will fund the medical aspect; the additional necessary health insurance is to be obtained through a network of government-approved nonprofit health insurance organizations. Medicare does not provide dental coverage, nor does it fund allied health services, which, of course, in actuality form an integral part of a modern health delivery system.

Role of State Government

The individual state governments have the responsibility of providing health services to their respective citizens. In doing this, their policies are influenced by national government health policy through its established funding mechanisms. Within the Medicare scheme, the states receive from the national government general revenue grants, which contain untied identifiable health grants as well as specific Medicare grants. These funds, together with funds generated by the state governments, enable the states to provide a wide variety of services.

Hospital and Mental Health Services. These services are available at no cost to public patients. All hospital facilities—both private and public—need to be approved by state authorities and are required to attain defined standards. Because of funding arrangements, all hospital beds are approved by both national and state authorities. Over recent years, governments have gradually reduced bed numbers to the present (1983) ratio of 5.9 acute hospital beds per 1,000 population, of which 22 percent are in the private sector. Nursing home beds are also regulated, with the present ratio being 4.8 beds per 1,000 population. Hospital occupancy rates of 67 percent are estimated, with the rate being much higher in the urban area and lower in the less populated inland areas where many "historical'' beds still exist and are retained because of political pressures relating to small-town economies.

Community Health Services. These are mainly support services, such as nursing and therapy.

Public Health Service. The environmental and occupational health agencies have a responsibility to formulate, regulate, and monitor policy related to this area of activity. Laboratories exist to support such services.

Children's Services. These services include baby clinics, school dental clinics, immunization programs, and school health services for screening purposes.

Aboriginal Health Programs. Both the state and national governments are involved in this service. The health status of the Australian aboriginal is often compared with the health status of the populations of many developing countries because of the high infant mortality rate (30.8 per 1,000 aboriginal births) and the reduced life expectancy (20 years less than the non-aboriginal population). Environmental and communicable diseases such as tuberculosis, sexually transmitted diseases, and parasitic infestations are more prevalent in this population, and these factors, together with dietary deficiencies, contribute to the lower health status of the aboriginal community as compared with the remaining Australian population. Authorities have only recently recognized the need to acknowledge aboriginal culture as a distinct entity with the Australian society. This has resulted in the national government's granting funds to aboriginal communities to plan, implement, and manage health-care programs, as the proponents of the health programs need to be cognizant of the beliefs, customs, and aspirations of the aboriginal people. This has not occurred historically and it resulted in the failure of many well-intentioned public health programs. The major problem presently being experienced is the shortage of health professionals willing to work in remote areas. These people are necessary to act as mentors for aboriginal health workers who, it is hoped, will be able to provide most of the health manpower for the aboriginal population in the future.

Regulation of Health Professionals. It is a state responsibility to regulate the medical and allied health professionals desiring to practice in the state. This function is undertaken by boards composed of members of the respective professions, who define the criteria acceptable for registration purposes.

Local Government Role. State legislation provides the framework in which local authorities maintain standards relating to water supply, sanitation, building codes, and noise and air pollution. These organizations also operate voluntary immunization clinics.

Clinical Practice

The present health system supports the concept that the family physician is the key player in the health system. It is this doctor who is best placed to assess the patient's needs and make decisions on future management. The government is investing significantly in educational programs for family physicians to ensure that their training is appropriate to their role in the health-care system. Most are located in private practice (fee-for-service medicine); a small percentage works in hospitals and community health centers (salaried practice).

If a patient is in need of specialist services, it is necessary for the patient to be referred by a family physician to a specialist. If this does not occur, the patient is not eligible for receipt of Medicare-funded benefits. The family physician has an important gatekeeper role for the more expensive specialist services. In practice, the indigent and those patients with chronic conditions attend hospital outpatient departments. The Australian national government does subsidize pharmaceuticals (the patient pays up to A$10 per item); however, the chronically ill cannot afford these charges and thus visit hospitals where pharmaceuticals are free.

This pattern changes when one considers inpatient services. Only patients who are privately insured are admitted to private hospitals, and usually for short-stay conditions. The public hospitals have traditionally been the locations of the facilities to treat the more serious medical conditions. However, because of lack of funding for equipment and inadequate staffing levels in public hospitals, this pattern is changing, and private hospitals are now developing facilities for the more complicated patient.

Public hospitals are staffed by a combination of full-time salaried staff and part-time visiting staff, as well as by a large number of junior medical staff undergoing supervised training. The method of remuneration of all medical staff in hospitals has been in dispute in recent years. The main point of contention is the relative value of different medical specialists—radiologists, pathologists, surgeons, cardiologists. The medical profession is insistent on fee-for-service payments, while the government prefers sessional payments where hospital facilities funded by the government are used by the specialists.

These problems are compounded by the actions of nurses within the hospitals. Nurses want to play a larger part in the decision-making processes relating to patients, as nurses become more involved in the delivery of more complicated medical processes. These inroads into clinical decision-making are not viewed favorably by the traditional conservative Australian physicians, who do not accept questioning about their role as health team leaders.

Education of Health Professionals

Medical Education

Tertiary institutions exist in each state and provide facilities for the education of medical and allied health students. Medical courses vary from five to six years in total length. This is followed by a one-year mandatory hospital internship prior to being granted registration by the state licensing board. Graduates desiring to attain specialist qualifications must satisfy the requirements of the appropriate "learned" college. The college system is modeled on the English system and is educational rather than medico-political in its objectives.

The Australian national government has funded the Family Medicine Program (FMP), and educational program organized by the College of General Practitioners. FMP involves both hospital and supervised practice training with the objective of ensuring that family physicians are adequately trained prior to their entry into private clinical practice. However, in Australia, there is no formal requirement for an individual to partake in such programs.

The present doctor to patient ratio of 1:521 will be reduced to 1:405 by the year 2001 if present projections of graduates (an increase of 63 percent) and population increase (27 percent) are realistic. The medical profession has been lobbying for reduced student intakes into medical courses for some time, as well as restrictions on the immigration of foreign doctors, but without success. The profession argues that reduced doctor to population ratios will create increased demand for services by the patient, and, to maintain economic viability, the doctor will overservice the patient population. Government, in contrast, expresses the view that additional doctors will increase competition and reduce costs, and, in the process, inefficiencies will be eliminated.

Nursing Education

In Australia, nurses have undertaken their training in the large hospitals to which is attached a school of nursing, which conducts a formal training program.

Over recent years, governments have started funding degree courses at tertiary institutions with the objective of making all training non-hospital based by the 1990s. The number of nurses completing training falls short of the needs of the health system, however, and it is expected that the change in the educational system will compound the problem during the transition period.

Allied Health Education

Therapists, social workers, pharmacists, and pyschologists complete an undergraduate course at the tertiary institution to gain qualifications acceptable to the licensing board. The number of graduates in all groups falls short of the needs of both the public and private sectors. Lack of educational resources is the main reason for the inadequate number of graduates.

Administrative Education

Several tertiary institutions offer courses at both a graduate and undergraduate level in health services administration. Ironically, these courses tend to be undertaken by professional health workers rather than individuals planning a totally administrative career. Many senior health administrators are appointed on the basis of experience, as seniority is a major factor in many public sector appointments.

Current and Future Problems

Every citizen of Australia has the right to health care irrespective of ability to pay for health care, and a substantial amount of service delivery, in particular public health, is undertaken by governments for the benefit of society as a whole. However, there are many aspects of health care which involve the individual citizen directly, and it is this aspect which generates significant questions. For example, does the government have the responsibility to ensure that every citizen has access to health care irrespective of lifestyle, financial means, or place of abode? Alternatively, does the citizen have the right to consume health care and not help meet its cost even though the individual may contribute to the problem? These issues structure the following discussion of current problems in the Australian health-care system.

Three key elements of the above questions deserve consideration: the role of government, the role of the provider of health-care services, and the role of the consumer and/or patient.

The Australian and state governments have become involved in health care from two related aspects: access to health care and the expenditure on health care. A large proportion of the population is now utilizing health services (both public and private) at direct cost to the government, due to the structure of the central government's Medicare reimbursement system. This has led to continuing increases in health-care outlays (Tables 2 and 3).

The medical profession in Australia, however, has been decidedly hostile to governmental attempts to introduce mechanisms to reduce costs. This reflects practicing doctors' fears concerning loss of clinical and economic autonomy due to increased regulation and monitoring of practice patterns. The government has been concerned about medical fraud and overservicing, and has established computer surveillance systems and professional review bodies. It clearly would prefer an alternative to the present fee-for-service system, which, the government argues, discourages internal medicine while promoting increased utilization of diagnostic support services and procedurally oriented specialties.

In similar fashion, the medical profession has not objected to treating the disadvantaged members of the community with reimbursement provided by the government if the remaining members of the community enroll in private medical insurance schemes free from government. The government, not surprisingly, does not share this view, believing it acts on behalf of the consumer (and taxpayer) as a regulator and supervisor of the health services since the patient lacks sufficient knowledge to ensure that quality of care is appropriate.

In 1976, the then Australian minister for health issued a challenge to the medical profession. If the medical profession did not develop programs for clinical review purposes, then the government would introduce a clinical review

Table 2
Estimates of Total Health Expenditure, 1982–1983 to 1984–1985 (Current Prices)

	1982-83	1983-84* ($ million)	1984-85
Recurrent Expenditure	12,199	13,609.5	14,879
Capital Expenditure	411	519.5	639
Total Health Expenditure	12,610	14,129	15,518
Percentage Increase over Previous Year	11.3	12.0	9.8
Total Health Expenditure as percent of GDP	7.6	7.6	7.5

*Medicare introduced during 1983-84 with its first full year in 1984-85.

Source: Australian Institute of Health, *Information Bulletin No. 1*, Canberra, 1986.

Table 3
Proportions of Total Health Expenditure, Financed by Sectors, 1982 to 1985

		Percentage	
Sector	1982-83	1983-84	1984-85
Commonwealth Government	27	31	39
Other Governments	34	34	35
Private Sector	39	35	26

Source: Australian Institute of Health, *Information Bulletin No. 1*, Canberra, 1986.

system as part of the health funding reimbursement scheme. In 1979, the Australian Medical Association and the Australian Council for Hospital Standards established the Peer Review Resource Centre, which was to be controlled by the forementioned bodies with operating funds to be provided by the national government. This center has acted as a stimulus for quality assurance programs, which have been introduced throughout the country on a voluntary basis. Hospital accreditation has also been widely accepted by hospital managers, although some state governments have not supported a concept they view as an intrusion requiring additional funds to achieve and maintain the defined standards. Despite this opposition, many hospitals in the public and private sectors have achieved the required standards.

Moreover, consumers are becoming more aware of health issues, particularly as a result of increased publicity relating to technological advances in diagnosing and treating disease. This awareness extends to challenging traditionally held attitudes of health professionals with patients or questioning advice given by professionals. Where conventional medicine does not fulfill the patients' needs, patients increasingly seek support from alternative providers of health care whose numbers are increasing significantly. Attempts are now being made to regulate these groups to ensure that patients are protected from potentially harmful practices.

A final area of concern is care for the aging population. This group is responsible for the consumption of a high proportion of each health dollar spent and for many of the demands which cannot be accommodated due to lack of resources. Australian society has not yet had the problem put before it since resources have not yet been restricted. However, in the near future, the issue of care for the aged in a technological era will need to be addressed.

References

Australian Bureau of Statistics. 1986. *Year Book Australia*. Canberra: Australian Government Publishing Service.

Australian Bureau of Statistics. 1983. *Australian Health Services 1983*. Canberra: Australian Government Publishing Service.

Dewdney, J. C. H. 1972. *Australian Health Services*. Sydney: John Wiley and Sons.

Director General of Health. 1986. *Commonwealth Department of Health Annual Report 1985–86*. Canberra: Australian Government Publishing Services.

Fenner, F. 1985. The Medical Research Institutes of Australia. *Med. J. Aust*. 142: 171–72.

Grant, C. and H. M. Lapsley. 1982. *The Australian Health Care System*. ASHSA Number 46. University of NWS: School of Health Administration.

Hospital and Health Services Commission. 1978. *A Discussion Paper on Paying for Health Care*. Canberra: Australian Government Publishing Service.

Leeder, S. 1985. Health for All by the Year 2000. *Med. J. Aust*. 142: 551–55.

Medical Journal of Australia. 1985. Aboriginal Health. *Med. J. Aust*. Special Supplement, Oct. 28, 1985, 143: 9.

Sax, S. 1980. *Medicine in the 80's. Can We Afford It?* ASHA Number 40. University of NWS: School of Health Administration.

Sax, S. 1984. *A Strife of Interests*. Sydney: George Allen and Unwin.

Tatchell, M., ed. 1984. *Perspectives on Health Policy*. Canberra: Australian National University.

Thame, C. 1974. Health and the State. Ph.D. thesis. Canberra: Australian National University.

BRAZIL

Marlow Kwitko and
Eleutério Rodriguez Neto

General Description of the Country and Existing Health Conditions

The Federative Republic of Brazil is divided into the following political-administrative units: 23 states, three territories, and the Federal District, where the nation's capital, Brasilia, is located. These units have been grouped into five major regions or regional divisions (Fundação Instituto, 1983, 1980).

Brazil's total population in 1985 was estimated at 135,564,000. The average geometric rate of annual growth of the population was 2.48 percent for the 1970–1980 period, having dropped from the 2.89 percent recorded for the previous ten-year period. In 1980, 67.59 percent of the population lived in urban areas, and it is estimated that over 160 million people will be living in cities in the year 2000. Of these, 80 percent will be living in agglomerations of over 20,000 persons, and approximately one half of these pepole will be living in the nation's ten metropolitan areas. A drop was registered in the under-14 age group, falling from 42.0 percent in 1970 to 38.2 percent in 1980; the over-60 age group, on the other hand, rose from 5.2 percent to 6.5 percent of the total population (Fundação Instituto 1983).

The gross domestic product (GDP) was US $226.72 billion in 1983, with a per capita GDP of US $1,768 (estimated on the basis of 128.2 million inhabitants). In the area of education, the rate of illiteracy was 29.9 percent for all persons over the age of five (1982 data). Six percent of the national budget was allocated to the education sector in 1984.

Tables 1 through 6 present data on health care: Table 1, life expectancy; Table 2, general mortality; Table 2, infant mortality; Tables 2 and 3, mortality by age

Table 1
Life Expectancy by Region and Monthly Family Income (1970)

STATE OR REGION	MONTHLY INCOME (cruzeiros)					Difference between Highest and Lowest Income Levels
	General Average	1 - 150 (1)	151 - 300 (2)	301 - 500 (3)	501 + (4)	
Amazonas	54,2	53,4	53,9	54,8	58,2	4.8
North Region	50,4	50,0	50,8	52,7	55,7	5.7
Northeast Region	44,2	42,8	46,1	50,3	54,4	11.6
Bahia	49,7	48,9	50,3	51,9	54,9	6.0
Minas Gerais	55,4	53,8	55,4	55,6	62,3	8.5
Rio de Janeiro	57,0	54,1	54,8	57,6	62,1	8.0
São Paulo	58,2	54,7	56,1	58,7	63,9	9.2
Paranã	56,6	54,8	56,5	59,3	63,7	8.9
South Region	61,9	60,5	61,2	63,4	66,9	6.4
Center-west Region	57,5	56,5	57,1	58,2	63,3	6.8
Brazil	53,4	49,9	54,5	57,6	62,0	12.1

Source: Carvalho, J.A.M., and Charles Hood, "Mortality, Income Distribution, and Rural-Urban Residence in Brazil," *Population and Development Review*, vol. 4, no. 3, September 1978. (Taken from a technical document of the CNRH/IPLAN/Planning Secretariat of the Presidency of the Republic, Brazil. Vitor G. Pinto and Líscio F. B. Camargo, July 1979.)

group and group of causes; Table 4, years of life potentially lost by group of causes; Table 5, vaccine-preventable diseases; and Table 6, endemic diseases.

With respect to the availability of health-care services, data are presented on basic sanitation services (Table 7) and health establishments and hospital beds (Table 8).

Statistics on professional health-care staff employed at public and private establishments across the country showed that, in 1980, the country had approximately 197,000 upper-level professionals (146,000 physicians, 17,000 dentists, 15,000 nurses, 5,000 pharmacists, 2,000 nutritionists, 4,000 social workers, and 8,000 in other categories), about 111,000 professionals with secondary education (technical and auxiliary staff), and approximately 265,000 with primary education (Fundação Instituto 1980).

Hospitalization, outpatient services, and dental care are provided mostly by the Social Security Fund's National Institute for Medical Care (Instituto Nacional de Assistência Médica da Previdência Social, or INAMPS), which covers approximately 90 percent of the population (Ministéro de Previdéncia 1983). In 1982, the institute directly or indirectly covered approximately 13 million hospitalizations, 206 million medical visits, and 39 million dental visits.

According to preliminary data provided by the secretaries of state for health

Table 2
Health Indicators by Major Regions (1980)

INDICATOR / REGION	Infant Mortality Coefficient (per 1,000 live births)	General Mortality Coefficient (per 1,000 persons)	COEFFICIENT FOR PROPORTIONAL MORTALITY						
			By Age		By Cause				
			Under 1 year	50 and over	Infectious and parasitic diseases	Tumors	Diseases of the Circulatory System	Diseases of the Respiratory System	External Causes
North	100.0	8.5	31.7	34.4	26.0	7.1	19.7	8.2	13.3
Northeast	130.0	12.0	34.7	39.1	31.0	7.4	24.3	9.3	12.3
Southeast	67.0	7.6	20.4	53.2	9.1	10.8	34.5	10.6	11.1
South	55.0	6.9	18.2	56.1	8.0	13.3	35.7	9.9	12.4
Center-West	85.0	7.5	21.6	42.8	14.8	8.7	26.1	9.3	17.2
BRAZIL	87.3	8.8	26.4	46.5	14.8	9.5	29.4	9.8	12.2

Estimated

Source: National Epidemiology Division, SNABS, Ministry of Health, Brazil.

Table 3
Proportional Mortality by Group of Causes* and by Age Group (1981)**

CAUSE	Under 1 year	1-4 years	5-19 years	20-49 years	50 and over	For all ages
Infectious and Parasitic Diseases	26.1	33.7	8.7	7.3	4.0	13.5
Neoplasms	0.2	3.9	7.4	10.6	16.1	9.7
Diseases of the Circulatory System	0.6	2.5	7.2	24.2	54.3	29.9
Diseases of the Respiratory System	15.4	25.0	7.1	5.3	8.4	9.8
Perinatal	41.3	0.1	0.0	0.0	0.0	9.8
External	0.7	13.0	51.9	35.0	4.6	12.4
Other	15.7	21.8	17.7	17.6	12.6	14.9
TOTAL	100.0	100.0	100.0	100.0	100.0	100.0
Unspecified	22.7	35.1	16.0	14.8	21.3	21.1

*Does not include unspecified causes.
**Does not include cases where age was not known.
Source: National Epidemiology Division, SNABS, Ministry of Health, Brazil.

Table 4
Years of Life Potentially Lost by Persons Between the Ages of 7 Days and 65 Years, by the 10 Major Groups of Causes of Death (Coefficients per 1,000 Persons, and Percentage of Total for State Capitals, 1980)

Nº	Group of Causes	Years Lost	Coef./1000 Persons	%
	All causes	4,394,366	153.5	100.0
1	Infectious Intestinal diseases	847,669	29.6	19.3
2	Pneumonias	526,941	18.4	12.0
3	Neoplasms	224,808	7.9	5.1
4	Nutritional Deficiencies and Anemias	206,167	7.2	4.7
5	Motor vehicle accidents	203,357	7.1	4.6
6	Homicides	164,985	5.8	3.8
7	Cerebrovascular diseases	115,120	4.0	2.6
8	Birth defects	112,748	3.9	2.6
9	Vaccine-preventable diseases	109,783	3.8	2.5
	(Measles)	80,829	2.8	1.8
10	Other Reducible Infectious	98,389	3.4	2.2
	Diseases (Tuberculosis)	58,138	2.0	1.3
	SUBTOTAL	2,609,968	91.2	59.4
	UNSPECIFIED	270,240	-	6.1

Source: National Epidemiology Division, SNABS, Ministry of Health, Brazil.

(related to the programs and standards of the Ministry of Health), approximately 3 million children under one year of age were immunized in 1984; vaccination coverage was 85 percent for measles, 69 percent for the triple vaccine (diphtheria-pertussis-tetanus DPT), and 78 percent for tuberculosis (Ministério de Saúde, 1984b).

Historical Overview and Current Structure of the Health-Care System

The development of Brazil's health-care services can be divided into three distinct periods on the basis of the general trends that characterize them.

Table 5

Number of Cases of Vaccine-Preventable Diseases and Coefficient per 1,000 Persons for Typhoid Fever, Meningococcic Diseases, and Meningitis (1980–1984)

YEAR / DISEASE	1980		1981		1982		1983		1984*	
	Nº of Cases	Coef.	Nº of Cases	Coef.	Nº of Cases	Coef.	Nº of Cases	Coef.	Nº of Cases	Coef.
Poliomyelitis	1,290	1.10	122	0.10	69	0.06	45	0.03	63	0.05
Measles	99,263	82.9	61,281	50.0	39,370	31.4	58,259	45.5	76,306	58.3
Diphtheria	4,646	3.9	3,846	3.1	3,297	2.6	3,369	2.6	2,968	2.3
Traumatic tetanus	...	...	...	...	1,977	1.6	2,098	1.6	2,177	1.7
Tetanus neonatorum	...	...	...	...	572	14.8	706	17.9	574	14.2
Tetanus - unidentified form	3,098	2.6	2,940	2.4	261	0.2	54	0.0	-	-
Pertussis	45,752	38.2	42,247	34.5	54,766	43.7	26,300	20.5	17,974	13.7
Typhoid fever	4,691	3.9	3,967	3.2	3,825	3.1	3,886	3.0	4,765	3.6
Meningococcic disease	1,568	1.3	1,229	1.0	1,220	1.0	1,448*	1.1	904	0.7
Meningitis in general	13,635	11.4	13,810	11.3	15,772	12.6	22,208*	17.3	19,374	14.8

*Preliminary data subject to modification.

Source: SNABS, Ministry of Health, Brazil.

Table 6
Number of Positive Cases by Endemic Disease (1970–1984)

YEAR / Nº OF CASES	MALÁRIA	YELLOW FEVER	PLAGUE	TRACHOMA	FILARIASIS	LEISHMANIASIS		SCHISTOSOMIASIS		CHAGAS' DISEASE	
						VISCERAL	TEGMENTARY	TESTS DONE	POSITIVE TESTS	TRIATOMAS EXAMINED	TRIATOMAS THAT TESTED POSITIVE
1970	52,469	2	101	64,856	8,371	209	2,481	1,798,558	58,696	44,652	1,377
1971	76,752	11	146	36,258	9,957	161	3,498	1,663,112	51,408	46,698	1,482
1972	82,421	9	169	30,160	12,636	198	3,064	1,819,255	56,300	88,487	6,072
1973	76,112	70	152	16,842	10,438	163	2,815	1,609,335	52,937	118,223	8,450
1974	64,320	13	290	17,493	7,362	192	3,056	988,998	54,847	108,858	3,972
1975	88,630	1	496	17,487	7,452	138	2,526	855,921	46,331	76,386	5,698
1976	86,437	1	97	12,752	8,042	93	5,561	1,018,496	51,718	99,090	4,989
1977	101,081	9	1	51,317	10,564	61	3,013	443,591	103,409	108,967	3,406
1978	117,267	21	11	68,975	8,628	93	2,557	626,657	86,111	135,137	5,637
1979	144,215	12	-	91,092	7,127	85	3,273	663,429	59,905	132,414	8,567
1980	169,871	27	107	81,944	9,435	177	3,942	1,684,619	164,860	141,495	6,159
1981	197,149	22	59	83,788	6,994	340	5,096	1,840,626	172,242	25,187	480
1982	221,939	24	151	128,048	6,541	1,092	4,821	984,181	80,868	38,043	1,579
1983	297,687	6	82	137,228	4,998	1,124	5,009	2,093,508	183,999	356,739	14,467
1984	176,816	41	17	49,845	1,671	762	3,093	73,097	3,634	176,289	5,169

Data as of June 1984.
Sources: SEST/DITEC/SUCAM/Ministry of Health/Brazil.

Table 7
Households with Basic Sanitation Services (1970–1980)

SANITATION SERVICE	YEAR	BRAZIL	URBAN	RURAL
a. Connected to general water supply services	1970	5,784	5,592	192
	1980	14,073	13,811	262
b. Connected to general sanitation system or having septic tank	1970	4,684	4,539	145
	1980	10,966	10,459	507
c. No sanitation facilities	1970	6,954	1,483	5,471
	1980	6,019	1,304	4,715

Source: IBGE, Statistical Yearbook for Brazil, 1981.

The first period ended in 1930 and was characterized, with respect to the manner in which health-care services were provided to the population, by the same institutional structure that was used in the last century. Individual medical care was provided by charitable institutions to persons who were not able to pay or by physicians who normally worked independently and provided services in exchange for direct remuneration at their own offices, at hospitals, or at the patient's home. In rural areas, where no health-care services were available, traditional methods of health care were used. Only medium-sized and large cities had hospitals, so health-care coverage was very low. Measures were taken to control major epidemics as well as health conditions in port cities. As early as the 1920s, when the first organized labor groups came into existence, health cooperatives began to appear. At first, they were financed exclusively by mutual aid societies; later, they gradually began to include employer contributions. Although health care was not their initial or principal motivation, these changes identified a new trend in the historical setting of the 1930 Revolution, when the rural oligarchy in power was replaced by populist rule. This brought about some positive changes, including new forms of health care for urban workers.

The period between the 1930s and 1960s was basically characterized by increased government involvement in medical care in the form of pension and retirement funds (Institutos de Aposentadorias e Pensões) established at the national level. Although oriented toward specific professions, these funds were supported by contributions from employees, employers, and the government and were governed by national standards for health care. Some of these funds adopted the strategy of creating their own services; others contracted medical care services from third parties. The early part of this period saw the gradual disappearance of the private practice of medicine and an increase in the number of salaried physicians and in government involvement in contracting for patient services. In the 1950s, the Ministry of Health was created; it was initially limited to

Table 8
Health Establishments and Beds by Classification and Region

HEALTH ESTABLISHMENT	CLASSIFICATION AND REGION											
	PUBLIC						PRIVATE					
	N	NE	SE	S	CW	BR	N	NE	SE	S	CW	BR
Health post	874	3,092	461	465	272	5,164	14	37	7	15	-	73
Health center	307	1,414	1,718	884	466	4,789	3	15	6	10	1	35
Medical care post or polyclinic	94	1,022	1,127	625	45	2,913	267	1,034	2,193	463	141	4,098
Emergency ambulatory unit	2	7	46	-	2	59	2	14	85	19	4	124
Mixed unit	123	222	20	1	29	395	12	17	21	2	3	55
Hospital	77	403	235	126	54	895	262	854	1,411	1,111	542	4,180
Hospital beds	7,140	29,312	47.490	16,463	7,792	108,197	11,758	55,396	168,163	76,431	25,965	337,713

N—North Region; NE—Northeast Region; SE—Southeast Region; S—South Region; CW—Center-West Region; BR—Brazil.

Source: Ministry of Health, Health Information System, 1983. Estimated populations and number of municipalities (1981): North—10.0 million persons and 276 municipalities; Northeast—32.0 million and 1,231; Southeast—53.0 million and 1,411; South—19.4 million and 733; Center-West—9.0 million and 367; Brazil—123.4 million and 4,018 municipalities.

formulating specific actions of a collective nature, such as the control of endemic diseases, the establishment of standards, the conduct of health inspection, the provision of medical care in special areas of interest to the government, and the maintenance of some hospitals and asylums for patients of tuberculosis, psychiatric treatment, and Hansen's disease. The state governments (State Secretaries of Health) operated within this same environment and had a relatively low level of involvement in medical care per se; city governments often were responsible for providing emergency treatment. In 1967, most of these funds merged to create the National Institute for Social Security (Instituto Nacional de Previdência Social, or INPS). The institute's principal strategy for providing medical care was to contract services from third parties, as well as maintaining services provided by some of the previously existing funds; this multiplicity created contradictions, conflict, and inefficiency. In addition, great disparities arose in the macroregions, owing to the fact that the states in the north, and in particular those in the northeast, had a lower level of coverage of services. In 1971, FUNRURAL was created, under the Social Security Institute, as a means to extend coverage to the rural population; however, the benefits and services it provides are quantitatively and qualitatively inferior to those provided to the urban population because of its particular financing structure.

The period beginning in the 1970s saw the consolidation of the Social Security Institute's now dominant role in providing health-care services in the country. Major administrative reforms in 1974 led to the creation of the Ministry of Welfare and Social Security and the National System for Welfare and Social Security in 1977, which included the National Institute for Medical Care (INAMPS). In 1975, the law establishing the National Health System was enacted, thereby institutionalizing the separation of collective/preventive actions and individual/curative actions, under the Ministry of Health/State Secretaries of Health and the Ministry of Welfare and Social Security, respectively. With the mandate of transferring health care to the private sector, these agencies grew very rapidly and unevenly, focusing mainly on the more developed regions. They were supported by federal funding provided through the Social Development Fund, used for hospital construction and equipment procurement, and the guarantee that the INAMPS would contract their services. In an attempt to reduce this macroregional distortion, the Ministry of Health began to work with the State Secretaries of Health in the northeast region in the late 1970s to establish a network of basic health-care services aimed specifically at the needs of the rural population.

Although the public subsector is the main source of financing for health-care services in Brazil today, private medical care institutions are the major service providers, particularly with respect to hospitals; approximately 75 percent of the available beds are located in private institutions. The health sector in Brazil also includes university hospitals and school-hospitals under the Ministry of Education and other institutions, in addition to the health-care services provided to specific groups (the Armed Forces, state social security programs, and so forth).

Due to their potential importance, two other institutions should be mentioned.

The first is the Central Office for Drugs (Central de Medicamentos, or CEME), an independent agency now related to the Ministry of Health, created in the early 1970s to handle the country's drug-related policies. At first, it was responsible not only for defining priorities and strategies, but also for distributing drugs through public health institutions. The second institution is the National Institute for Food and Nutrition (Instituto Nacional de Alimentação e Nutrição, or INAN), an independent agency, also related to the Ministry of Health, which establishes guidelines and channels funds for the sector in the area of food and nutrition, carrying out its specific programs in conjunction with the State Secretaries of Health.

The area of sanitation services involves a number of institutions, such as the Ministry of Urban Development and the Environment, the Ministry of Health, and the state and municipal governments. Of these, the Ministry of Urban Development and the Environment plays a particularly important role inasmuch as it is responsible for coordinating the National Plan for Sanitation, which implements government policy in this sector and receives the largest share of financial resources, dealing principally with urban areas.

Given the multiplicity of agencies in the health sector in Brazil and the duplication of efforts for a given population, the Interministerial Committee on Planning (CIPLAN) was created in 1980 to allow interinstitutional coordination at the federal level. Within the area of social security, the Consulting Council of the Bureau for Medical Care (Conselho Consultivo da Administração de Saúde Previdenciária, or CONASP) was instituted in 1981, increasing the level of representativeness in the management of medical care services, with the goal of restructuring the activities of the Social Security Institute with respect to health-care services.

More recently, in May 1984, CIPLAN approved a new strategy for interinstitutional coordination in the sector, entitled "Comprehensive Health Action," which, through the establishment of agreements, involves the federal, state, and municipal governments and creates state and municipal management committees for the respective levels of the health-care system.

Current Problems of the Health-Care System

Health conditions in Brazil vary greatly, as can be seen by the coexistence of morbidity and mortality patterns that are characterized by the "diseases of development" (degenerative diseases, occupational diseases, diseases related to work accidents, traffic accidents, violence, etc.) and "diseases of poverty" (malnutrition, diarrheal diseases, infectious/contagious diseases, etc.).

The impact of socioeconomic factors on the population's health is also noteworthy: Table 1 shows the variations in the risk of becoming ill or dying as reflected by the life expectancies for different social classes (classified in accordance with their position in the labor market) for various regions of the country. There is a difference of approximately 24 years between the life expectancy of persons of lower income levels in the northeast region and the higher income populations in the country's south region. Similarly, regional imbalances with respect to mortality are evident in Table 2, which shows higher rates for general and infant mortality in the north and northeast regions with respect to the other regions; furthermore, in the north and northeast regions, the mortality rate for the 50 and over age group is only slightly higher than the rate for children under one year of age, unlike the other, more developed regions, where the spread is considerably larger. Table 2 also reveals significant differences in the regional distribution of mortality by group of causes, with "diseases of poverty" being more common in the lesser developed regions and "diseases of development" prevailing in the regions that are more economically privileged.

Differences are also visible between rural and urban populations. The 1980 figures for life expectancy at birth were 56.3 years for men and 62.8 for women in Brazil: 57.5 and 64.1 years, respectively, in urban areas, but only 54.6 and 61.0 years, respectively, in rural areas. Studies sponsored by the Ministry of Health revealed a malnutrition level of 66 percent in rural areas and 58 percent in urban areas of the northeast region for children between the ages of one and five; in some states of the southeast region, the ratio was 52 percent for rural areas and 38 percent for urban areas. The major endemic diseases present in Brazil (Table 6) are concentrated mainly in rural areas along the internal migration routes and in areas involved in projects for territorial penetration. There is no doubt that the precarious status of basic sanitation in rural areas (not to mention living conditions and income profiles) contributes to the existence of such disparities. This is shown in Table 7, which reveals a trend toward the implementation of new basic sanitation services in rural areas; however, no significant improvements were achieved in the 1970–1980 period, contrary to the results in urban areas.

An analysis of the data on the years of life potentially lost (Brazil, 1980) according to the ten major groups of causes of death (Table 4) shows that infectious intestinal diseases are the major cause, followed by various kinds of pneumonia. An analysis of this kind by region shows that these two groups of diseases predominate in every case, with the former being more common in lesser developed regions (north and northeast) and the latter showing a slight predominance in the economically privileged regions.

It is estimated that, for Brazil, approximately 100,000 cases per year involve diseases that could have been prevented by immunization.

With respect to environmental conditions and in addition to the above-mentioned imbalance between urban and rural areas, there is also a considerable lack of basic sanitation services overall; the 1980 census showed that approximately 50 percent of Brazilian households did not have these services. Even in urban areas, according to 1976 data, about half of all private homes have inadequate water and sewage facilities or were built with rude construction materials. In regard to living conditions, special attention should be given to those areas in which Chagas' disease is endemic: The precarious conditions of approximately one million households favor the transmission of this disease. Deficiencies also exist in the area of protecting the environment from pollution caused by chemical and physical contaminants, principally in urban and industrial centers, where protection against work-related accidents is also very limited. With respect to this kind of accident, the country spends a considerable amount on treating and caring for workers who have been injured on the job or who are carriers of occupational diseases, but it invests relatively little in the application of available preventive measures.

The precarious profile of personal income in Brazil is certainly a determining factor in the structure and risk of morbidity and mortality (shown in part in Table 1); furthermore, the great majority of the population is not able to assume directly any material responsibility for its own health care.

With respect to the problems related to the current organization of the health sector, the law that established the National Health System in 1975 but was never implemented made the institutional separation of technically indivisible actions more or less official by disassociating preventive/collective actions (under the responsibility of the Ministry of Health and the state and municipal Secretaries of Health) from individual/curative health care (under the responsibility of the Ministry of Social Security and the public and private institutions contracted by the ministry) and activities involving sanitation, prevention/inspection of occupational health, and the training and development of upper level human resources (under the responsibility, respectively, of the ministries of Urban Development and the Environment, Labor, and Education).

Furthermore, although the law establishing the National Health System attributed the responsibility for formulating policy to the Ministry of Health, it did not establish any connection between the health-care services provided under Social Security, which are unevenly distributed in the sector, and the National Health Policy; nor did it give the Ministry of Health the power to allocate sectoral resources. This, added to the fact that the other elements of the system at the federal level, with the exception of the Ministry of Labor, are financially more powerful than the Ministry of Health, makes this agency, in regard to the formulation of policy for the sector, merely an instrument for drawing up normative documents that it cannot always enforce. As a result, the efforts to establish interinstitutional coordination by means of specialized groups or the coordinated development of programs have not been able to bypass these disassociations and balance the health care system. The system also suffers from the following distortions:

- Major discrepancies in the distribution of health-care services among different regions and social groups, with preference being given to urban areas and populations; it is estimated that one-third of Brazil's population does not have regular access to health-care services.
- Discrepancies between actual needs and the health-care services provided, with services being biased not only in their distribution, as pointed out above, but also in the pre-

dominance of specialized and curative hospital services, thereby interfering with the new comprehensive aspect of health activities (which should also include basic, efficient activities for the control of environmental pollution, endemic diseases, nutritional status, and occupational health) and a broader, more even distribution of services.

- Excessive overlapping of resources and multiplicity of costs based on the lack of interinstitutional coordination mentioned above.
- Overcentralization of decision-making powers and financial resources, leaving little margin for political, financial, and technical action by state and municipal health agencies.
- Low level of utilization of the installed capacity of government health agencies, particularly outpatient services (estimated at 60 percent).
- Insufficient preparation of managers to administer government health agencies and lack of availability of human resources and materials for these services.
- Limited impact of collective programs, implemented directly by the Ministry of Health and the State Secretaries of Health, on the general health of the population.
- Harmful separation of institutional responsibilities with respect to occupational health activities by means of preventive measures and compliance with legislation, with the Ministry of Labor being responsible for inspection and the Ministry of Social Security being responsible for medical care and rehabilitation.
- Major problems with respect to the health-care services provided by Social Security, health-care services in rural areas, funding for the sector, and its current policies on human resources and drugs, which will be examined later in this chapter.

In regard to health-care services provided under Social Security, it should be pointed out that this system has had to treat an ever-growing number of patients, leading it to expand its treatment capabilities. It virtually tripled its coverage capabilities in the 1970s, using government services and, to a greater extent, private services contracted by the government. The public subsector was unable to handle the growth in demand, primarily because there was no political support for it to grow at the required pace. The Social Development Fund, created in the 1970s, seemed to be the best alternative to subsidizing resources for investment in the urban and rural networks of federal, state, and municipal health-care services; these subsidies, however, were channeled mostly into the private urban hospitals. This fact, along with the policy adopted by the medical care activities of the Social Security Institute in 1974 to increase the contracting of private services, consolidated the position of the private subsector as the main vehicle for providing medical-hospital services to the population and resulted in a greater concentration of these resources in urban areas to the detriment of rural areas.

The Social Security Institute, as the institution responsible for almost all medical care services throughout the country and which, as such, incorporates widely varying methods of organization for these activities, consolidated its current methods for operating on this basis. It is true that it has expanded coverage to new levels (approximately 87 percent of Brazil's population), but, by the same token, it has also accumulated the wide variety of distortions described above.

Special mention should be made of the health-care problems in rural areas, where approximately one-third of the country's population lives. If we include the residents of cities with fewer than 20,000 inhabitants and those who live in small towns around the large cities, this number represents over half of Brazil's total population. It should be pointed out here that this population group's ability to apply pressure through representative organizations and institutions to obtain access to health-care services is very limited; as a result, they receive little consideration in the health policy decisions that affect them.

Health-care services in the rural areas of Brazil are governed by two different strategies, both of which have major flaws. One of the strategies is to provide care under Social Security, thereby spreading resources thinly without having a defined program of support; the second, developed mainly by the State Secretaries of Health under the auspices of the Ministry of Health, establishes a program for primary health-care actions, but suffers from an insufficient level of institutional coordination as well as major operational deficiencies. To provide a clearer idea of the deficiencies in health care in rural areas, 1981 data from the Social Security Institute show that the services provided in urban areas exceed those provided in rural areas by approximately 9 times with respect to medical visits, 15 times for related services, 2.7 times for dental visits, and 4.5 times for hospitalization.

In regard to financing problems in this sector, Brazil assigns only 4 percent of its GNP to the health sector each year, and it has a low level of per capita disbursements (US $77 in 1982).

A very concentrated (regressive) pattern has been identified in the process of collection, circulation, and distribution of financial resources for health-care services. Nearly 50 percent of the health sector's available funds comes from withholdings from paychecks; consequently, work-intensive firms are penalized, pushing the cost of labor up and contributing to unemployment. Furthermore, this cost is then included in the final price for goods and services consumed by the population, placing an excessive burden on the purchasing power of lower income groups. Approximately 10 percent of these resources are provided by indirect state taxes, which show the same regressive features as described above. Only slightly more than 10 percent of these resources are provided by government funds taken from more progressive sources, such as income tax. With respect to spending in the private subsector, costs for personnel represent at least half of this area (15 percent of the health care budget); here, there is the unique feature, also regressive, that income tax is deducted as well. Similarly, the participation of employer schemes in the sector's budget also shows regressive features, being characterized by firms that provide health-care services to their employees, but pass the additional cost for these services on to the market, while they receive at the same time subsidies from Social Security, when agreements exist, or from the government in the form of income tax deductions for employees and employers. A health budget that is funded by different sources with different structures of political and economic support and the need to decentralize from federal sources (which currently provide over 60 percent of all governmental funds for health care) to state and municipal sources are two key obstacles to unifying the health-care system and to coordinating its various institutions.

In regard to the flow of financial resources within the health sector, federal government resources are transferred to state and municipal institutions through a variety of specific projects; this results in overlapping efforts, particularly by the State Secretaries of Health, which expand their technical and bureaucratic structures without producing a proportional effect on improving local health-care services and programs. In addition, the transfer of financial resources for projects from the federal government to state or municipal governments takes a long time, thereby limiting the planning capabilities of the receiving institutions and often putting them behind schedule in the implementation of projects, since they have to rechannel resources for other purposes. In this same area of problems related to the intrasectoral flow of financial resources, it must be noted that large subsidies are granted to some private producers. For example, hospitals that are recognized as being philanthropic or charitable receive subsidies in the form of exemptions from employer contributions to Social Security, reduced rates for public services, exemption from income tax, and so on. This gives them a financial advantage over other private hospitals that provide services to Social Security. Other types of subsidies to private providers also exist, and these can be seen in relationships between private and public providers, particularly with respect to the siting of private establishments near large government agencies. Patients with complicated conditions are sent to government services whereas the more lucrative ones are retained by the private services; there is also higher utilization of specialized diagnostic and therapeutical facilities and more permissiveness in observing work hours at government agencies.

There is, furthermore, evidence showing that the higher-income groups are turning more to using free public services in relation to the other social groups due to the relative drop in their purchasing power; this aggravates the already precarious coverage of the lower levels of the social pyramid and increases the phenomenon of concentration in the distribution of resources.

Other problems pertaining to financing can also be identified. The public health subsystem, which is financed by general taxes, has been shrinking gradually with respect to the subsystem of medical care provided by Social Security. With reference to public spending on health matters, the share of the first subsystem fell from 87.1 percent in 1949, to nearly 30 percent in 1975, and then to 15 percent in 1982. Of the total for federal spending, the share of the Ministry of Health has also been falling: from 1.8 percent in 1978, to 1.6 percent in 1982, and to 1.5 percent in 1984, although real growth is projected for the Ministry's 1986 budget. As to the control of endemic diseases, one of the Ministry's principal programs, costs for malaria and schistosomiasis control programs dropped between 1978 and 1981, in real terms, by 35 percent and 80 percent, respectively. In 1981, the real costs for controlling communicable diseases were 43 percent lower than in 1978. Spending for the Ministry's four priority programs—basic health care services, food and nutrition, control of communicable diseases, and drugs—represented only 7 percent of the Ministry's total costs in 1978 and 12 percent in 1982.

With respect to Social Security, the system as a whole, which includes medical care (INAMPS), has changed since the 1970s, when it grew faster than the economy as a whole. This is a result of the current unfavorable economic conditions which are reflected in an increase in Social Security payments and the trend toward exponential growth in the system. Beginning in the 1980s, the hospital-medical care subsystem has had to face constraints on resources as a result of this crisis. Consequently, INAMPS' share in the system's budget (SINPAS), estimated at approximately 25 percent, has dropped gradually. In the 1970s, it was constantly above 26 percent. As of 1980, however, when it was at 27 percent, it began to fall, with values of 24.3 percent, 23.0 percent, and 22.3 percent for 1981, 1982, and 1983, respectively. In 1984, however, it reached 25.4 percent. This drop over recent years was caused basically by the pressure created by benefits paid in cash by the system, which could not be reduced, and these gradually depleted the available resources for medical care and forced the INAMPS to apply measures to contain and rationalize its expenses. Such measures, due to their inadequacy and insufficient application, have not been able to obtain the desired control of expenses and have contributed to the existence of a deficit in the Social Security system. In addition, it is expected that growth in the revenue of the Social Security Institute and the National Treasury (general taxes) will remain below the growth of overall health-care costs. This means that these costs will have to be covered by other sources of financing. Hence, the Social Investment Fund (FINSOCIAL), created in 1982, has as one of its objectives to act as an additional source of financing for the health system; it may, however, become merely a substitute source for funds.

Note should also be taken of the low level of participation of the Ministry of Education in paying for its university hospitals, which are financed to a great extent by resources provided, through agreements, by Social Security; the depletion of state and municipal levels, caused by the current centralized tax policy, making it impossible for them to earmark more resources for health care (their total amount currently accounts for less than 40 percent of public financing in this sector); and the progressive difficulty of the middle-level strata of the population to pay directly for their own health care, thereby increasing the demand for services paid for by the state, in particular, by Social Security.

Rural areas present special financing problems, which are characterized by an unavailability of resources that is even more acute than it is in urban areas. In 1980, for example, Social Security spent almost five times less on hospitalizations in rural areas than in urban areas and almost thirteen times less on outpatient services. The programming of rural health-care services under Social Security shows a deficit, with expenses exceeding incoming funds by about 10 percent in 1981.

With respect to investment problems in the sector, recent estimates have indicated that the needs for reinvestment in the public and private service network, particularly hospital services, would be approximately 2 billion dollars each year until the end of this century, and this would merely be to maintain coverage levels existing at the beginning of the 1980s (adjusted for population growth during the period). This figure, which represents approximately 10 percent of the country's gross capital formation, is probably not within the health sector's reach. The public subsector has been investing a very low amount, concentrating mostly on expanding the network of peripheral outpatient units. The number of public hospital beds has risen only by two-thirds since the 1950s. These hospital facilities, as well as the network of basic units, which has been expanding more recently, need larger allocations in order to recover their operational capacity and avoid, at the same time, any significant reversal in the structure. The private subsector, on the other hand, has invested considerably in the expansion of its installed capacity, particularly in hospitals; over the past 30 years, its capacity has grown from a level of having 54 percent of the nation's hospital beds to 80 percent. This growth, which was concentrated in the southeast region and which has been slowing down since the end of the 1970s, occurred mainly at the expense of small and medium-sized units which were funded, as mentioned above, by credit from the Social Development Fund (FAS) and supported by the fact that Social Security contracted its services. There have been indications, however, of deterioration in the private hospital situation, in the form of a slower rate of growth, as mentioned, or based on the progressive devaluation of the prices that Social Security pays for services provided. As a result, there is a need for more investment to facilitate their recovery; these investments, however, are progressively less viable for most small and medium-sized private investors, making it possible to foresee a possible, gradual deactivation of part of the nation's hospital network, bringing about a major reorganization.

It is surprising to note the inadequacy of policies regarding health-care personnel with respect to the development of human resources as well as working conditions and remuneration, thereby contributing to the low level of quality of health-care services. Furthermore, the training of upper level human resources does not correspond, particularly in the area of medicine, to the population's real health-care needs. Educational institutions (universities), besides their own inadequacies, are totally incapable of remedying the situation by reorienting the expectations created in the training of professionals. This is due to the prevailing medical care model existing in the country, which favors technological sophistication and specialization to the detriment of technologies that are better suited to meeting priority health-care problems. Programming is still precarious for continuing education programs for upper level and auxiliary personnel in public and private health-care services, in the area of providing services as well as in the managerial training of the personnel responsible for administration. Moreover, the institutional pluralism in the health sector implies the existence of salary patterns that, for a given professional category, differ from institution to institution, and this is one of the elements that complicate efforts aimed at intrasectoral coordination.

With regard to physician income, it should be noted that exclusive private practice has dropped considerably in Brazil over the last decades, owing to the lack of a market (currently, approximately 95 percent of all physicians receive some kind of salary). Private practice was replaced by semiprivate practice, where physicians who are accredited by the Social Security system (INAMPS) work in their offices or in a hospital and are remunerated according to the volume of services they provide. This format, however, not only does not satisfy the physicians' desire for private practice, but also shows great distortions and masks a series of touchy issues at the corporate level. In the first place, the expectation that all physicians can be accredited by the INAMPS is not viable, owing to economic constraints and lack of need. Furthermore, the provision of medical services for Social Security is concentrated in the hands of a very limited number of professionals in each of Brazil's states; in the state of Rio de Janeiro (southeast region), for example, about 5 percent of the practicing physicians receive 36 percent of the payments made by the INAMPS for professional services (1982 data). As a result, the distribution of income in this category became highly distorted, leading to the undesirable (because it is underpaid) practice of subcontracting services. Moreover, the Social Security Institute's current logic for remunerating the physicians it has accredited places much higher value on specialists who use sophisticated technology, thereby benefiting professionals who are "equipment dependent" rather than general practitioners who are "work dependent."

The health sector also shows considerable distortions in its lack of proper planning for the training of upper level professionals (particularly physicians, dentists, and nurses) for the geographic distribution and the absorption capacity of the labor market.

With regard to Brazil's national policy toward drugs, the marketing strategies of producing firms greatly overstate the population's need for pharmaceuticals. These companies follow a basic strategy of constantly putting new products on the market, accompanied by insistent advertising campaigns aimed at the middle class and the general population. Moreover, access to most drugs, including antibiotics, is not regulated, thereby encouraging indiscriminate use.

Although the country today has the technology to produce special pharmaceuticals (final products), it depends to a great extent on external sources for raw materials and intermediate products. Approximately 80 percent of the raw materials required for producing drugs are imported, which represents about 50 percent of Brazil's overall imports in the chemical sector, i.e., materials for the pharmaceutical industry (around US $300 million in 1982). This dependency is not based on technological considerations, but rather on politics. Brazil is capable of producing almost all the materials it needs for producing drugs, but the decision depends on the government. The major economic interests involved in the health sector have, however, always opposed this in the past. Consequently, the CEME, created in 1971 to establish a public and private system for handling drugs domestically as well as providing the low-income population with essential drugs, operates at a very low level today. Without the necessary resources to meet its obligation to supply the public service network, the CEME is reduced to the role of a distributor, and, even at that, it has marked inadequacies.

The Social Security Institute included the Plan for the Reorientation of Health Care in its official policy in August 1982, and, considering the predominant role of the institute in the sector, the plan has the weight of a real national policy for health care. Even though it has not been able to advance further in its efforts to democratize the health sector, the plan presented significant and important proposals for the rationalization and reorientation of the existing health-care model based on an analysis of the existing distortions. However, in the three years following its approval, the plan was not implemented to the extent hoped for, owing to implications and hindrances of a political and administrative nature; hence, the model that was used up until that time remained in force. The coordination proposed between the agencies of the health sector, involving mainly the INAMPS, the Ministry of Health, and the State Secretaries of Health, considered to be the axis of the plan, led to the establishment of agreements with most of the states in Brazil and the adoption of general structural standards at the national level. It was not able, however, to obtain from INAMPS the level of financial resources sufficient to achieve the desired structural reorientation.

Trends in the Health-Care System

In light of the financial and economic difficulties experienced in the health sector, considerable thought has been given in recent years to identifying alternative approaches and solutions. The proposed alternatives have been based on a variety of concepts, in accordance with respective political-ideological perspectives on society in general. Over the last decade, certain patterns have arisen in the attempts to fill the holes in the actual model—holes that were caused mainly by the crisis in the Social Security system. These proposals can be classified into three general categories: the conservative proposal, the modernist/private proposal, and the rationalist proposal.

The Conservative Proposal

The conservative proposal basically preserves the current pluralist model, based on the public subsectors, particularly Social Security, purchasing services from the private subsector. The Ministry of Health and the Secretaries of Health would encourage the promotion of collective activities to provide health care to the population that is not covered.

According to this approach, the inadequacies of the present system are the result of current economic conditions, which have led to a contraction in the health-care budget, and technical deficiencies in controlling services by the government, which has been accused of ineptness. This proposal is supported by two segments: hospitals and producers of equipment and materials, on the one hand, and, on the other, neo-liberal professionals who, although they defend individual patient-physician relationships, believe that the only way to make this project financially viable is for the government to contract physicians and dentists under Social Security.

The Modernist/Private Proposal

This proposal aims for the modernization of the health sector, structuring it more in accordance with the rules of the market. It calls for more independence in competition among providers in the private sector, on the assumption that this will improve cost/benefit relationships in the health sector overall. This approach recommends less involvement by the government in the provision of health-care services to the employed urban population. The government would be responsible for collective activities and provision of services to the rural populations and the populations that are not covered since these groups, owing to their low-income levels or location, would not be able to provide the profitability that a business organization would require. This proposal has some variations, too. One of these is the concept of "Group Health" or "Company Agreements," a structure that was used by Social Security as early as 1964, but was halted in 1979; today, it accounts for approximately 5 percent of Social Security coverage. This type of agreement, established with a private company, delegates to the company responsibility for the medical-hospital care of its employees in the form of a per capita subsidy granted to the company by Social Security. The company provides care directly or, as is more often the case, contracts for services from a firm that provides "group health services." The employee relinquishes his right to any other kind of care under Social Security, with a few exceptions, such as very costly treatment or chronic diseases. Another variation is that of organizing the population independently, in the form of unions or other kinds of organizations, to provide the necessary health-care services through cooperative contribution structures. Some of these variations could be implemented rather quickly, particularly if they were to use the private health insurance industry, which has been trying to move in as an alternative in the sector.

The Rationalist Proposal

The theory behind this proposal is that health care is the right of every citizen and consequently implies:

- Responsibility of the state for the health-care system, with the private sector acting to supplement in a subordinate manner;

- Interinstitutional integration;
- Organization of services under a single network, regionalized and structured with mechanisms for the referral and cross-referral of patients;
- Full and equal health coverage for the entire population, ensuring access to all care levels;
- Decentralization of planning and implementation, giving an essential role to states and cities;
- Participation as a mechanism for social control over the sector (definition of needs and quality control);
- Planning of activities based on epidemiologically determined needs;
- Comprehensive health actions and elimination of the dual system (at the institutional level as well) for individual/collective and preventive/curative actions;
- Structure of concepts, programs, and methodologies between the sectors of training (education) and utilization (services) of health workers.

Different versions of this third model have been presented in various government and private proposals in recent years. On the various occasions when financial crises have arisen in Social Security, this model has been identified as a possible alternative. It is the one that is identified with the Strategy of Primary Health Care to achieve Health for All by the Year 2000, as proposed by the World Health Organization. The Plan for the Reorientation of Health Care under Social Security, as approved by the government in August 1982, theoretically contained these elements, despite some incoherencies and inconsistencies owing to its broad composition as well as the economic recession that triggered this plan. Even so, its most outstanding element, which came to be known as the strategy of "Comprehensive Health Actions" and which was approved as a policy for sectoral reorientation, identified the mechanisms required for its viability, but did not have the necessary political and financial support to become fully effective, owing to the lack of concern of the government and to the imbalances in the sector's financing structure.

Brazil's current political situation, characterized by a period of transition toward the democratization of its institutions, makes it possible to conclude that genuine priority will be given to government programming in social areas. In light of the evidence in the health sector, in particular, it may be possible to implement this rationalist proposal, considering its greater identification with the principles of universality and equality in health-care service delivery.

References

Carvalho, J. A. M. and C. Hood. 1978. Mortality, Income Distribution, and Rural-Urban Residence in Brazil. *Population and Development Review* 4: 3.

COPAG. 1985. *Government Program of Action—Health*. São Paulo, Brazil: Comissáo de Programa de Agáo de Governo—COPAG.

Fundação Instituto Brasileiro de Geografia e Estatística. 1980. *1980 Census*. Rio de Janeiro: IBGE/BRASIL.

Fundação Instituto Brasileiro de Geografia e Estatística. 1983. *Statistical Yearbook for Brazil–1983*. Rio de Janeiro: IBGE/BRASIL.

McGreevey, W., L. P. M. Baptista, V. G. Pinto, S. F. Piola, S. M. Vianna. 1984. "Política e Financiamento do Sistema de Saúde Brasileiro : Uma perspectiva internacional." Series: Planning Studies, no. 26. Instituto de Planejamento Econômico e Social. Brasilia: IPEA/SEPLAN/BRASIL.

Ministério da Previdência e Assistência Social—MPAS/BRASIL. 1982. "Plan for Reorienting Health Care under Social Security." Official MPAS Document no. 3026, 23 August 1982.

Ministério da Previdência e Assistência Social—MPAS/BRASIL. 1983. Data obtained from the National Institute for Medical Care under Social Security: INAMPS.

Minnistério de Saúde—MS/BRASIL. 1984a. "Draft Project for Health in Rural Areas of the Northeast." Presented to the World Bank (IRDB).

Ministério de Saúde—MS/BRASIL. 1984b. Data obtained from the National Secretariat for Basic Health Actions—SNABS and the Superintendency for Public Health Campaigns—SUCAM.

Pinto, V. G. 1984. "Saúde para Poucos ou para Muitos: O Dilema de Zona Rural e das Pequenas Localidades." Series: Planning Studies, no. 26. Instituto de Planejamento Econômico e Social. Brasilia: IPEA/SEPLAN/BRASIL.

PMDB. Programa de Saúde. Partido do Movimento Democrático Brasileiro; A Nova República, Assessoria Parlamentar—Saúde. December. Brasilia: PMDB.

Política Econômica. 1984. In *Revista Brasil em Exame*, pp. 63–74. June. São Paulo: Editora Abril.

Rodriguez Neto, E. 1984. *Subsídios para a Definição de uma Política de Atenção à Saúde para um Governo de Transição Democrática*. Rio de Janeiro, Brazil: n.p.

Vieira, C. A. B. 1984. *Apontamentos para a Análise do Financiamento das Políticas Nacionais de Saúde*. Brasília, Brazil: n.p.

COLOMBIA

Francisco J. Yepes Lujan

The Country

Colombia is a country of 27,800,000 inhabitants with a democratically elected government and a centralist constitution. Politically, it is divided into 23 departments (states), a special district (Bogotá), and 9 special provinces (intendencias and comisarias). Each department is run by a governor who is appointed by the president. The governor, in turn, appoints the municipal mayors. Geographically, Colombia is divided into four regions: the grasslands or ''llanos'' and jungles on the east; the highlands of the Andes in the center, where most of the population is concentrated; the Pacific coast in the west, with tropical forest and a low population density; and the plains on the Atlantic coast in the north. Per capita income was US $1430 in 1983.

Historic Overview

At the time of Colombia's discovery by Europeans, the native population had its own health institutions with magic, herbalistic medicine, and even surgical practices (Avila 1986). The conquerors, for their part, brought health institutions and practices current in fifteenth-century Spain.

After Pope Alexander VI donated the new lands to Fernando V, the king promulgated a bill establishing hospitals for both Spaniards and Indians. The first hospital in Santa Marta del Darien was built in 1513, as was San Lazaro hospital in Cartagena for leprosy (Hansen's disease) patients. In 1530, a hospital was established in Santa Marta and another in Cartagena by 1553. In 1564 the San Pedro hospital was established in Santa Fe de Bogotá as a diocesan institution. It later evolved to become the San Juan de Dios hospital as it is known today.

Spanish law in 1798 established hospitals in each province. These hospitals were to include surgeons, auxiliary personnel, and a pharmacy. Hospitals were administered by religious orders and were financed through tithes and donations by government officials and wealthy citizens. In 1636 the first medical school was established in the Colegio Mayor y Seminario de San Bartolome de Santa Fe de Bogotá.

The Boards of King's Physicians (Protomedicatos), Spanish institutions charged with directing and controlling health activities, were transplanted to the New World. They were abolished in 1822 by Fernando VII.

In 1639, the first physician to the king arrived at Santa Fe. He was in charge of regulating physicians' work, giving licenses, inspecting titles, controlling lay practitioners and pharmacies, and collecting and administering funds. In 1763 the first public pharmacy, owned by a religious order, was opened in Santa Fe de Bogotá.

In 1825 the Juntas de Sanidad (Sanitation Boards) for the provincial capitals were created to administer cemeteries, vaccines, sanitary regulations, sanitation inspectors, and leprosy hospitals. In 1848 the Department of ''Beneficencia y Recompensas'' (charity and rewards), attached to the Secretary of Foreign Relations, was assigned responsibility for leprosy and slave hospitals, hospices, and asylums as well as retirement and old-age pensions.

In 1856 the National Vaccination Office was created as part of the Secretary of the Interior. In 1887 Bill 30 created the Junta Central de Higiene (Central Board of Hygiene) as well as the state boards administered by the Ministry of Public Institutions. In 1913 Bill 33 created the ''Consejo Superior de Sanidad'' (High Sanitary Council), which replaced the boards. It was in charge of regulating, inspecting, and controlling private and public hygiene.

In 1938 the Ministry of Labor, Hygiene, and Social Provision was created. In 1946 the Ministry of Hygiene was established; it later changed its name to Ministry of Public Health and then the Ministry of Health as it is today.

General Health Statistics

According to the last census (1985), Colombia had 28 million inhabitants (DANE 1986, vol. 1), 67.2 percent urban, and 17.7 percent illiterate (DANE 1986, vol. III). The four largest cities have more than 1 million inhabitants each, which, together, account for one-fourth of the total population. The small and intermediate-size cities (50,000–500,000) account for another quarter of the population.

The crude birth rate for 1985 was 30.7 per 1,000, and the average annual growth rate between 1980 and 1985 was 1.9 percent (SENALDE 1986), which resulted from important declines in fertility and mortality during the seventies. About half of all couples currently use contraceptives.

Figure 1 shows the age structure in 1973 alongside the structure expected for

Figure 1
Age Composition by Age and Sex, 1973–2003

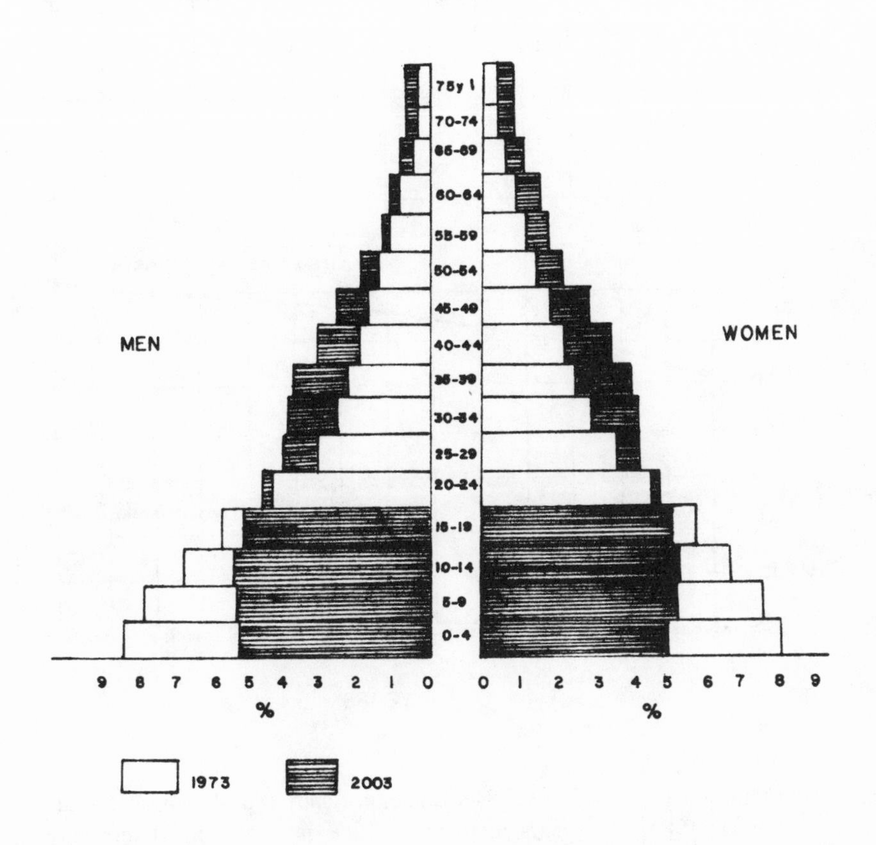

2003. The proportion of children under fifteen dropped from 46.6 percent to 41.4 percent in the late 1970s and was expected to drop to 39 percent by 1984.

Health conditions have been improving in general as reflected by traditional indicators. Epidemiologic transition is present; infectious diseases progressively are giving way to cardiovascular diseases, cancer, and accidents. Two-thirds of the population has access to piped water, and over two-fifths have sewer connections. Geographical and socioeconomic disparities, however, remain large.

Mortality

General mortality was 5.8 per 1000 inhabitants in 1982. Infant mortality for the same year was 57 per 1,000 newborn, and maternal mortality 1.17 per 1,000

Figure 2
Infant Mortality Rate and Life Expectancy at Birth

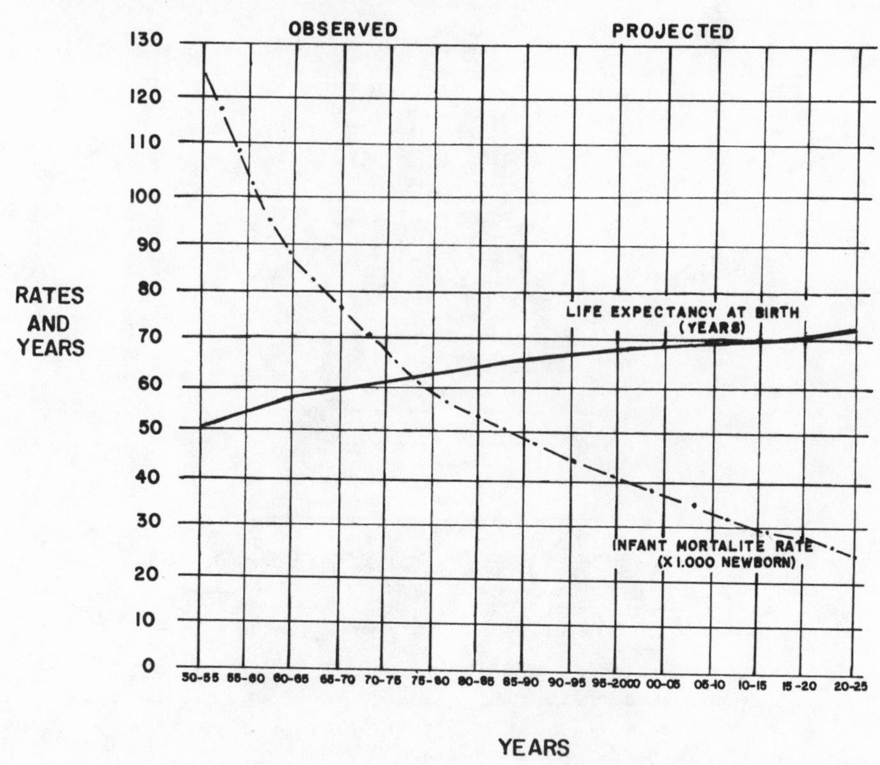

newborn (Ministerio de Salud 1983–84). Life expectancy at birth was 62.1 years in 1981 (Ochoa 1986), 3.5 years more than it was in 1966. Infant mortality ranged from a low of 28 for the city of Cali to a high of 100 for the states of Cauca and Narino in 1981. Families where the mother had six or more grades of education presented infant mortality rates of 34 per 1,000; mothers with no education presented rates of 92 per 1,000 (Ochoa 1983) (Fig. 2).

Cancer, heart disease, strokes, and homicides were the primary causes of death in 1981 for the population as a whole (Tables 1 and 2). For children under the age of one, the primary causes of death were perinatal diseases, gastrointestinal and acute respiratory infections, respiratory failures, and nutritional deficiencies. For those age one to four, gastrointestinal diseases, acute respiratory infections, and malnutrition were the primary causes of death. Accidents and cancer were the primary causes of death for children age 5 to 14; homicides and accidents, for adults 15 to 44; and cancer, isochemic heart disease, and cerebrovascular accidents, for adults 45 and over (Ministerio de Salud, Subsistema de Información 1984).

Table 1
First Five Causes of Death—All Ages, 1970

DIAGNOSES	IDC (150 list)	Order	% of all
Enteritis and other diahrreic	5	1	9.4
Other pneumonia	92	2	7.9
Other hearth diseases	84	3	6.4
Ischemic hearth diseases	83	4	5.0
Bronchitis, emphysema, asthma	93	5	4.8
The Rest			66.5

Table 2
First Five Causes of Death—All Ages, 1981

DIAGNOSES	IDC (170 list)	Order	% of all
Other diseases from the heart and pulmonary circulation	097	1	7.5
Acute miocardyal inf.	095	2	6.0
Cerebrovascular diseases	098	3	5.8
Homicides, lessions by other	168	4	5.7
Enterits, other diahrreic	006	5	5.1
The Rest			69.9

Source: Ministerio de Salud, Subsistema de Información, *Macroindicadores en Salud*, Bogotá, 1984.

Morbidity

According to the National Health Survey, 41 of every 100 Colombians felt sick in a period of two weeks; of those who felt sick, only 11.5 percent consulted a health provider. Illness perception varied with age, sex, urban-rural distribution, and socioeconomic characteristics. It was positively associated with age, and negatively associated with urbanization, income, and education. Women had larger rates of illness perception than men. On the other hand, consultation rates were positively associated with income, education, and urbanization. Women had also larger consultation rates than men. Of those who felt sick in the population over six years of age, 34.1 percent had at least one day of disability in the two-week period and, of these, 75 percent had at least one day in bed (Pabón 1983).

The first five causes of outpatient diagnoses in 1982 were ''other diseases of the genital organs,'' enteritis and other diarrheic diseases, other helminthiasis, diseases of the skin and subcutaneous tissues, and acute respiratory diseases. The first five causes of hospital discharges were normal deliveries (one fourth of all), abortion, enteritis and other diarrheic diseases, complications of labor, and complications of pregnancy (Ministerio de Salud, Subsisteme de Información).

According to the compulsory reporting system on communicable diseases, enteritis and diarrheic diseases were by far the first cause of morbidity. Incidence of malaria has been increasing during the last fifteen years, selvatic yellow fever is a significant problem in colonization areas, and dengue is present in epidemic form (Ministero de Salud, Subsisteme de Informacion 1984). (Table 3.) Sexually transmitted diseases have been shown to be highly prevalent, but, even so, they are grossly underreported by official registries (Bersh 1985).

Nutrition

The nutritional status of the Colombian population has improved significantly in the last twenty years, with a reduction in the prevalence of malnutrition. The reduction, however, has been more marked in instances of moderate malnutrition than in instances of severe malnutrition. In the period between 1965 to 1966 and 1977 to 1980, overall malnutrition decreased by 20 percent and growth retardation decreased by 25 percent. The improvement was greater in rural areas and in low-income groups. In large cities, however, the situation deteriorated. On the other hand, the prevalence of obesity increased (Mora 1982).

The Health-Care System

Colombia's health sector is divided into three major parts: the official subsector, the social security subsector, and the private subsector. Each subsector

Table 3
Incidence Rates of Some Communicable Diseases (per 100,000 inhabitants), 1972 and 1982

	1982	1972
Diahrreas and enterits *	1757.6	6324.0
Malaria	209.6	113.0
Gonococal infección	155.0	167.7
Syphilis (All Forms)	63.2	84.2
Tuberculosis	45.0	52.7
Measles	34.4	116.8

*Children under 5 years.
Source: Ministerio de Salud, Subsistema de Información, *Macroindicadores en Salud*, Bogotá, 1984.

has different constituencies, different administrative schemes, and different financing arrangements, although both population and personnel crossovers occur.

Currently, it is estimated that 10 percent of the population has access to the private sector. The different social security schemes, including the armed forces, cover 18 percent of the population. The remaining 72 percent is the responsibility of the official Ministry of Health sector, which is unable to provide universal coverage.

There are important regional disparities in health conditions and services as there are disparities among the different schemes. The average expenditure per person in 1978 was US $28 in the official sector; it was US $108 in the social security programs (not including the armed forces). Per capita expenditure in health, including household expenditures, was US $46 for the country, amounting to 5.4 percent of the gross domestic product.

Official Subsector

This sector has, by far, the largest network of health facilities with 644 hospitals in 1982 with almost 29,000 beds and approximately 3,000 health centers and posts. Under the National Health System legislation enacted in 1975, this subsector is divided into four administrative levels. The national level, which sets policies, norms, and standards, is administered by the Ministry of Health; the departmental level for each state, or special province and the district of Bogotá, which adapts national policies and norms to the regional characteristics;

Figure 3
Organization of the National Health System in Colombia

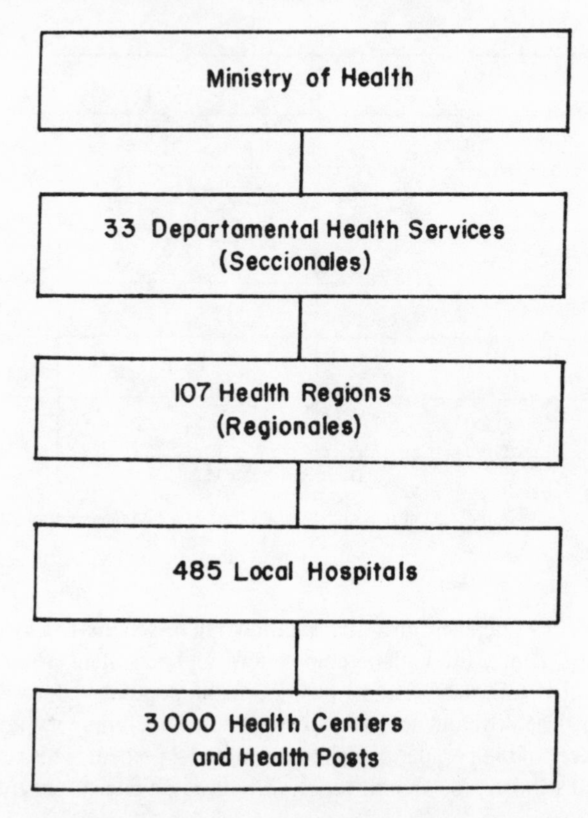

and the regional and local levels, which are operational (Fig. 3). There are 107 health regionals, 97 of which have a regional hospital, and 990 local units with 485 (in 1981) local hospitals and 3,000 health centers and posts.

The service is centralized for policy formulation, normatization, and standardization; however, it is decentralized for actual administration and execution of operating activities. The departmental health services operate under contracts subscribed between the Ministry of Health and departmental (state) administration. They are administratively autonomous within the boundaries set by the National Health System legislation, but they must comply with the policies, norms, and standards set by the ministry. Overall policy is vested in a departmental health board, the members of which include the governor, health-related agency representatives, and citizens.

Policy matters and overall internal management are the responsibilities of the director, who, depending on the terms of the contract between the ministry and the state, is appointed either by the governor or by the minister from a list of three names presented by the health board. The director is supported in the day-to-day management by a technical coordinator who must be a career officer. Departmental, regional, and local units have three operational units: medical care, environmental sanitation, and administration.

Regionalization. Health services regionalization was officially proposed in 1969 and was legally created with the National Health System in 1975. It has two components, one administrative and one of service delivery. The health post, health center, and local and regional hospital are responsible for both the administrative and the service components of their activities; however, at the department level, the administrative component rests with the departmental health service, and the service component lies with the university or departmental hospital or departmental laboratory.

With regard to services, regionalization consists of three levels: university, regional, and local, represented by 12 university hospitals, 97 regional hospitals, and 485 local hospitals, along with some 3,000 health centers and health posts. Patients are expected to be referred from the less sophisticated peripheral services toward the center.

With regard to administration, regionalization consists of the above-mentioned four levels: national, departmental, regional, and local. Besides setting policies, norms, and standards, the Ministry of Health supervises and controls the other levels as do, respectively, the departmental health services and the health regionals.

The local level is located in the municipalities where there is either a local hospital or a health center. The health center is an outpatient facility with a permanent physician, an auxiliary nurse, a sanitary inspector, and, in many instances, a dentist. Health posts are also outpatient facilities, which are located in smaller settlements; they are staffed with auxiliary nurses and periodically visited by a physician. At the community level, mainly in rural but also in some urban areas, there are the *promotoras de salud*, or community health workers who have three months of training and who mainly perform health promotion (health education, child growth and development control, vaccination, and referral).

Hospitals. Local hospitals are small units with an average of 20 beds, staffed by general physicians; the 485 local hospitals account for 10,100 beds. Regional hospitals are medium size, ranging from 50 to 150 beds with at least the four basic specialties (surgery, internal medicine, pediatrics, and obstetrics), although some have not been able to maintain this minimum. The 97 regional hospitals account for 9,107 beds. There are 12 university hospitals with 4,483 beds and 45 specialized hospitals with 5,063 beds (Ministerio de Salud, Oficina Panamericána de la Salud 1984).

The regional hospital at the department or province capital, which is usually more developed, serves as the center for care of referral patients in places where there is no university hospital. Patients in need of more sophisticated care usually are referred to university or specialized hospitals in neighboring departments.

Population Coverage. Government programming for the official subsector is done on the basis of an assigned (target) population of 70 percent, on the assumption that the rest is covered either by the private subsector or by social security. Coverage, however, varies considerably depending on region of the country, age, sex, urban-rural distribution, and type of service. It is highest for vaccination but much lower for medical visits.

Official figures showed that by 1984 real coverage for the assigned (target) population was 31.6 percent for medical visits, and 3.4 percent for nursing control. On the other hand, vaccination coverage for all children under four was 78.8 percent for polio; 87.2 percent for BCG, the tuberculosis vaccine; 76.6 percent for diphtheria, pertussis, tetanus (DPT); and 79.6 percent for measles. For all children under the age of one, coverages were 61.1 percent for polio, 67.7 percent for BCG, 60.3 percent for DPT, and 52.9 percent for measles (Ministerio de Salud, OPS/OMS, PNUD 1984).

Environment. Environmental activities, including water supply, sewage disposal, waste management, vector and food control, and control of air-water-noise pollution, are the responsibility of the official sector through the national, sectional, regional, and local levels. However, the responsibility for the execution of many of these activities is shared with other extrasectorial institutions. Water supply and sewage disposal in the larger cities are the responsibility of autonomous enterprises depending on municipal governments; waste collection and disposal are the responsibility of municipal governments; and some environmental protection activities are also the responsibility of the National Institute for the Protection of Renewable Resources (INDERENA).

Vertical Campaigns. Malaria, dengue, and yellow fever control activities are carried out by a vertical organization dependent on the Ministry of Health which extends throughout the country to the field level.

Decentralized Institutes. Five decentralized institutes are linked to the Ministry of Health. The National Institute of Health (INS) is responsible for biologicals, epidemiological and public health research, laboratory quality control, and water supply and sewage in towns with up to 2,500 inhabitants. The National Municipal Development Institute (INSFOPAL) handles water supply and sewage for larger towns. The Colombian Family Welfare (ICBF) is responsible for preschool nutrition programs, child-care facilities, and protection of minors. The Cancer Institute is in charge of the National Cancer Control Program, and the National Hospital Fund (FNH) allocates funds for and approves and supervises hospital investments for construction, remodeling, equipment, and maintenance.

Financing. The official sector is financed from national, departmental, and municipal sources and from sales of services.

National contributions, in 1982, represented 35.7 percent of the total official budget. Departmental and municipal contributions, which included beer and liquor as well as lottery taxes, represented 22.3 percent. Sales of services, primarily derived from the multiple insurance schemes which buy services from the official subsector institutions, represented 11.9 percent. The remaining 30 percent came from returns on investments, leasing of property, donations, endowments, external and internal credit, and miscellaneous (Ministerio de Salud, Organizacion Panamericana de la Salud 1984).

According to the National Health Study (Velandia and Yepes 1986), in the 1977 to 1980 period, Colombians spent an annual average of Col $2,686.11 (pesos of December 1980) per individual and Col $14,477.9 per family totalling Col $66,249 million in out-of-pocket health expenditures for the whole population. Forty-six percent of the out-of-pocket health expenditures was spent on drugs, 21.8 percent on dental services, 17 percent on visits to physicians and other health providers, 8.4 percent on hospitalization, and 6.9 percent to others (e.g., fees and laboratory X-rays). Composition of health expenditure by these components varied depending on income, education, and urbanization. Drugs represented 68 percent of the total health expenditures in the lower income group but only 26.5 percent in the higher income groups. Dental expenditure, on the contrary, represented only 9 percent for the low-income group but 30 percent for high-income groups.

Health expenditure was 12.1 percent of the family income, ranging from 8.1 percent for high-income groups to 25.5 percent for low-income groups. Women spent 31 percent more than men, but families with a female head of family spent 53 percent less than those with a male head of family. (Families with a female head had lower incomes.)

Social Security

The social security sector consists of almost 300 institutions at the national, departmental (state), and municipal levels. They may be grouped into four main categories, which operate independently and under separate regimes and cover different but specific segments of the population.

As a whole, the social security subsector covers 18.4 percent of the population, basically urban, and with higher levels of income and education, as compared to the rest. Between 1965 and 1980, the coverage provided by social security schemes doubled; however this growth has been very slow compared to the need.

Social Security Institute (ISS). Provides services for the employees of the private sector and covers 10 percent of the total population. Besides health services it provides retirement, disability, and life insurance. Predominant schemes cover only workers, their children under one year of age, and maternity benefits for spouses. Experimental and limited schemes are offering family coverage. The ISS owns 37 hospitals with 4,195 beds plus a network of outpatient facilities. In addition, it contracts services with both the official and private sectors. Financing comes both from employee and employer who, together, contribute 7 percent of the payroll.

"Cajas de Prevision." The *Cajas de Prevision* operates approximately 210 separate entities at the national, state, and municipal levels for government employees. They have different financing schemes: some jointly by employer and employee, others by employee contributions and allocations from the budget

of the nation, state, or municipality which do not necessarily reflect actuarial predictions and lead to major financial problems in some instances. The services provided (health, retirement, disability, and life insurance) are similar since set by law, but family coverage varies.

"Cajas de Subsidio Familiar." The *Cajas de Subsidio Familiar*, or Family Subsidy, is financed by a compulsory contribution of 4 percent of the payroll. These 74 institutions are run under the private regimen but are supervised by the government. Besides giving cash allowances for each child, for workers within certain salary categories they provide recreation, education, and health services. The health services are provided basically to children and spouses not covered by the Social Security Institute or the *Cajas de Prevision*.

Armed Forces. The armed forces health services as a whole cover 2.6 percent of the population under two schemes, one for the military (army, navy, and air force) which has three hospitals with 920 beds and 44 dispensaries, and the other for the police which has eight hospitals with 458 beds and 4 dispensaries. Health services for the military cover both active and retired personnel, as well as their families and contract civilian personnel. Family coverage includes the spouse, a maximum of four children until they are eighteen years of age if male or until married if female, and handicapped children for their lifetime. Active military do not make any individual contribution, although retired military and civilian personnel contribute 5 percent of their salaries.

Private Sector

This sector is made up of the private hospitals, private offices of physicians and dentists, private laboratories, and a shrinking number of domiciliary nursing services and charitable health services run by the churches or voluntary, nonprofit organizations. There were 190 private hospitals with a total of 8,892 beds in 1982, but there is no available information on the number and distribution of physicians, dental offices, or laboratories. Private insurance covered only 1.5 percent of the population by 1980.

Miscellaneous

There are other health services, some of which are provided by the government, for example, those for prisoners under the Ministry of Justice or those that cover the colonization areas under the Land Reform Institute (INCORA). Coverage is minimal.

Human Resources

Health manpower supply depends on the educational sector through universities and technical institutes. Since 1977 there has been a National Council of

Human Resources composed of the ministries of Health, Education, and Labor; the directors of the Institute for Development of Superior Education (ICFES); the Association of Medical Schools; and representatives of the National Planning Office, the Institute of Social Security, the Colombian Association of Nursing Schools, and the Pan Americn Health Organization.

The council provides overall policy direction for human resources development and deals with the minimum requirements for the establishment of new schools of medicine, dentistry, and nursing and with the training of nonprofessional personnel and curricular changes.

Colombia has observed an increase in the ratio of health personnel to population over the last thirteen years (Ministerio de Salud, Organización Panamericana de la Salud 1984), basically due to the creation of new schools. Medical schools increased from 9 in 1973 to 21 in 1982 with an increase of about 400 percent in the number of graduates. Dental schools increased from 4 to 9, increasing the annual output by 480 percent in the same period; nursing schools, from 9 to 23, increasing the annual output by about 600 percent (Ministerio de Salud, Dirección de Recursos Humanos 1984).

By 1981 there were an estimated 17,999 physicians, 6,609 dentists, and 4,710 professional nurses, which meant 6.67, 2.45, and 1.55 per 10,000 inhabitants, respectively, compared to the 1968 rates of 4.3 physicians, 1.3 dentists, and 0.65 nurses per 10,000 inhabitants (Ministerio de Salud, Organizacion Panamericana de la Salud 1984).

There are about 20,000 auxiliary nurses and 15,000 nursing aides. Auxiliary nurses, whose number has more than doubled since 1970, are the backbone of the services provided in the rural health centers and posts and fulfill many of the nursing needs in other health institutions. They are mainly females, with at least two years of high school plus a year and a half of training at an auxiliary nursing school.

Promotoras de salud are women who are trained for three months and are usually assigned to the communities surrounding their homes, under the supervision of auxiliary nurses, to perform basic health education, health promotion, and first aid. There are approximately 5,000 of them.

There are problems of geographic distribution, basically of the professional personnel, who are concentrated in the urban areas. As a partial solution, compulsory social service was required for physicians in 1959; later, dentists, nurses, and bacteriologists were included. These professionals must serve one year in places assigned by the government before they are licensed. They are salaried while in service but under a special regimen.

Currently, there are signs of oversupply, particularly for dentists and physicians who are experiencing problems in finding employment. The principal employer is the official sector, 62 percent; followed by the Social Security Institute, 22 percent; the Caja de Prevision, 10 percent; and the private sector, 6 percent (Ministero de Salud Dirección de Recursos Humanos 1984).

National Health System

A series of laws enacted in 1975 established the legal basis for the so-called National Health System. Under this legislation (Orejuela Bueno 1978), the Minister of Health was clearly defined as the ultimate authority for setting policies and standards, as well as for supervising and evaluating all institutions involved in health delivery (except in the armed forces).

This legislation grouped all health institutions into two categories: "adscribed" which includes all public institutions, and "vinculated," which includes all private institutions providing health services to the community. In this form, the law gave the Ministry of Health the capacity to supervise, control, and, if necessary, to intervene in any health institution be it private or public.

The 1975 law also defined hierarchical levels and established six subsystems as a basis for sector coordination: planning, information, human resources, research, investment, and supplies (Orejuela Bueno 1978). It was initially envisioned that the six subsystems would apply to all subsectors (official, private, and social security, except the armed forces). However, it has provided an excellent legal and administrative basis for improved operation and management modernization of official health services. Currently, a project to consolidate the National Health System and further improve management with innovative approaches is under way. It centers on managerial development of health regionals, reinforcement of administrative decentralization, development of instruments for local planning and programing, and targeting of operational objectives based on avoidable deaths, diseases, and disabilities (Ministerio de Salud 1985).

Future Development

Primary health-care actions have been an important activity of government institutions since the 1960s. The *promotoras de salud* were created through a university program in 1958, with persons from rural communities given intensive training for carrying out health education activities, first aid, and health promotion.

This program was subsequently extended to the whole country through the Ministry of Health. Today, there are almost 5,000 *promotoras de salud* officially recognized as the bottom line of the Colombian health services. They receive three months of training, are natives of the community in which they work, and periodically visit the families in their assigned area, house by house, performing health education, vaccination, prenatal control, and family planning. They also attend deliveries and provide first aid.

Besides the governmental *promotoras*, many kinds of alternative primary health-care programs are carried out by universities or private institutions. Starting in 1985, a massive national primary health-care program focused on children under the age of five years is being implemented. The Child Survival and Development Plan, as it is known, centers on house-by-house visits to identify health risks, perform health education, and promote opportune intervention to avoid preventable deaths caused by diarrhea, upper respiratory infections, perinatal causes, malnutrition, and immunopreventable diseases. Moreover, it contemplates a component to educate parents on appropriate ways to care for the psycho-affective development of children. The objective is to reduce infant mortality from 57 to 40 per 1000 newborn in a period of five years.

In order to carry this program out, a massive social mobilization is under way with participation of all fourth-year high school students, Red Cross volunteers, and police and church volunteers as health guards or sentinels. Mass media and interpersonal educational techniques also will be used to reinforce health education messages.

References

Avila, Néstor. 1986. *Historia de las Instituciones de Salud en Colombia.* Authorized abstract from a thesis for the Master in Health Services Administration. Bogotá. Javeriana University.

Bersh, David. 1985. Personal communication.

Consejo Nacional de Política Económica y Social. 1984. *Plan Nacional de Supervivencia de la Infancia.* Bogotá.

DANE (Departamento Nacional de Estadística), *XV Censo Nacional de Problación y Vivienda de Colombia.* Julio 1986. Bogotá. Vol. 1.

DANE, *XV Censo Nacional de Problación y Vivienda de Colombia.* Julio 1986. Bogotá. Vol. III.

Ministerio de Salud. 1984. *Cambio con equidad - Políticas y realizaciones 1983–84.* Bogotá: Empresa Editorial Universidad Nacional de Colombia.

Ministerio de Salud, Dirección de Recursos Humanos. 1984. *Planificación de Recursos Humanos en Salud para el año 2,000.* Estudio preliminar. Bogotá.

Ministerio de Salud, Oficina de Planeación, División Financiera. 1985. *Análisis Financiero del Sector Salud—Nivel Institucional 1982.* Bogotá.

Ministerio de Salud, OPS/OMS, PNUD, Unicef. 1984. *Jornadas Nacionales de Vacunación.* Bogotá.

Ministerio de Salud, Organización Panamericana de la Salud. 1984. *Colombia, Diagnóstico de Salud, políticas y estrategias.* Bogotá.

Ministerio de Salud, *Proyecto de Consolidación del Sistema Nacional de Salud.* 1985. Mimeo, internal document. Bogotá.

Ministerio de Salud, Subsistema de Información. 1984. *Macroindicadores en Salud—Colombia 1970–83.* Bogotá.

Mora, José Obdulio. 1982. Estudio Nacional de Salud: *Situación nutricional de la población Colombiana en 1977–80.* Vol. I: "Resultados antropométicos y de laboratorio—comparación con 1965–66." Bogotá.

Ochoa, Luis Hernando et al. 1983. Estudio Nacional de Salud: *La Mortalidad en Colombia: 1970–1982.* Vol. II: "Tendencias y diferenciales 1963–1983." Bogotá.

Ochoa, Luis Hernando et al. 1986. Estudio Nacional de Salud. *La Mortalidad en Colombia.* Vol. VI. Bogotá.

Orejuela Bueno, Raúl. 1978. *Informe al Honorable Congreso de la República de Colombia 1974–1978.* Bogotá.

Pabón, Aurelio. 1983. Estudio Nacional de Salud: *Población y Morbilidad General*. Vol. I: ''Morbilidad sentida 1977–1980.'' Bogotá.

SENALDE (Servicio Nacional de Empleo), *Transición demográfica y oferta de fuerza de trabajo en Colombia*. 1986. Bogotá: Colección Biblioteca Senalde.

Velandia, Freddy and Francisco J. Yepes. 1986. Estudio Nacional de Salud: *Gasto privado (de bolsillo) en Salud*.

Yepes, Francisco J. et al. 1970. *Niveles de atención médica para un sistema de regionalización en Colombia*. Bogotá: Canal Ramírez.

EGYPT

Julius B. Richmond and
Jeremiah Norris

Historical Review

Contemporary Egyptian health services, both public and private, are rooted in political, social, and economic conditions specific to the country and to its history. The development of health-care delivery systems reflects the machinations of internal and international power relations—European rivalry and colonial intervention—including the establishment of private medical practices, socialism, and state expansion. It also reflects a pronounced growth in the last twenty years of the demand for personal health services in the private sector.

Through the nineteenth century, British and French rivalry in Egypt was manifest in their efforts to shape the development of public and private medical services. Professional medical training was entirely in the hands of the state and was centered at Qasr al 'Aini medical school. In 1831, the European consuls in Egypt organized a special health administration, *L'Intendance de Santé*, to check the spread of a cholera epidemic. Only later, in 1840, as a countermeasure, was a *Conseil de Santé* organized made up entirely of Egyptians. Together, these institutions constituted Egypt's sanitary and medical administration until the British occupation at the end of the century (Kuhnke 1971).

Meanwhile, foreign physicians set up private medical practices and established a number of hospitals. While the Suez Canal was being built, the Canal Company established several hospitals and dispensaries, and, after the canal had been completed, the company sold its health facilities to the government. By 1905, Cairo alone had ten private hospitals run by foreigners. At the time that Britain occupied Egypt (1882), Egypt had 25 government hospitals (with 2,273 beds), all but two of which were in the provinces outside Cairo (Tignor 1960).

Under the British, the sanitary services and medical school were reformed.

English replaced French and Arabic as the language of instruction. The British authorities, stressing clinical (rather than academic) training and the necessity of reducing government expenditures, shortened the curriculum from six to four years in 1887. Not until 1929, did an Egyptian again head the faculty at Qasr al 'Aini. Additional medical schools were not built until 1942 in Alexandria and 1947 in Cairo ('Ain Shams University) (Sonbol 1981).

In anticipation of Egypt's formal independence in 1936, a Ministry of Public Health (MOH) with very limited functions was founded. In the following decades, the ministry gradually grew by bringing the country's disparate health delivery services under its control and by developing new services.

For example, in 1939, a health insurance program was established for children attending a limited number of government schools in Cairo. In 1945, the scheme was extended to governorate capitals. The ministry established a Department of Rural Health in 1943. It original plan proved overly ambitious: the development of 860 rural centers—one for every 15,000 villagers—was never realized. At the time of the 1952 revolution, only a total of 270 such centers had been built.

In the National Charter presented to the nation by President Nasser in May 1962, the "basic rights" of citizens articulated included medical care, education, employment, minimum wages, and insurance benefits in sickness and old age. In 1962, private associations (*jama'iyyat*), many of which provided health-care services, were brought under central government regulation and control. Since then, all such associations have been required by law to register with the Ministry of Social Affairs. Hundreds of associations at present offer health care at fixed rates through private group practice.

A private association (the *Jama'iyya Mobara al-Marat al-jadida* or Charitable Association of the Modern Woman), founded in 1919 by a group of wealthy Egyptian women, eventually became responsible for a network of twelve major hospitals and eighteen outpatient clinics throughout Egypt. President Nasser placed these facilities under the direct administration of a new agency, the Curative Care Organization (CCO). The CCO operates as a fee-for-service institution under MOH review. Other private hospitals, mostly maintained by resident foreigners, were also nationalized and placed under the newly formed Health Insurance Organization (HIO). The HIO was established in 1964, also under MOH auspices (Mayers 1984).

In the last twenty years, the Arab Republic of Egypt (ARE) has experienced dramatic and pronounced changes in socioeconomic structure. The economic effects of the 1967 and 1973 wars, and the direct impact of worldwide price inflation, created serious imbalances in both Egypt's trade accounts and government budgets. In response to these and other factors, President Sadat announced a new economic policy, *El-Infitah* (The Opening), in his *October Working Paper* in 1973. The changes in strategy and direction were meant to accelerate economic growth by encouraging foreign investment and greater private sector participation within a planned framework (Richmond 1982). At the same time, the socioeconomic changes of the past two decades—the rapid expansion of the industrial, manufacturing, and service sectors—have removed a growing portion of the population with disposable income from the need to seek free health care through the MOH.

The outlines of an incipient public and private fee-for-service health industry, oriented toward curative care in fixed facilities, began to emerge in 1964, accelerated with the new economic policy initiated in 1973, and continues at an increased rate today. Since 1973 the number of private clinics and hospitals has increased in response to an increased demand for nonpublicly provided services.

Current Policy

Development planning and strategy are still based on three critical assumptions articulated in the policy of 1973:

1. Acceleration of economic growth is the basic element in the modernization process—this implies changes in the roles of different sectors and the development of "an outward looking economic policy."
2. "Contradictory policies" of the past that inhibited maximum production by the private sector should be eliminated.
3. Social goals should not be neglected since "economic development cannot proceed soundly unless accompanied by a social development at compatible rates" (Richmond 1982).

The government has endeavored to bring health services to the largest possible proportion of the population, given economic constraints, and has attempted to improve health care through (Richmond 1982):

1. A commitment to equity in health services and affordable medications, with the MOH playing a central role.
2. The construction of hospitals and rural health facilities.
3. A commitment to extend safe water supplies and provide for proper sewage disposal.
4. The expansion of training programs for the health professions.
5. The development of a high degree of pluralism in the delivery of health services, which includes an active private sector and a public sector in the form of the Health Insurance Organization, the CCOs (in Cairo and Alexandria), voluntary health agencies, and private fee-for-service practices.
6. The development of a national pharmaceutical program.
7. The initiation of a full employment policy, which has had major program and budgetary implications for the efficient operation of health programs today.

Current Health Status

Over the past 30 years, the ARE has implemented a governmental health program infrastructure that many countries would do well to emulate (Table 1).

Table 1
Summary of Statistical Profile of Egypt[1]

Per Capita GNP (U.S. $) (1985)	610
Population (January 1985)	49 million
Land Area (thousands of sq. km.)	1,001
Agricultural land area (feddans) (2)	6 million*
Crude birth rate per thousand population (1982)	35
Percentage change in crude birth rate since 1960	-22.1
Crude death rate per thousand population (1982)	11
Percentage change in crude death rate since 1960	-44.6
Urban population as percentage of total population	46
Infant mortality rate (1960)	128
Infant mortality rate (1985)	93
Child death rate (aged 1-4) 1960	23
Child death rate (aged 1-4) 1985	11
Life expectancy at birth, 1960	46
Life expectancy at birth, 1985	61
Population per physician, 1985	760:1
Population per physician, 1960	2,550:1
Population per nursing person, 1985	790:1
Population per nursing person, 1960	1,930:1

* 1 feddan = 1.04 acres.

1. All data, except where noted, are from The World Bank's "World Development Report, 1987," Washington, D.C., 1987.

2. The Futures Group, "The Effects of Population Factors on Social and Economic Development," Washington, D.C., 1982.

This achievement has not, however, been reflected in a commensurate improvement in the health of the people. It is apparent that significant health problems remain (Richmond 1982):

1. Rates of mortality and morbidity from largely preventable diseases continue to be very high.
2. Infant, early childhood, and maternal mortality rates remain unacceptably high.

3. Immunizations are either lacking or are inadequately administered. This is reflected in the prevalence of preventable common infectious diseases.
4. Despite massive efforts to treat schistosomiasis and to prevent it through snail control, perhaps two-fifths of the country's 47 million people now harbor these parasites—a public health burden of staggering proportion (Buck 1982).
5. Adequate water supply and sanitation services continue to be unavailable to a large majority of the people.
6. The health programs for the poor in rural and urban areas often lack the professional skills and/or resources necessary to carry out their missions effectively.
7. Educational and training programs are largely directed at preparing health workers for the curative and private health-care sector. Relatively little effort has been directed to developing programs to prepare health professionals for community health programs, public health practices, and administrative and management careers in public health.

Despite the fact that some morbidity indicators are unacceptably high—relative to the national investment in health—preventive strategies have had an impact on health status, particularly on that of infants and children. As development has moved forward, the disease mix (excepting schistosomiasis) has gradually changed from one with predominantly acute and infectious conditions to one with more chronic conditions. Furthermore, this development has enabled individuals to experience and survive diseases that once were commonly fatal, and more chilldren have survived to adulthood.

Recent epidemiological studies showed that diseases of the digestive system were the leading cause of death among both sexes until the mid–1970s when the category of "other diseases" became the leading cause. Deaths caused by diseases of the circulatory system have shown the most consistent increase among both males and females. Deaths from infectious and parasitic diseases seem to have decreased quite significantly between the late 1940s and early 1970s (Buck 1982). The leading causes of hospitalization in Egypt are accidents, poisonings, and violence (National Academy of Sciences 1978).

Between 1960 and 1982, urbanization increased from 38 percent to 45 percent of the total population. During this same period, the infant mortality rate (aged under one) dropped from 128 to 104; the child death rate dropped from 23 to 14; and life expectancy increased from 46 to 57 (Richmond 1982). Fertility rates have been difficult to calculate due to inconsistent reporting procedures. Recently, the ARE released figures to show that in Upper Egypt, the fertility rate averages 6.3 children per woman in a lifetime compared with 3.5 in Cairo and Alexandria (Richmond 1982). The World Fertility Survey reports, in the period between 1960 and 1965, that the national rate was 7.09, and in the period between 1975 and 1980 that it was 5.27 (Richmond 1982). Both data sets support the contention that fertility rates are declining rather substantially.

Fertility decline (rather than increased life expectancy) is the main determinant of population aging. Successes in treating and preventing infectious and parasitic illnesses and in reducing fertility through effective family planning programs have produced changed patterns in mortality and morbidity as well as in the population structure of Egypt.

The changes in these basic health status indicators are altering patterns of demand from government-provided services to nongovernment and private services. In large part, this demand is generated through lower fertility among wage-based earners in highly concentrated urban centers and the shift in morbidity and mortality from parasitic and infectious diseases to the more chronic diseases: the epidemiological transition.

Effects of the Epidemiological Transition on Government Policy

The past two decades have seen impressive changes in the lives of Egyptians. Policymakers are faced with perplexing questions about the optimal ways to organize and finance efforts to maintain and improve health. The answers that have been accepted in the past have been based on a social and economic reality that is changing rapidly. In the forefront of changing indicators is the epidemiological transition. In Egypt, as elsewhere, the consequences of this phenomenon are proving difficult for health planners to manage effectively.

Egypt, like other nations in the Third World, is striving to attain a goal of an average life expectancy of 60 for its population by the year 2000. Predicted decreases in mortality, particularly if they coincide with ARE's renewed resolve to conduct an effective family planning program, will have a profound effect on the health-care sector, its organization, and its priorities. Not only will the focus shift to chronic disorders found among older individuals but also the burden for treatment will fall on the nongovernment and private sectors where per capita expenditures have been increasing. This will increase total gross national product (GNP) expenditures for health.

Organization of the Health Sector in Egypt Today

The Egyptian health sector has great diversity and pluralism, and it is not easily understood in western terms. To simplify matters, the following descriptions will be used throughout the text to identify its major actors (Richmond 1982):

1. The governmental sector (MOH, Ministry of Education, etc.)
2. The public sector (Health Insurance Organization, CCO, etc.)
3. The private sector (Medical Syndicate, traditional practitioners, religious and community groups, private practitioners, etc.).

Since the government sector is overextended, the public sector is seen, and is beginning to be used, as an agent to relieve the MOH of some of its operating liabilities. At present, two main public entities act in this role:

1. The Health Insurance Organization, which now had over 3 million subscribers.
2. The CCO, which serves approximately 5 percent (2.4 million people) of the total population.

Both of these groups report to the Minister of Health (rather than to the ministry) and hire and reimburse personnel on what may be considered, in the Egyptian context, a "private" sector competitive basis.

In addition to these public sector groups, there are four main private sector entities in operation (Richmond 1982):

1. Private practices in urban and rural areas, though many of these practices are conducted by physicians who hold concurrent appointments with the MOH and have MOH approval to operate as private practitioners in the afternoon.
2. The Medical Syndicate, which has formed a Medical Professions Corporation for Investment (MPCI) in accordance with Law 43 for development in the medical professions field.
3. Traditional practitioners (approximately 20,000) and religious groups, which operate health facilities on grounds contiguous to mosques.
4. Privately owned and operated hospitals, mainly in Cairo, which are constructed with private funds and charge patients on a fee-for-service basis (e.g., the Arab Contractors).

Ministry of Health

Since 1936, the MOH has evolved through a series of reorganizations associated with critical events in Egypt's history: World War II, independence from British colonialism, the change from monarchy to socialism in the 1952 revolution, the deterioration of a one-crop cotton economy which generated most of the foreign exchange, three Arab-Israeli wars, nationalization, the 1962 National Charter, and the 1973 *El-Infitah*. By 1984, the ministry employed over 16,000 people.

The premises that gave impetus to MOH expansion in 1952 did not apply in 1984. The land upon which every MOH health facility was constructed in rural areas was donated by the communities. Then, the population was predominantly rural in nature. By 1977, the MOH had a total of 3,500 units, 2,300 of which were located in rural areas (Richmond 1982). However, with rapid urbanization, the ministry now has most of its infrastructure capital in areas experiencing emigration and lower economic growth rates as a percent of gross domestic product. Moreover, land is at such a premium in Cairo and in Alexandria as to put it out of reach both of the ministry and of the community, given current budget decisions of the ARE.

Private Health Sector

There are approximately 280 private hospitals (37 percent of which are in Cairo and Alexandria), 478 licensed polyclinics (59 percent of which are in Cairo and Alexandria), and 12,210 clinics (60 percent of which are in Cairo and Alexandria) in the private sector. Ministry of Health statistics place the number of beds in these facilities at 7,005; other sources have estimated that figure to be 5,000. Ministry data also document 363 private laboratories in Egypt, 80 percent of which are located in Cairo, Alexandria, and Port Said.

It has been estimated that between 30 and 45 percent of Egypt's outpatient visits are accounted for in the private sector, exclusive of visits to private pharmacies. The ministry estimates that 70 percent of these visits were for general medical services, although the majority of private physicians have specialist training.

Whatever the exact number of personnel and facilities and the level of utilization, it is clear that the private sector in Egypt is growing rapidly. Some estimates place the annual private investment in health facilities, equipment, and space at L.E. 50 million (US $60.5 million), almost double the annual rate of governmental sector investment in health (Raymond 1983).

Estimates from the MOH indicate that there are now about 12,000 private physicians in practice, of whom about 4,000 are located in rural areas. Comparisons to the number of publicly employed physicians are misleading, since many of these private physicians are government-employed physicians with part-time private practices. In rural areas, this process of "privatization" has been speeded not only by economic need, but also by changes in government regulations which now officially allow government physicians to carry on private practices in government facilities. This regulatory change, combined with the medical saturation of the urban market and high start-up costs of urban practices, has resulted in more than 50 percent of young physicians, after completing their one-year required rural service tour, choosing to remain in rural systems (Raymond 1983).

Results of Social and Economic Changes

Given the health investments of the past, one might have expected a more favorable outcome on health status. The capacity of the ARE to meet national health objectives has changed over time. Although the public sector share of total governmental expenditures for health has remained relatively stable during the past sixteen years, the MOH's share of total expenditures has declined precipitously, from 8.6 percent in 1970 to 1.8 percent in 1983 (Badran 1984). Rapid and sustained urban migration has had a serious, negative impact on the quality of urban life; local governmental authorities in urban and rural areas have been unable to keep pace with the provision of adequate public services, such as water, sewerage, and the collection of solid waste. Meanwhile, industrialization, urbanization, the expansion of the service sector, and the increase in per capita income have altered expectations about the government's role in providing health services and increased public demand for alternative health services.

The government has a public health program infrastructure that reaches most of the population. Currently, a public health facility exists within 3 kilometers of every village of 3,000 people; the physician to population ratio is 1:1090; and the nurse to population ratio is 1:800 (based on provider registration figures, in Richmond 1982).

In terms of health facilities and personnel, Egypt has in place today a primary health-care system. It does not work well. Its efficiency is at a level inconsistent with the level of national investment.

Decline in Governmental Health Resources

The amount of resources the MOH has at its disposal, as a percentage of total government expenditure, has declined precipitously. This may be in response to low utilization rates of ministry facilities. Perhaps more significantly, the government has shifted health resources from the MOH to the private and other public sectors. The government has set price controls for pharmaceuticals and pharmaceutical materials and has allowed their importation, at whatever rates are necessary, to satisfy the demand. Laws 79 and 32 established a legal mechanism to finance health insurance of wage-based workers, including civil servants, through government-subsidized premium payments.

Decentralization

The process of decentralization is picking up momentum across all sectors. As this process advances yet farther, the management support needs of the public health services delivery system will change. Already, in the past five years alone, the management support structures of the MOH have been altered dramatically. Centralized functions have been transferred to local governments at district levels. The ministry plays increasingly programmatic roles, such as planning, measurement of utilization and cost effectiveness, monitoring and evaluation, and the organization and analysis of information (Richmond 1982).

Changes in Demand for Health Services

Changes within the MOH system are taking place at a time when the public's demand for alternative health services is increasing. Since 1972, the scale and diversity of available health-care services have expanded rapidly. The capacity of the governmental health sector to respond to national health objectives has been constrained, slowly at first and now more dramatically, by dynamic forces acting on an expanding and changing economy. Expectations on the part of the public and the central government have altered the roles of each. There is no longer a need for the MOH to provide, free of charge, health services to all the people. The ministry system, which was organized to fulfill that role, now finds itself with an enormous infrastructure that it is unable to maintain. It is overextended and underfinanced. Health resource allocation decisions by the central government favor investments away from MOH services toward employed wage earners in socially financed health schemes (HIO) or those who can afford private fee-for-service health care (CCO).

Changes in Private Sector Services

In urban areas, the number of specialists in private facilities has always been considerable, but in recent years their proliferation has been extraordinary. This development does not seem to be confined to the growing middle class. In some areas, such facilities increasingly draw factory-level and services industry personnel. For example, in a June 1981 Helwan Zone Study, covering an area of 600,000 people with a ceiling income of L.E. 50 monthly for a family of five, 309 physicians were found in private practice, a ratio of one physician to 1,942 people. Rural area private practice expansion, judging by indicators such as sales of drugs and supplies and registration figures has also accelerated quickly (Richmond 1982).

In recent years, small, cooperative, and joint sponsorship arrangements have arisen between selected physicians and various groups—neighbors, religious organizations, or members of a company or profession. Certain fixed fees for services are established, and the physicians are retained by the group on a salaried (or a salary/commission) basis. These arrangements are a growing resource in major urban areas. Many are arranged by religious groups that house the health-care facilities (mostly outpatient but with planned expansion to inpatient) contiguous to a mosque or church.

Tensions in the Health Sector

In the past three decades, substantial progress has been made in the development of health infrastructure, particularly in rural areas, though major health problems remain for the people. The rapid rate of industrialization, of urbanization, and of the expansion of health-care education has served to increase tensions within the entire health system, as noted below (Richmond 1982).

Curative vs. Preventive Medicine

The Egyptian health training system focuses on curative medicine. This characterizes both the public and the private sectors in the health-care system. There are some encouraging trends, however. The decision to introduce the teaching of community medicine in all years of the medical curriculum is one example. Development of the new medical curriculum oriented toward community and preventive medicine at the University of the Suez Canal is yet another. It is discouraging to note, however, that at the High Institute for Public Health in Alexandria, where there are 2,000 students studying for masters' degrees, only 300 are in the field of public health. This means that the 26 governorates and the positions in the MOH are short of trained and experienced people in public health practice. It means that there is a clear shortage of epidemiologists to work throughout the country in order to provide the kind of data and surveillance that is so necessary for the mapping of new preventive and public-health-oriented activities.

In a sense, the dominance of curative medicine over prevention and health promotion is the reverse of what the priorities for Egypt should be. The inevitable question is, "Should public health be a part of medicine, or medicine a part of public health?" The physicians who dominate the curative sector would never permit medicine to become a part of public health.

The problem is further highlighted by the fact that approximately 65 percent of the hospital beds in Egypt are in MOH facilities. In these facilities, the ministry has extensive outpatient clinic responsibilities that keep it focused heavily on curative medicine. Although any society must provide appropriate care of the sick, it seems clear that, if both the public and the private sectors are heavily involved in this manner, little attention will be given to preventive activities.

Hospital and Clinic Facilities Construction vs. Program Improvement

There are inordinate MOH demands for the completion of some 21 hospital buildings and the construction of new facilities which compete for funds for improving existing programs in both urban and rural areas. The bed to population ratio is not as favorable as it is in many other countries; however, there is reasonable access to beds (although there is some geographic maldistribution) when Egypt is compared to many other developing countries. There is evidence that both inpatient and outpatient facilities have undergone considerable deterioration, and the question arises whether resources could be better employed to improve existing facilities and their programs prior to undertaking new construction.

It should be observed that there has been considerable expansion of the number of hospital beds in the private sector. Many small hospitals (mainly under the aegis of individual physicians or groups of physicians) have been expanding as have some larger ones, such as the Arab Contractors. There are considerable concerns about the extent to which the country can afford expenditures for this new and relatively high cost capital development.

The growing expenditures for private health services are raising questions concerning the extent to which the country can afford them. There is increasing pressure on the MOH and on the Parliament to exert some regulatory constraints on the patient charges that may be generated through these sources. The new law which requires all physicians' offices and hospitals to be registered with the MOH may well be a prelude to some kind of regulatory activity.

Employment Policies: Universal Employment and Motivational Problems

It is apparent that the 1952 revolution and the "full employment policy" have created many problems. Stipends in government health service are low and have resulted in considerable measure in an attitude anecdotally described as "the government pretends to pay us, and we pretend to work."

There are also certain inequities in assignments. Medical students, for example, with better academic records are retained for specialty training; those with lower grades are assigned to rural areas and urban clinics. Apparently, the less desirable assignments go to the students with lower academic records. As a consequence, there is widespread unhappiness about service with the MOH, and members of Parliament are reported to complain about the unhappiness of people who are assigned to work in their areas. The result is inadequate performance, high turnover, and what seems to be relatively low productivity. Many of the people assigned to the rural areas, in particular, are very junior and often are inadequately trained to meet the responsibilities assigned to them.

The recent trend for some physicians to elect to stay in rural areas because of housing and private practice opportunities may be encouraging. However, it is important to add that this is occurring because of limits in opportunity (high costs of establishing a practice) for private practice in the cities. The resentment over this seems to be widespread.

The Medical Syndicate and the Ministry of Health

Because of the increase in the number of medical school graduates in recent years and the limited opportunities for private practice, there is considerable disenchantment among the younger members of the Medical Syndicate concerning professional opportunities. One should add to this the reduction in the number of opportunities for practice abroad. As the Gulf States have developed new medical schools, the need to draw on Egyptian physicians is decreasing as is the potential for practicing in the United States as a consequence of recent Congressional immigration legislation.

The president of the syndicate has been developing a program to finance the establishment of individual and group practices, particularly outside of the major cities, in an effort to alleviate these problems. In addition, he is a very strong proponent of opening up the clinics of the MOH to private practice for the physicians who are serving in those facilities. Some 80 percent of the physicians practicing in the governmental sector conduct concurrent practices in the private sector (Richmond 1982). In effect, this puts them in a conflict of interest position.

With the increase in class size of the medical schools in recent years there will be a predominance of younger physicians—in terms of numbers—in the Medical Syndicate before long. As these people reach maturity and come into positions of power, if the opportunity system remains rather limited, some problems of crisis proportions could develop, since the expectations of young physicians have been that they will in one way or another have reasonable and adequate incomes. What form this discontent may take is difficult to predict; however, it is a real possibility sometime in the next decade.

The Universities and the Ministry of Health

As it is true in many countries, the schools for health professionals are largely under the Ministry of Education, and the health services are under the Ministry of Health. Thus, there is a basis for considerable tension. The increase in the number of students has certainly created problems for the medical schools, because it appears that the schools have not been given adequate resources with which to accommodate the extra students. It may be that the decision made recently to reduce class size will improve morale among faculty and students, but this will take time. As a result of the expansion, many students have a considerable concern about the quality of their education.

Part of the tension is associated with the university recruiting students with the best academic records for training as specialists. This includes approximately 1,500 physicians out of the 5,400 who graduated in 1982. These students, in addition to receiving more favored staff training, are also spared the responsibilities of serving in the rural areas. Thus, there is destined to be a significant number of graduates who feel that the training opportunities for them have been severely limited.

The recent development of the general practice specialization track through a master's degree program, which has been accepted by the Egyptian Medical Association, may minimize this problem. There are, however, many skeptics who feel that in the Egyptian system, the general practitioners, even if they are designated specialists, will not have the status and power of other specialists.

Perhaps the greatest source of tension is the need within the MOH for staff to develop training programs for health professionals in the field. The leading professionals to do the training are in the universities. Ministry funds to support these people for additional tasks are relatively limited. More significantly, the long-term qualitative improvement of services would depend upon drawing into the service system the people in the universities who have higher professional qualifications.

Without such an infusion of some of the most qualified people in the country into the service system, the potential for improving performance may be low indeed. In an informal way, these relationships do exist to some extent. For example, the HIO has consultants from the medical schools who participate in its service program, presumably to the advantage of both. However, university faculty members are probably spreading themselves rather thin, and it may well be that their teaching potential and certainly their research potential are not being fully developed as a consequence.

Drug Expenditures: Too Low or Too High?

Among the priorities announced by the prime minister and the minister of health, the commitment has been made to provide drugs to the population at reasonable costs. The officials responsible for the development of policy concerning pharmaceuticals have suggested that, on a per capita basis, expenditures for drugs are lower than in many other countries of comparable levels of development. However, it is important to note that 40 percent of total health expenditures are for drugs. This seems to be a relatively high figure for one segment of the health sector (in the United States, for example, 40 percent of all health expenditures go for hospital care; 10 percent, for drugs and appliances [Richmond 1982]). There seems to be considerably more prescribing of drugs and self-medication than is appropriate or desirable. For instance, in the HIO, patients have become aware of the fact that they are permitted a maximum of four prescriptions. As a consequence, the patients often demand four prescriptions from the physicians, and it is not uncommon for them to trade some of the drugs so obtained for cosmetics and other desirables in pharmacies.

This is a difficult public policy problem. Instead of accepting the fact that per capita expenditures should rise for drugs, it may be more appropriate to move toward some gradual constraints. Self-medication and the extensiveness of prescribed medications are not good health practices.

Some Consequences of These Tensions

The economic policies of 1952, 1962, and 1973, especially those dealing with the expansion of private sector activities, may well have shaped actions and events now being played out in the health sector. One can argue, on the basis of a considerable body of evidence, that the pluralism and diversity found in the health sector today are the direct result of past policies adopted by the ARE, namely, to provide no more than modest resources to the MOH. In Egypt, as in many other countries, the response to underfunded MOH systems which offer ostensibly free services, which are increasingly unreliable, has been the growth of social security type schemes and a vigorous private sector. These things are the result of basic underlying budget decisions rather than of policy initiatives.

The significance of growth in the public and private sectors and the decrease in government outlays to the MOH are major factors affecting current operations within the health sector at large, particularly in the following four areas: water and sanitation, organization and financing of health services delivery, health manpower, and public health practices and health services delivery.

Water and Sanitation

Environmental health conditions are poor and deteriorating. The lack of basic sanitary services for a large portion of the population and the precarious state of those available to the remainder cast a shadow over all aspects of public health in the country. The most alarming aspect is the growing deficit in water supply and sanitary waste disposal services. The present method of financing and administering the water and sewer utilities is chaotic. The heart of the problem is the current system of grant financing from the central government and inadequate user service charges to provide for proper operation and maintenance. Unless this issue is faced squarely, by putting water and sanitation on a self-supporting fiscal basis, there is no hope of significant progress, and there can be no hope for an improvement in the health status of the great majority of the people (Richmond 1982).

Organization and Financing of Health Services Delivery

The government-financed MOH system delivers preventive/promotive services as well as curative services. The latter take the major portion of its budget and personnel. Because of the high costs for curative services and reduced funding from central government, this impairs the capacity of the MOH system to discharge its preventive/promotive functions and responsibilities adequately. National health policy cannot rely upon private financing alone to secure efficient rates of resource allocation to preventive/promotive activities.

The MOH system is severely underfinanced. There appears to be little or no prospect that the MOH will, in the foreseeable future, enjoy substantial increases in the funding available to it from general tax revenues. Yet, even if it were to receive adequate financing, there remains a fundamental structural problem with the system as it is now constituted. The pressures from consumers for increases in the quantity and quality of the curative services delivered by the system are powerful and difficult to resist. The curative services' claim upon scarce MOH resources tends inevitably to displace the claim of the preventive/promotive activities, particularly since it undertakes to deliver these services at zero price.

The ARE is not committing levels of funding sufficient to maintain and operate an essentially physician-dependent MOH health services delivery system. Of the L.E. 10 billion that was to be expended on improvements of the public sector during 1978–1982 Five-Year Plan, less than 1 percent went to improvements in the health sector. This figure drops even farther in the 1983–1987 Plan. When the numbers are adjusted for inflation, the health sector investment ratio to other investments drops to 0.85 percent.

Every day, the population increases by approximately 3,300 persons—an annual rate of 1,200,000. The expansion of population is not matched by comparable rates of employment in publicly operated health-care facilities or with rising rates of efficiency in the deployed facilities and personnel.

Increases in hospital bed capacity have been in the private sector. In 1976 the MOH had 69.8 percent of total bed capacity; in 1980, it had 65.3 percent. The private sector had 4.6 percent in 1976; in 1980, it had 5.8 percent (Richmond

1982). All other providers, such as university hospital complexes, declined relatively in hospital bed capacity.

Health Manpower

The ARE has a relatively high number of trained health providers available, as well as a high capacity for producing physicians and nurses. Since achieving independence in 1952, there has been a policy of equity and full employment. The growth in population has led to increasing job division. Now there are more and more health workers to do parts of the same job. Every person trained is guaranteed a job, and very are refused admission to training if they have the required academic preparation. However, once they are formally trained, there are few opportunities for continuing education. For those programs that do exist, the high drop-out rate signals that they may be ineffectual in meeting professional needs (Richmond 1982).

Following graduation, the need for income supplementation pushes health-care providers into a multiple employment pattern, through a combination of public and private sources of income. This pattern leads to divided job loyalties, minimum commitment to a place of work, and a pitting of public service against the possibility for private gain.

The government has made a substantial investment in the training of health manpower. Medical schools are producing approximately 5,000 graduates a year, and the nursing schools (including both MOH and university-operated schools) now graduate over 5,000 annually. However, the maintenance of this production level is inconsistent with the country's capacity to absorb graduates.

Egypt's health system has nearly achieved the recommended World Health Organization standards of physician population ratios and population coverage of health facilities. Still, with the availability of this extensive infrastructure, one to two of every ten infants died before reaching one year of age, including 2,000 deaths from tetanus neonatorum in 1982 (Richmond 1982).

The successful implementation of this infrastructure has failed to keep pace with changing expectations and preferences of a society in transition. This highlights the necessity to "rethink" standard prescriptive formulas for manpower and facilities development in the MOH subsector of health. These are seen now as static solutions to dynamic and evolving conditions in the health sector at large.

Public Health Practices and Health Services Delivery

Preventive and public health services are likely to be, for the foreseeable future, contained largely within the domain of the Ministry of Health. The populations most in need and potentially most affected by these services are the rural and urban poor. Although the thrust of national health policy in Egypt is toward a shifting of personal health services away from the "free" MOH modality to the private and public sectors, the two parts of the health sector (MOH vs. all other providers) are linked and interdependent. The major problems of quality (both effectiveness and efficiency) have common roots in the manpower training system which feeds into both subsectors. The shift of population from the MOH to other elements of the health system without attention to these quality issues would only displace, rather than solve, many of the problems cited herein.

Mortality and morbidity data suggest that the health status of the population worsens as one moves from lower Egypt to upper Egypt. The Physician Quality of Life Index also suggests that the well-being of the population deteriorates from lower to upper Egypt. However, there is little evidence (apart from increased employment in rural services as one moves away from upper Egypt) that the distribution of health personnel reflects need. In fact, such personnel are scarce where health status is lowest. The emphasis appears to be on geographic equity of distribution and not on services focused on epidemiologically determined priorities. There is no coordinated system for the recording, compilation, analysis, and publication of information about disease patterns in Egypt. The institutional fragmentation with the MOH and its isolation from other service providers make it barely possible to guess at the prevalence, incidence, case fatality, and geographic distribution of even the most important diseases.

The prospects for substantial near-term qualitative improvements in MOH-managed health services are rather slim. This is due to resource scarcity, lack of discipline, inadequate supervision, low pay and motivation of provider staff, and to the expanding availability of alternative health delivery systems to meet increased consumer demand for curative services. These problems can be summarized as follows (Richmond 1982):

1. There is a large cohort of young nurses and physicians with training ill fitted to the epidemiology of diseases in Egypt.
2. The health system is curative in focus, hospital-based, and physician dependent, with emphasis on specialized nonintegrated services. Preventive care is the sole responsibility of the Ministry of Health.
3. It appears that existing government facilities are underutilized and need a better focused set of treatment priorities.
4. The accessibility of services is a major factor in utilization; current health practices in Egypt demonstrate that the content of services delivered (i.e., availability and acceptability in terms of quality and consumer expectations) is probably a stronger determinant of service choice. Geographic access to preventive and curative facilities is only the first step to achieving coverage and utilization.
5. Most villagers, according to rural physicians, visit government facilities to get the free drugs and not to be examined. Since the examination is cursory and the attending physician usually prescribes a double list of drugs (those that are in the clinic pharmacy and those that must be purchased), villagers regard the free drugs as a net "gain" to them.
6. Consumer health behavior seems to affect the demand for secondary care in two ways: Those who are ill wait much too long, in general, before seeking medical

care. Then, they feel they need or actually do need more specialized care and go directly to the specialists and specialized clinics without first seeking guidance from general practitioners.

7. Urban, publicly supported secondary health services are varied in distribution, content, and organization. As in the case of urban primary services, they tend to be fragmented by specialty and function. The specialized clinics of district and general hospitals appear to be increasing in numbers, and there is an increasing demand for urban polyclinics.
8. Current types of health services consumer options seem to be curative and stabilizing for somewhat complicated and diagnostically demanding medical care. Patients are seeking more personalized care, with improved equipment and facilities, with stress on ambulatory care. In response to this growing demand, the public sector seems to be augmenting specialist staffing at hospital outpatient clinics, establishing special clinics and developing a network of polyclinics.
9. The private sector, at certain economic levels of the population, seems even more vigorous in expanding resources and organizational coverage for a secondary system. This is the case in the larger and more middle-class urban settings, but it is also said to be occurring in high-volume, specialized clinics in poorer neighborhoods.
10. Self-referral to secondary and tertiary facilities is clearly one of the major problems facing health services delivery. Conversely, the relatively low utilization of primary care services is rather discouraging.
11. The health status of people in Egypt is not in keeping with the amounts of health services available, and preventable diseases constitute the majority of all health problems.

Conclusion

The assumption on which the provision of free health services is based in Egypt has been nullified by recent events. The change in the structure of production from agriculture to manufacturing, services, and industry has altered expectations, both about the government's traditional role in the provision of health services and the public's incipient demand for a role in seeking alternative services. The change in the composition of morbidity and the decline in fertility (a precursor to increased life expectancy) represent a dynamic shift in the distribution of diseases needing treatment/cure, of causes of death, and of resources devoted to health.

Policy officials and health planners face a major challenge in meeting the needs of a population whose age structure will change between now and the year 2000. In Egypt, as elsewhere, the number of people with chronic conditions will rise, and the utilization of health services, especially hospital facilities, will increase markedly (Davis 1984). The Ministry of Health is underfunded now; it cannot be expected to continue to provide free services to an expanding population demanding expensive curative care in highly concentrated urban settings.

The ARE has recently formulated a plan to extend health insurance to cover the great majority of the population. In the main, the extension of health insurance coverage will be accomplished by increasing enrollment in the Health Insurance Organization of employed groups, pensioners, and dependents. The government feels that it can extend coverage in the HIO to 60 percent of the population by the year 2000. This would leave 20 percent for free government services and 20 percent for the private sector. The implementation of such a policy would relieve the Ministry of Health of the burden of services now financed by declining general tax revenues, allowing the ministry to devote more of its fiscal and technical capacity to its primary role in fostering public health activities (Badran 1984).

References

Badran, Ahmed. 1984. "Structural Factors/Requirements in Utilizing Cooperative Concepts: A Perspective from the Consumer and Producer Viewpoints." In *Alternative Health Delivery Systems: Can They Serve the Public Interest in Third World Settings*. Washington, D.C.: The National Council of International Health.

Buck, Alfred. 1984. "Health Status and Categorical Disease Research and Control in Egypt." Cairo: Office of Health, USAID, 1982 Health Sector Assessment.

"Health in Egypt: Recommendations for U.S. Assistance." January 1979. Washington, D.C.: National Academy of Sciences, Institute of Medicine.

Davis, Karen. 1984. "Computer Assisted Planning: Applications to Health of the Elderly by the Year 2000." *World Health Statistics*. Vol. 37, No. 3. Geneva: World Health Organization.

Kuhnke, Laverne. 1971. "Resistance and Response to Modernization: Preventive Medicine and Social Control in Egypt, 1825–1840." Ph.D. diss. University of Chicago.

Mayers, Marilyn. 1984. "A Century of Psychiatry: The Egyptian Mental Hospitals." Ph.D. diss. Princeton University.

Richmond, Julius et al. 1982. "A Report on Health Development in the Arab Republic of Egypt: A Sector in Transition." For AID, the American Public Health Association.

Sonbol, Amira. 1981. "The Creation of a Medical Profession in Egypt during the Nineteenth Century: A Study in Modernization." Ph.D. diss. Georgetown University.

Tignor, Robert. 1960. "Public Health Administration in Egypt under British Rule, 1882–1914." Ph.D. diss. Yale University.

Ueber Raymond, Susan. 1983. *Beyond the Public Prescription: Private and Public Roles in Near East Health*. New York: Center for Public Resources.

FEDERAL REPUBLIC OF GERMANY

Fritz Beske

Historical Overview

The development of the health-care system of the Federal Republic of Germany has been greatly influenced by the compulsory health insurance system introduced in 1883. Before that time, social benefit associations or cooperative societies had existed on a voluntary basis. They were probably the oldest mutual benefit societies in Europe. However, even earlier, in 1838, official regulations had been introduced in Prussia requiring employers to make specific contributions toward the costs of health care for their workers. Both the mutual benefit societies and the contributions of employers in Prussia provided sickness benefits, disability and funeral benefits, and pension to widows. In 1854, a Prussian law made membership in mutual societies compulsory for miners.

In 1871, Bismarck founded the German Empire. A subsequent economic crisis—the result of rapid industrialization during the mid-nineteenth century—created serious social unrest. In an effort to defuse this social problem, Chancellor Bismarck responded with a program of social legislation. The three laws then passed—together with the unemployment law and the social welfare law of later times—remain the backbone of the Federal Republic's overall social security system: in 1883, the compulsory health insurance law; in 1884, the accident insurance law; and in 1889, the disability and old-age pension insurance law.

In the beginning, the compulsory health insurance law, the first law of its kind in Europe, applied to manual industrial workers only. The main purpose of this law was to provide their members with cash benefits during episodes of illness and with a limited range of medical services.

In the following century and up until now, the insurance system has gradually evolved in two directions. First, emphasis has shifted from cash benefits toward comprehensive medical benefits in kind, including the whole range of modern medical and dental service. Cash benefits for illness are now paid for the first six weeks by the employer, with subsequent benefits the responsibility of the health insurance system. Second, an ever-larger proportion of the population has come under compulsory membership or has been granted the right to join the statutory system. As a result, in 1987, about 90 percent of the population belonged to the compulsory health insurance system.

Health Status of the Population

In 1986 the Federal Republic of Germany had 61.1 million inhabitants. The life expectancy for males at birth in 1900 was 45 years; in 1985, it was 71.2 years. The figures for females were 48 years and 77.8 years, respectively.

The birth rate, which was about 18 per 1,000 population in 1960, has decreased continuously, reaching 9.6 in 1985. It currently is among the lowest in Europe. According to forecasts, this low birth rate will cause the population of the Federal Republic to drop to 45.8 million by the year 2030 (Table 1). Table 1 indicates that the percentage of children under twenty will, in 2030, be only 15.4, whereas the percentage of people 60 and older will increase from 20 percent in the period 1970–1990 to 37.3 by 2030.

The death rate was 11.4 in 1984. The infant mortality rate decreased from 55.3 in 1950 to 9.6. in 1985. The leading causes of death are cardiovascular diseases, cancer, diseases of the respiratory system, diseases of the digestive system, and accidents and poisoning.

Health System Structure

Administrative Organization of Health Services

No specific federal health law governs the structure or functioning of health services in all of Germany, since the constitution specifies that health responsibilities are to be divided between the federal and the state (*Länder*) levels. There is also no comprehensive national health plan, nor are there comprehensive health plans on the state level. There do exist, however, special programs to meet needs in individual problem areas, e.g., handicapped or cancer registries. In general, the German health-care system is extremely complex and complicated, with many participating parties. It also is a health-care system with a very high standard and full coverage of the population.

At both federal and state levels, authority is divided among various ministries, but their area of responsibility differs from state to state. At the federal level, certain responsibilities pertaining to health are dealt with by the Ministry of Youth, Family Affairs, Women, and Health: human medicine, veterinary medicine, the professions in the health field, medicament, pharmacy, foodstuffs, and consumer protection. Other responsibilities are dealt with by the Ministry of

Table 1
Forecast of the Population According to Age Groups (Germans and Foreigners)

Age Group	1970[1)]	1982[1)]	1990[2)]	2000[2)]	2010[2)]	2020[2)]	2030[2)]
				in millions			
Under 20	18.2	15.9	12.4	11.7	9.8	7.8	7.2
20 to 60	31.3	33.7	35.4	33.2	31.0	27.9	22.2
60 and older	12.0	12.1	12.4	14.8	15.5	16.1	17.5
Total	61.5	61.7	60.2	59.7	56.3	51.8	46.9
				in percent			
Under 20	29.6	25.8	20.4	19.6	17.4	15.3	15.4
20 to 60	50.9	54.6	58.3	55.6	55.1	53.7	47.3
60 and older	19.5	19.6	21.3	24.8	27.5	31.0	37.3

1. Berichtüber die Bevölkerungsentwicklung in der Bundesrepublik Deutschland, 2. Teil (BT Drucksache 10/863), S. 139.
2. Modellrechnungen zur Bevölkerungsentwicklung in der Bundesrepublik Deutschland, aktaulisierte Fassung (Hrsg. vom Bundeminister des Innen, Bonn 1987).

Labor and Social Affairs: social security including health, medical, and dental care under the statutory system; hospitals; rehabilitation; and labor protection. The Ministry of Environmental Protection, Nature Protection, and Nuclear Safety is responsible for environmental protection.

The federal level has no general legislative power in the health field, but it has specific legislative power in relation to the control of infectious diseases and diseases constituting a public danger, the health professions, pharmaceuticals, narcotics, toxic substances, foodstuffs and other substances for human consumption, social insurance including health, labor protection, hospital financing, and public welfare. Insofar as the federal level has not been given or does not exercise jurisdiction, responsibility lies with the states. The states also implement the federal laws. Coordination of activities in the field of health is achieved by means of the Conference of Health Ministers and the Conference of Social Ministers, both federal and state, and through working groups of head administrators, e.g., the directors of the state health departments or for specific subjects.

At the federal level, there are a number of agencies, offices, or institutes for advice or research; the most important of these is the Federal Health Office which is located in Berlin. Both the federal level and the states have advisory bodies such as the Federal Health Board or the health boards of the states, which are composed of experts in the different fields of health.

Public health is primarily the responsibility of the states and it is carried out predominantly at the intermediate (region) or local level of administration, in counties and in communities. Each county has a public health office directed by a public health physician staffed with physicians, dentists, sanitary engineers, nurses, and social workers.

The most important law is the Federal Public Health Law of 1934 (*Gesetz über die Vereinheitlichung des Gesundheitswesens*, 3 July 1934), which is still the framework for many public health activities. In the meantime, some states have replaced the Federal Public Health Law through state health laws. There is now some danger that separate state public health laws may disrupt the existing unity of public health in Germany. The main responsibilities of public health authorities concern infectious diseases, hygiene, environmental protection, supervision of health institutions and health personnel, health education, maternal and child health, school health, and care for the handicapped and the aged.

Hospitals

The present structure of the German hospital system reflects a long history that started in the middle ages with hospitals for the poor run mainly by churches. Since the beginning of this century, many additional hospitals have been built by public authorities (states, counties, and communes), by churches, by voluntary organizations (e.g, the Red Cross), and by private owners.

The development of acute and special hospitals since 1960 is shown in Table 2. Since 1960, the number of hospitals has continuously decreased from 3,604

Table 2
Hospitals and Hospital Beds, 1960 to 1985, Acute Hospitals and Special Hospitals

	Total of hospitals and hospital beds			Acute hospitals			Special hospitals		
	No. of hospitals	No. of beds	Beds per 10,000 pop.	No. of Hospitals	No. of beds	Beds per 10,000 pop.	No. of Hospitals	No. of beds	Beds per 10,000 pop.
1960	3,604	583 513	104.6	2,678	406 022	72.8	926	177 491	31.1
1970	3,587	683 254	112.0	2,441	457 004	74.9	1,146	226 250	37.1
1980	3,234	707 710	114.8	1,991	476 652	77.3	1,243	231 058	37.5
1985	3,098	674 742	110.6	1,825	462 124	75.7	1,273	212 186	34.9

to 3,098. The number of beds had, during the first decades, increased from 583,000 to 707,000, but then it decreased to 674,742. The sharpest decline of hospitals occurred with acute hospitals where the number decreased from 2,678 in 1960 to 1,825 in 1985. Mainly small hospitals with from 20 to 50 beds have been closed.

The ratio of 75.7 beds per 10,000 population in 1985 is very high compared with other highly industrialized countries. According to the opinion of most experts, there is a considerable surplus of acute hospital beds resulting in high investment and operating costs. This fact is of great concern to those who worry about the ever-increasing cost of medical care and especially of hospital care. There is no easy solution, however, since local politicans typically resist hospital closings.

Until 1972 there was almost no hospital planning in Germany. The deficit in running costs per year of all acute hospitals was about 2 billion DM. This situation prompted the federal government to introduce a hospital financing law, which was passed in 1972. The 1972 hospital law regulated not only the financing of hospitals but also the scope and conditions of regional hospital planning.

For the financial support of hospitals, the law provides for investment subsidies for building new or renovating old hospitals. The federal government distributes its financial aid among the states on the basis of approved hospital plans. The states divide this financial support together with their own financial aid among individual hospital projects that are in conformity with the state hospital plan. The hospitals have to negotiate the per diem with the sickness funds and with private health insurance but are granted by law a per diem to meet running costs based on need and efficient operation of the hospital.

The 1972 Hospital Financing Law resulted in a great deal of expensive hospital building, a considerable increase in hospital running costs, and consequently in higher per diems. This, in turn, led to a strong opposition from the sickness funds, and the law is now in the process of being revised. It is expected that, in the future, there will be more freedom for individual hospitals to cut their running costs, as well as more influence for the sickness funds in the hospital planning process.

Health Professions

There is a great variety of professionals working in the health field, with new professions developing almost every year, and with increasing numbers. The most important professions and their numbers in 1986 are shown in Table 3.

Of great importance to the health-care system in general and to the statutory system specifically is the increase in the number of physicians (Table 4).

The number of physicians increased from 79,350 in 1960 to 165,015 in 1985. Accordingly, the ratio of physician to population decreased from 1:703 to 1:360. In the year 2000, there will be as many as 257,000 physicians, and, by then, there will be a 1:200 ratio for physicians to inhabitants (Brenner 1986). Since

Table 3
Medical and Other Health Personnel, 1986

Occupation	Number
Physicians	160,900
Dentists	38,820
Pharmacists	36,500
Nurses	278,720
Medical laboratory technicians and X-ray technicians	30,620
Masseurs and bath attendants	22,050
Pharmaceutical technicians	25,100
Physiotherapists	12,740
Midwives	5,730
Dietitians	3,150
Occupational therapists	3,715
Disinfectors	2,250
Speech therapists	931

Table 4

Number of Physicians, Dentists, Pharmacies, 1960–1985

	Physicians		Dentists		Pharmacists		Pharmacies	
	Number	Inhabitants per physician	Number	Inhabitants per dentist	Number	Inhabitants per pharmacist	Number	Inhabitants per pharmacy
1960	79,350	703	32 509	1,716	15,803	3,530	8,832	6,276
1970	99,654	612	31 175	1,956	20,866	2,923	11,218	5,406
1980	130,431	442	33 240	1,855	28,674	2,150	15,877	3,883
1985	165,015	360	36 853	1,656	33,702	1,811	17,705	3,550

there is no indication that the number of students admitted to medical schools will be reduced, the forecast for the year 2000 can be considered reliable. The potential impact, especially on the statutory system, is tremendous.

The number of dentists was nearly stable between 1960 and 1982. This will change now since the number of student places in dental schools has been increased considerably. Thus there will be in the coming years a surplus of dentists in addition to the surplus of physicians which is already evident.

Pharmacists have experienced a similar situation to that of physicians: Their number increased from 15,803 in 1960 to 33,702 in 1985. As a result, the average number of inhabitants served by a pharmacy went down from 6,276 in 1960 to 3,550 in 1985, and an increasing number of pharmacies have economic difficulties.

Health System Financing

Expenditures for Health

In 1982 the overall expenditures for health including preventive and curative medicine, rehabilitation, cash benefits, education, and research amounted to 215 billion DM, or about 14 percent of the gross national product. This is three times the comparable figure in 1970, when the overall expenditure was 70 billion DM. During this same period, the gross national product only doubled: from 679 billion DM in 1970 to 1,750 billion DM in 1984. Hence, expenditures for health are increasing at a substantially greater rate than the gross national product.

Particular concern focuses on the increase of expenditures in the statutory system, which in 1983 spent more than ten times as much as it did in 1960. Table 5 presents the development of the statutory system from 160 to 1986.

Total expenditures increased from 9.5 billion DM in 1960 to 113.8 billion DM in 1986, with almost one-third of the overall expenditures absorbed by the acute care hospital sector. Private health insurance paid in addition 13.4 billion DM in 1986.

Health Insurance

Almost everybody in Germany is a member of a health insurance system, compulsory or private, or is covered by social welfare. Out of 100 persons, 90 percent belong to the statutory system, 8 percent have private insurance coverage, and 2 percent receive free medical services (armed forces, police, or social welfare); less than 0.2 percent (exclusively well-to-do people) have no coverage.

About 7 percent of the population, who are members of the statutory system, also carry private health insurance, usually to allow for choice of physician, for more comfortable accommodations in hospitals, or for cash benefits in case of illness.

The statutory system operates on a decentralized base within federal statutes

Table 5
Expenditure of the Statutory System, 1960 to 1986 (in Billion DM)

Year	Total	Index	Outpatient medical care		Dental care excluding dentures		Drugs and other products from pharmacies		Drugs and other products not from pharmacies		Artificial dentures		Hospital care		Cash benefits	
			Total	Index	Total	Index	Total	Index	Total	Index	Total	Index	Total	Index	Total	Index
1960	9.5	1.0	1.9	1.0	0.5	1.0	1.1	1.0	0.2	1.0	0.2	1.0	1.6	1.0	2.7	1.0
1970	25.2	2.7	5.4	2.9	1.7	3.7	4.2	3.9	0.7	3.1	0.8	3.1	6.0	3.8	2.4	0.9
1980	89.8	9.5	15.4	8.2	5.5	11.8	12.6	11.5	4.9	22.6	7.4	27.3	25.5	16.2	6.6	2.5
1986	113.8	12.0	20.4	10.7	7.1	14.2	17.6	16.0	7.1	35.5	6.9	34.5	37.5	13.4	6.9	2.6

(*Reichsversicherungsordnung*, or RVO). There are 1,194 individual sickness funds (1986), which are governed by boards of 50 percent employers and 50 percent employees (workers' sickness funds) or 100 percent employees (white-collar sickness funds) and which are organized into state and national associations. Benefits offered in kind include outpatient medical and dental care, hospital care, drugs and other pharmaceuticals, physical rehabilitation, artificial dentures, sanatory curative care, sanatory preventive care, home care, home nursing, orthopedic appliances, pregnancy care, preventive health screening for children up to four years of age, preventive cancer screening for women and men, sickness pay, and burial allowance. For some benefits, there is a modest amount of copayment, e.g., artificial dentures, drugs, hospital care, and transport. There is a choice of physician in ambulatory care, including specialists. Ambulatory care is delivered almost exclusively through private practice. This is also true for dental care.

The statutory system is financed through contributions shared equally between employer and employee. The contribution differs according to the individual sickness fund, but the average contribution in 1985 was about 12.2 percent of income.

Ambulatory medical care is provided by sickness fund doctors (*Kassenärzte*), and ambulatory dental care is provided by sickness fund dentists (*Kassenzahnärzte*). By law, they must be members of a state association of registered doctors or registered dentists. These associations have statutory responsibility to tax, supervise, discipline, fine, and expel members. They guarantee to the patient and to the sickness funds the standards of their members' medical practice.

The sickness fund doctors usually work in solo practice, although there is a certain trend recently toward group practice, typically two physicians in the same specialty. Although members of the statutory system have free choice of physician, this applies only to physicians working in ambulatory care in private practice. Hospital physicians in general are not allowed to care for ambulatory patients, and hospitals have no outpatient departments. This does not apply to university hospitals, where outpatient departments exist in almost all disciplines for teaching and research purposes.

The associations of sickness fund physicians and the associations of sickness fund dentists negotiate their remuneration on a fee-for-service basis with the sickness funds on the federal and on the state levels. The sickness funds pay the associations a lump sum, which, in turn, is distributed to the members by the association according to their work load for the sickness fund. Hospitals are paid a per diem by the sickness funds which again is the result of negotiations between the sickness fund and the individual hospital. In case of disagreement, the state ministry of health has the right to determine the per diem; however, there is always the option to appeal a decision in court. Every physician and every dentist has the right to work for the statutory system if he or she fulfills certain requirements, e.g., a qualified specialist or a general practitioner who has worked in medicine for eighteen months after graduation. The sickness funds and the associations of sickness fund physicians and dentists are supervised by federal and state ministries, respectively.

Major Problems Confronting the Health Sector

The central problem facing the Federal Republic's health system is the increase of expenditures in the statutory system and of growing efforts to halt measures that increase these expenditures. The situation is likely to continue to deteriorate as the overall population decreases while the relative number of aged people increases.

The causes for increased expenditures have been widely discussed. No single cause appears to be responsible for this development. Among others, the following causes have been suggested: life-styles with increasing consumption of alcohol and tobacco, obesity, inadequate physical exercise, road traffic accidents, demands of a fairly wealthy society for comfort in health services, a higher proportion of older people with a greater need and demand for health services, a surplus in hospital beds, advances in medicine and especially in high and expensive technology, an increase in the number of physicians and in other health professions, and the 1972 Hospital Financing Law. Additionally, some point to the responsibility of the statutory system to provide care for certain groups of the population (e.g., handicapped persons and students) without recouping the full expenditure for these groups from public funds. Similar responsibilities have also been given to the statutory system for purely social reasons, e.g., cash benefits for leave from work for the mother or father of a risk child, sterilization on social grounds, and cash benefits in case of maternity, again without full remuneration of expenditures by the public. Finally, some commentators point to the constant enlargement of benefits up to a point where virtually everything possible in medicine is granted to members of the statutory system. This factor may well be most important for the increase of expenditures in the statutory system.

In an effort to bring expenditures under control, two cost control laws have been passed, one in 1977 and one in 1981. Besides minor changes in the statutory system (e.g., some copayment or broadening of the responsibilities of review boards for physicians and dentists), the Concerted Action for Health Affairs was established (*Konzertierte Aktion im Gesundheitswesen*). The Concerted Action for Health Affairs has some 60 members including representatives of sickness funds, private health insurers, physicians, dentists, hospitals, pharmacists, pharmaceutical manufacturers, trade unions, and employers. The states, the municipalities, and the counties are also represented in this group.

The Concerted Action was convened by the Minister for Labor and Social Affairs, in order to develop recommendations concerning the global budgets for ambulatory medical care, dental care, drugs, and hospitals; to discuss major problems of health connected with the provision of medical care; and to make recommendations as to the efficacy and efficiency of medical service delivery.

The Concerted Action has been successful to some extent. For several years now, increases on the statutory system's expenditures have been less than before. At present, however, there is new growth in expenditures, and it is questionable whether the Concerted Action will be able to cope with this resurgent problem.

Possible Future Developments

If the stabilization of health expenditures is to be achieved—and there is a widespread consensus that this is necessary—important changes in the Federal Republic's health-care system must be anticipated. These could include reducing benefits, enlarging copayments, publishing lists of drugs including quality assessment and price, increasing the number of drugs no longer paid for by the statutory system (the existing list of such drugs, called the "negative list," includes drugs for minor ailments), limiting the number of physicians who work for the statutory system, giving priority for ambulatory care including home help and home nursing in order to reduce hospital care, limiting the number of medical and dental students, changing the fees for the service system, cutting down hospital beds, and changing the per diem system in hospitals toward a more differentiated system, e.g., diagnostic related groups (DRGs). Some of these changes may be introduced without too much opposition, but most will meet strong responses from interested parties. It will also be difficult to find a majority in parliament for a number of these changes. It should also be mentioned that there are proposals to change the medical care system completely and to introduce a system similar to a nationalized health-care system.

WHO Concept of Health for All

The WHO concept of Health for All is rarely discussed in Germany. Only the "Greens" (*Die Grünen*) have proposed to introduce the Health for All concept in Germany. This concept, which is in essence the outcome of the 1978 WHO/UNICEF Conference on Primary Health Care in Alma Ata, is seen in Germany as pertaining mainly to developing countries. Much of this primary health-care concept is already a reality in highly industrialized countries, e.g., sanitation and food supply. On the other hand, primary medical care has been strengthened in Germany in recent years, e.g., the general practitioner as the family physician, home nursing, and health education. Nevertheless, the WHO primary health-care concept is an incentive to reconsider the aim, the functioning, the outcome, and the value of the present medical care system in the Federal Republic of Germany.

References

Beske, F. 1982. "Expenditures and Attempts of Cost Containment in the Statutory Health Insurance System in the Federal Republic of Germany." In G. McLachlan and

A. Maynard (eds.), *The Public/Private Mix for Health*. London: Nuffield Provincial Hospitals Trust.

Blanpain, J. 1978. *National Health Insurance and Health Resources: The European Experience*. Cambridge, Mass.: Harvard University Press.

Brenner, G. 1986. *Medizinische und Okonomische Orientierung*. Sachver-Ständigenrat für die Konzertieste Aktion in Gesundheitwesen.

Deppe, H.-U. 1983. *Gesundheitssysteme und Gesundheitspolitik in Westeuropa*. Frankfurt/New York: Campus Verlag.

Glaser, W. 1978. *Health Insurance Bargaining. Foreign Lessons for Americans*. New York: Gardner Press.

"Health Services Systems in the European Economic Community." Seminar Proceedings. Seminar Proceedings. DHEW Publication No. (HRA) 76–638. Washington, D.C.: U.S. Department of Health, Education, and Welfare.

Krauskopf, D. 1986. *Soziale Krankenversicherung*. München: Verlag C. H. Beck.

Maynard, A. 1975. *Health Care in the European Community*. London: Croom Helm Limited.

Peters, H. 1987. *Handbuch der Krankenversicherung*. Stuttgart: Verlag W. Kohlhammer.

Prins, R. 1984. *Socio-medical Services and Labour Incapacity. An International Comparative Study*. Amsterdam: Stichting CCOZ.

Schriftenreihe des Bundesministers für Jugend, Familie und Gesundheit. 1983. *Daten des Gesundheitswesens - Ausgabe 1985* -. Band 154. Stuttgart: Verlag W. Kohlhammer.

Statistisches Jahrbuch 1986 für die Bundesrepublik Deutschland. 1984. Stuttgart: Verlag W. Kohlhammer.

Steuer, W. 1974. *Sozialhygiene*. Stuttgart: Georg Thieme Verlag.

Stone, D. 1980. *The Limits of Professional Power: National Health Care in the Federal Republic of Germany*. Chicago: University of Chicago Press.

World Health Organization. *Health Services in Europe*. 1981. Third Edition. Volume 2: "Country Reviews and Statistics." Copenhagen: Regional Office for Europe.

GERMAN DEMOCRATIC REPUBLIC

Jürgen Grosser

Introduction

The German Democratic Republic (GDR) was founded on October 7, 1949, as a response to the merger of the American, British, and French occupational zones into the Federal Republic of Germany in September 1949. The GDR is the first socialist state on German soil, with a national economy based on state ownership of the means of production.

The GDR is located in Central Europe. It borders Poland in the east (460 kilometers), Czechoslovakia in the south (454 kilometers), and the Federal Republic of Germany in the west (1378 kilometers). In the north, the Baltic Sea forms a natural frontier. The country had a population, in late 1985 of 16,640,059—7,877,669 males and 8,762,390 females. Of this population, 3,098,804 are children below the age of fourteen and a half (18.6 percent); 10,786,493 are people of working age (64.8 percent); and 2,754,762 (16.6 percent) are people at retirement age (men over 65 and women over 60).

Historical Overview

At the end of World War II in 1945, a very difficult health situation existed in what is now the GDR. Many towns and villages had been entirely or partly destroyed. As a consequence of the war, hundreds of thousands of people were starving, homeless, and suffering from such diseases as typhoid fever, dysentery, and diphtheria. The number of people with tuberculosis increased dramatically. The achievements of the GDR's health system since 1945 must be judged against this background.

The Communist Party of Germany's appeal of 11 June 1945 and the principles of the health policy of the Socialist Unity Party of Germany (formed in 1946 when the Communist Party of Germany and the Social Democratic Party of Germany merged together) of 1947 initiated a fundamental transformation that included the health-care system. The development of the socialist GDR health system is based on the following principles:

1. Medical facilities are under governmental supervision.
2. Medical care and treatment are free for everyone.
3. The health system is developed on the basis of governmental plans.
4. Primary attention is attached to preventive options for health protection. Responsibility for this is shouldered not only the health system but also by enterprise managers and heads of state authorities. This applies particularly to industrial safety and environmental protection.
5. Attempts are being made to synthesize theory and practice, as soon as possible. This means a rapid translation of scientific findings into practice for the benefit of the people.
6. Direct involvement of the citizens is encouraged in questions of health protection.

Based on these principles, a socialist health system was established in the GDR. Important stipulations are fixed in the GDR constitution in Article 35:

1. Every citizen of the GDR shall have the right to the protection of his health and working capacity.
2. This right shall be guaranteed by the systematic improvement of working and living conditions, public health measures, a comprehensive social policy, and the promotion of physical culture, school and popular sport, and outdoor recreation.
3. Material security, medical aid, drugs and other medical services shall be provided free of charge in the event of illness or accident on the basis of a social insurance system.

State of Health of the Population

Demographics

The GDR's demographics were strongly influenced by both world wars. There were sharp drops due to losses, especially among men, and subsequently falling birth rates. Children make up 18.6 percent and pensioners 16.6 percent of the total population. The working population amounts to 64.8 percent. More than two-thirds of the work force are employed in industry (including construction industry and transportation). The number of people employed in agriculture has steadily decreased. It totalled 2.2 million in 1949 and only 22,000 in 1985. Almost 6 percent of the working population are employed in the health-care system (Staatliche Zentralverwaltung 1986).

Comparative data on the average life expectancy of children in Germany and

Table 1
Life Expectancy at Birth According to Sex (in years)

Year		Male	Female
1871-81	)	35.58	38.45
1901-10	) Germany	44.82	48.33
1924-26	)	55.97	58.82
1952	)	63.90	67.96
1970	) GDR	68.10	69.09
1984		69.64	75.42

in the GDR are shown in Table 1. In 1984, a boy had a life expectancy of 69.64 years and a girl of 75.42 years in the GDR.

During and after World War II, the birth rate dropped considerably. When general living and working conditions normalized, the number of live births grew and reached its highest point in 1960. By then, the losses caused by World War II had been roughly made up.

In the interest of true equality for women, interruption of pregnancy within the first twelve weeks was legalized in 1972. This led to a temporary decrease in the birth rate (see Table 2), with second children being born later, and third and additional children becoming ever more scarce. Due to a comprehensive system of social benefits for young couples, expectant and young mothers, however, the number of births subsequently rose to the current level of 230,000 per annum. The legalization of an interruption of pregnancy did entirely away with illegal abortions, which had amounted to between 50,000 and 70,000 annually before 1972. Cases of death among women after illegal abortion also vanished.

Infant and Maternal Mortality

The rate of infant and maternal mortality is, to a considerable extent, an expression of the socioeconomic situation—of the general working and living conditions and of the level of medical care. In 1946 the infant mortality rate amounted to 131.4 in 1,000. By 1985, this rate was down to 9.6 (10.7 for boys

Table 2
Live Births in Absolute Terms

Year	Total	per 1,000 population
1949	274,022	14.5
1955	293,280	16.3
1960	292,985	17.0
1965	281,058	16.5
1970	236,929	13.9
1975	181,798	10.8
1980	245,132	14.6
1985	227,648	13.7

and 8.3 for girls). There are no differences betweeen children of married and single mothers, or between town and countryside or other socioeconomic conditions. Perinatal mortality of women also took a favorable turn. From 20.6 per 10,000 live births in 1950, it had dropped to 1.2 in 1982. Apart from a general rise in living standards and the extension of the health and social services as a whole, these results can be related to intensive prenatal care and the wide extension of obstetrics and pediatrics, especially neonatology.

Child Mortality

In 1982 the number of infant deaths totalled 2,741. Of the children between the ages of one and four, 598 died; between the ages of five and nine, 314 died; and between the ages of ten and fourteen, 242 died. Substantial changes have not taken place in this field in recent years (Table 3). The main causes are injuries and poisoning, inborn abnormalities, and diseases of the nervous system and the sense organs, followed by tumors and diseases of the respiratory system. The share of contagious diseases in the mortality rate dropped to 0.5 percent of all death. This result was achieved as a result of the consistent implementation of the immunization program introduced by the government.

Diphtheria, poliomyelitis, and tetanus were conquered in children years ago. Whooping cough has become a rare disease (Figure 1). Also, hepatitis and

Table 3
Children Deceased per 10,000 of Same Age and Sex

Year	1-4 Years Male	1-4 Years Female	5-9 Years Male	5-9 Years Female	10-14 Years Male	10-14 Years Female
1950	37.0	31.0	15.0	10.0	11.0	7.0
1960	18.6	14.8	6.1	4.4	4.6	3.3
1970	9.7	7.5	5.0	3.2	4.5	2.6
1980	7.6	5.7	4.1	2.6	3.7	2.2
1982	7.0	5.7	4.4	2.3	3.2	1.9
Cases						
1982	331	258	208	106	191	106

measles have been successfully fought (Figure 2). With other contagious diseases, progress is still lacking. The number of incidences of typhoid and paratyphoid fever, and dysentery has also clearly decreased (Figure 3). This last reflects the constant improvement of general living conditions (housing conditions, nutrition, drinking water supply, and sewage disposal). In 1950, 927,660 people contracted this disease in the GDR; in 1983, only 3,390, mostly adults, contracted the disease.

Major Causes of Disease and Death

As in other advanced industrialized nations, general mortality has decreased in the GDR over the past 30 years. In the aftermath of World War II, it was not until the mid-1950s that death characteristics from the 1930s were reached again. The structural change in mortality especially related to a decrease in contagious diseases. The number of accidents also dropped. Chronic diseases (e.g., cardiovascular diseases, respiratory diseases, and malignant neoplasms) have increased as causes of disease and death.

The number of deaths per 10,000 people was 130.03 males and 142.32 females in 1982. The sequence of the ten diseases causing death is listed in Table 4. Diseases of the cardiovascular system, malignant tumors, and diseases of the respiratory system are also prominent causes of death.

Figure 1
Incidence of Diphtheria, Poliomyelitis, Pertussis, and Tetanus, per 100,000 Population, to 1984

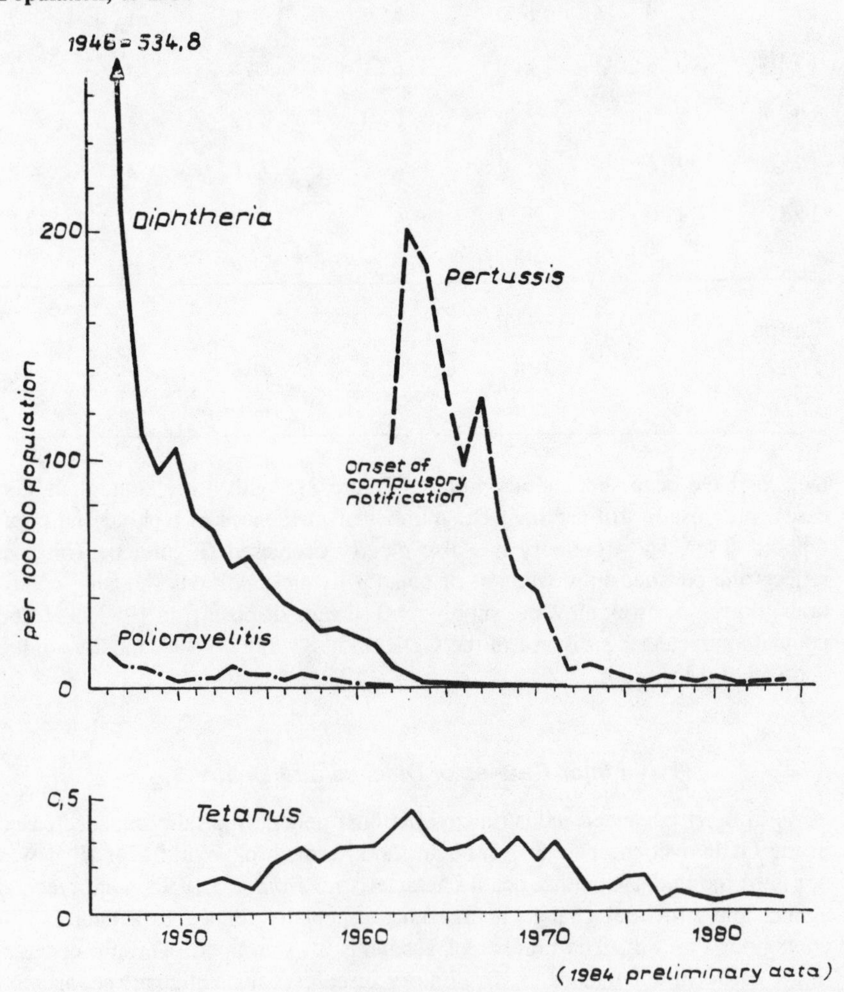

Figure 2
Incidence of Infectious Hepatitis, Measles, Mumps, and Scarlet Fever, per 100,000 Population, to 1984

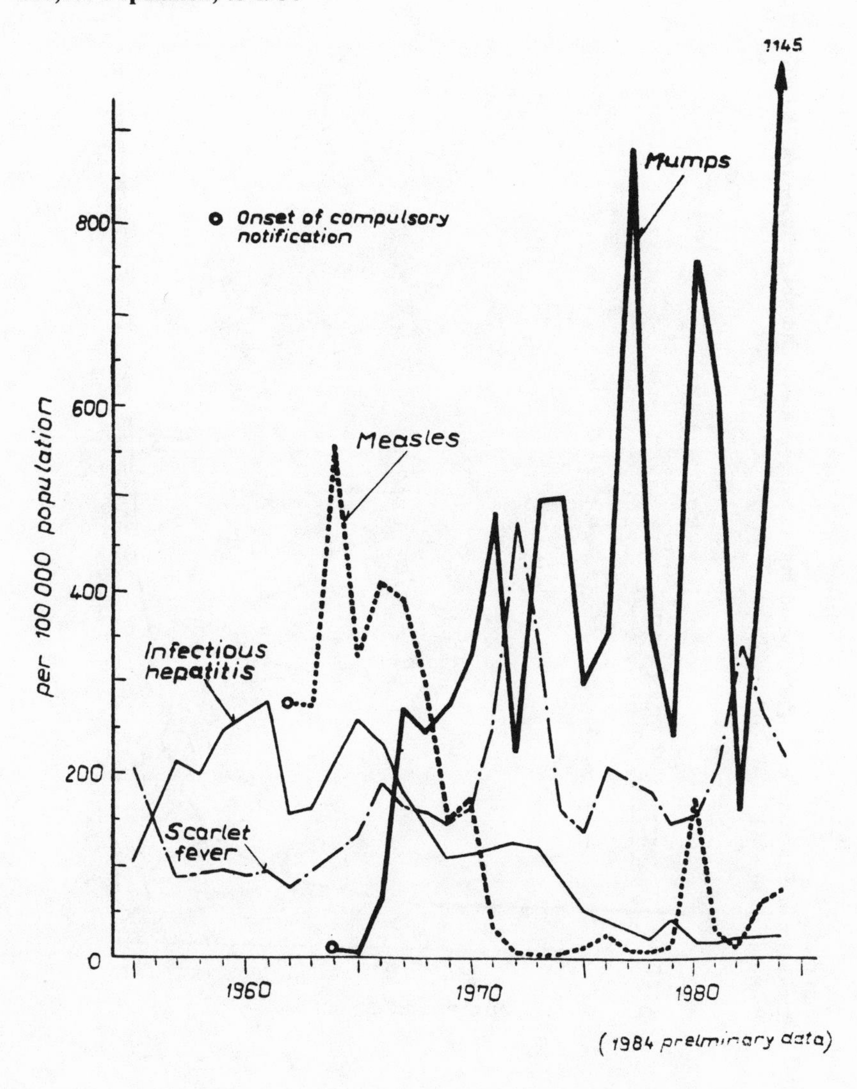

Figure 3
Incidence of Typhoid Fever, Paratyphoid Fever, Salmonellosis, and Shiggellosis, per 100,000 Population, to 1984

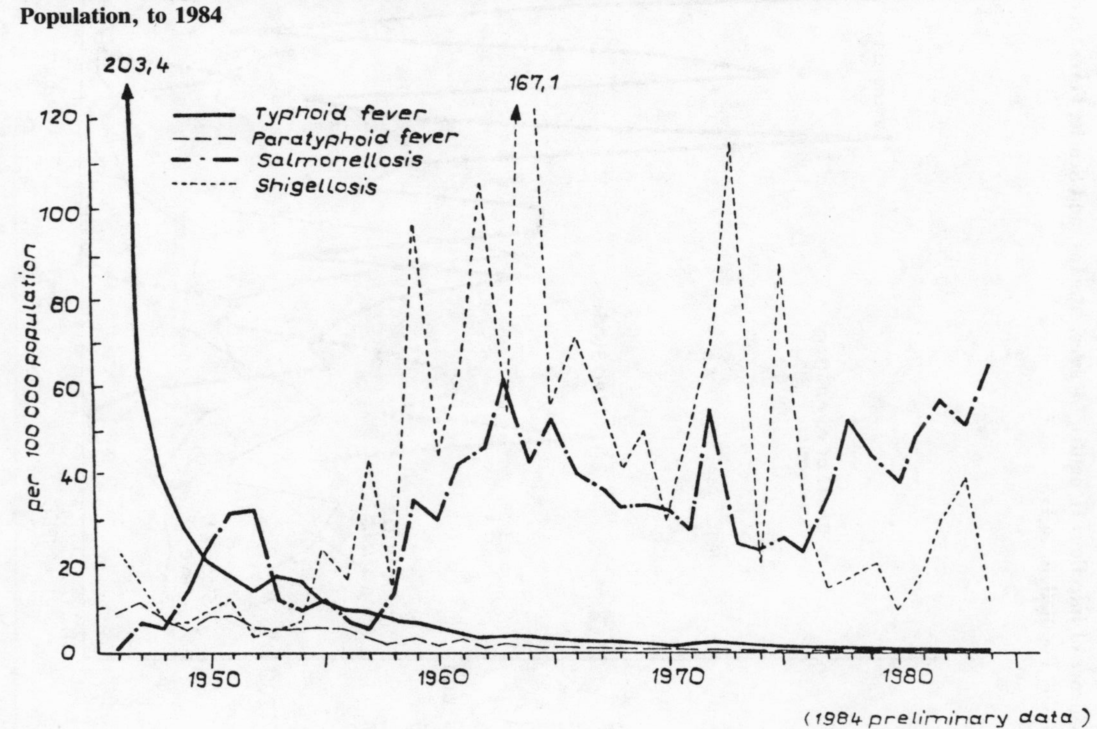

Table 4
People Deceased per 10,000 According to Top Ten Causes by Sex, 1982

No.	Male persons Diagnosis (ICD-No.)	Female persons Diagnosis (ICD-No.)
1	Arteriosclerosis (440) 21.41	Arteriosclerosis (440) 31.30
2	Ischemic heart disease (410-414) 12.88	Cerebrovascular disease (430-438) 14.61
3	Cerebrovascular disease (430-438) 9.26	Ischemic heart disease (410-414) 13.42
4	Hypertension (401-405) 7.51	Hypertension (401-405) 13.28
5	Bronchitis, emphysema and asthma (490-493) 6.90	Diabetis mellitus (250) 4.09
6	Acute myocardial infarction (410) 6.62	Acute myocardial infarction (410) 3.47
7	Malignant neoplasms of the tracheas, bronchi and lungs (162) 6.61	Malignant neoplasms of the female mammary gland (174) 2.92
8	Malignant neoplasms of the stomach (151) 3.03	Pneumonia (480-486) 2.63
9	Pneumonia (480-486) 2.42	Malignant neoplasms of the stomach (151) 2.36
10	Chronic liver disease and cirrhosis (571) 2.13	Bronchitis, emphysema and asthma (490-493) 2.35

Organization of the Health-Care System

Administrative Structure

The health system and part of the social services in the GDR are supervised by the Ministry of Health, the structure of which is shown in Figure 4.

Each of the 15 County Councils and 227 District Councils has a department of health and social care, which is headed by health officers who are elected by the respective county and district assemblies, the supreme local authorities, and who bear the responsibility for the supervision of health and social care in their territories. The people working in these departments of health and social care

Figure 4
German Democratic Republic, Ministry of Health

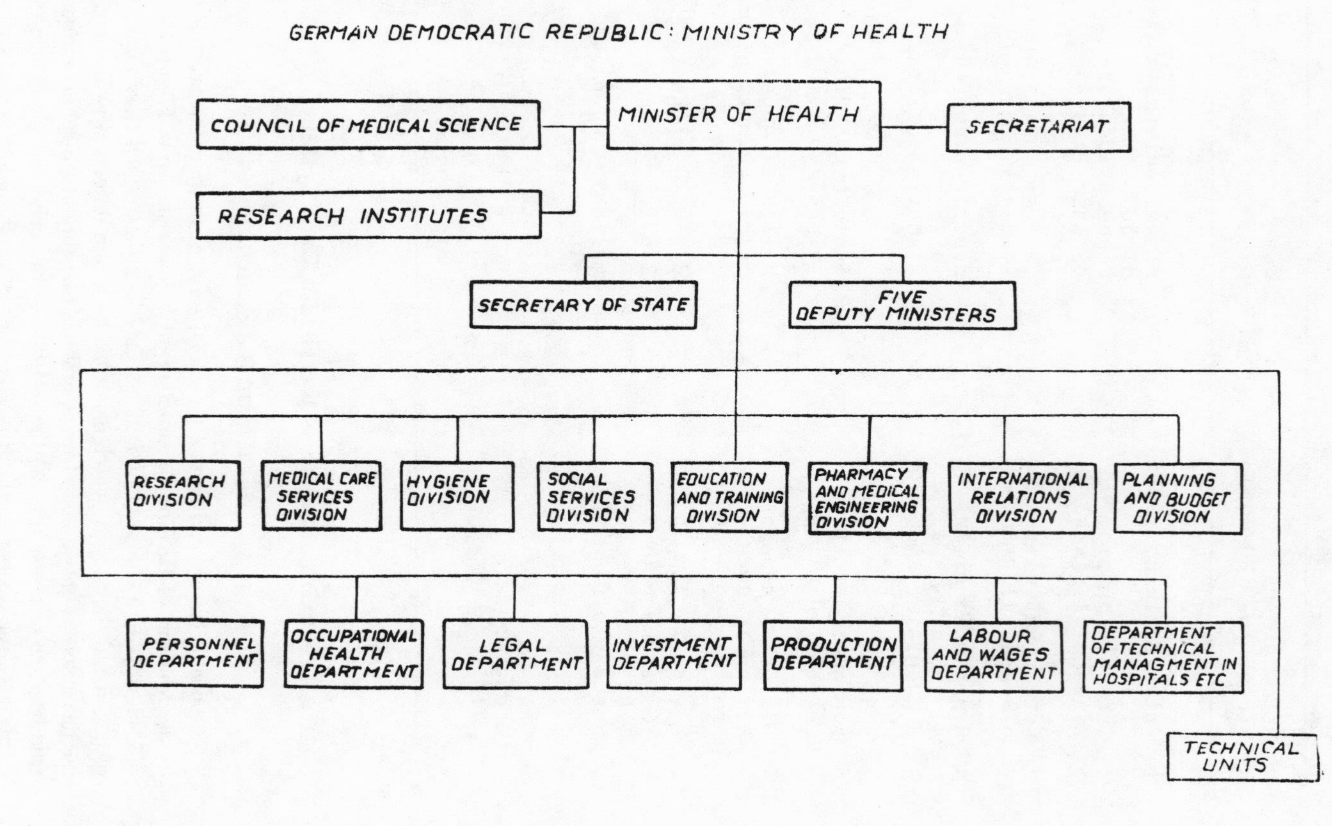

are full-time employees. They are assisted in their work by advisors from the medical and social facilities.

There are divisions of the public health inspectorate and the industrial hygiene inspectorate within the frame work of the Ministry of Health and at the county and district levels. They give guidance and supervise work in the fields of prevention of infections, environmental protection, food, nutrition, and industrial hygiene.

Hospitals

In 1982, the GDR had 545 hospitals of all types, with a total of 171,280 beds. Thus, 102.6 beds are available per 10,000 population. A total of 12,278 doctors work in these hospitals—one doctor to fourteen beds, on the average. The state runs 463 of the hospitals mentioned, with 159,321 beds; the Protestant and Roman Catholic churches operate 78 hospitals, with 11,615 beds; and private establishments operate four hospitals for inpatients with 344 beds. Hospitals are subordinated to local, district, county, and central levels of control. Among the latter are the nine medical schools. The average stay in all hospitals under central supervision in 1983 came to 16.1 days and that in local hospitals to 19.2 days (Staatliche Zentralverwaltung 1984).

Due to historical conditions, hospitals were scattered somewhat randomly over what is now the GDR. After 1945 they were specialized according to a central plan and merged to reduce their number. Reductions also have occurred in the number of hospital beds, a trend which reflects increasing specialization, improvement of conditions for bedside care, and changing needs. As a result of reduced incidence of tuberculosis, approximately 30,000 beds were either closed or shifted to other functions.

Outpatient Facilities

After 1945 a network of state-run health centers and other health facilities was set up to provide outpatient treatment. Currently there are 580 outpatient clinics, almost 1,000 ambulatory clinics, and more than 2,500 state-run medical and dental practices (Institute für Sozialhygiene 1983).

Over 50 percent of the physicians work in outpatient facilities. They hold more than 150 million consultations and conduct 7 million home visits annually. These physicians in outpatient service ensure that every citizen can be treated by a family doctor. This outpatient service also includes district nurses and about 1,500 doctors and dentists, who hold private consultations.

Outpatient Emergency System

In order to provide better treatment to people with acute illnesses, an outpatient emergency system has been developed. This includes hospitalization by emergency ambulance and urgent home visits.

In cases of serious acute illness, especially if there is danger to life or a need for hospitalization, emergency call ambulances with special equipment are sent. These ambulances are capable of carrying out fluid infusions and minor operations on the spot. Urgent home visits also are provided for acute illnesses occurring outside normal consultation hours of local health centers. In some areas, this has been introduced as a separate service for children. The outpatient emergency service made 475,000 runs in 1982 (Institute für Sozialhygiene 1983).

Health Care for Pregnant Women, Infants, Children, and Young Persons

Mothers, children, and young people enjoy special protection in the GDR. All pregnant women undergo medical checkups periodically prior to delivery in one of almost 900 special prenatal clinics. Ninety percent of these women go to the prenatal clinics during the first sixteen weeks of pregnancy; 99 percent of all children are born in hospital obstetric departments.

Mother and child are looked after in one of 9,900 postnatal clinics. Mothers receive guidance on correct nutrition and proper care for their babies. Regular examinations are carried out, and physical handicaps or metabolic disorders are monitored and treated. During this time, infants also get scheduled vaccinations, and vitamin D is administered orally. During their first year of life, children, on the average, are examined seven times by physicians.

Rehabilitation centers look after disabled children and youths. Once they join the workforce, young people enjoy special protection as to working hours, physical strain, and exposure to physical and chemical noxious substances.

Industrial Health

The constitution of the GDR ensures every citizen the right to work in conditions free from health hazards. Managers and their governmental supervisors bear the responsibility for enforcing this right.

Starting in 1947, a network of industrial health facilities was established in the GDR, by the then Soviet military administration. These health facilities are budgeted separately from the enterprises they service. In 1982 there were 130 health centers, 319 outpatient clinics, and about 3,400 first-aid posts with a medical staff of 22,000 of whom 4,400 were doctors (Institute für Sozialhygiene 1983).

In these industrial health facilities, about 70 percent of all employees receive medical care, particularly in case of acute illneses. These facilities also are responsible for industrial hygiene, medical examination prior to employment, and monitoring various groups of people such as young people, pregnant mothers, and those exposed to physical and chemical noxious substances. They also monitor hygiene at work jointly with representatives of the trade unions. Additionally, a medical staff of some 2,200, located in fifteen county health inspectorates for enterprises affiliated to county councils and over 200 industrial hygiene inspectorates affiliated to district councils, exercises various advisory and monitoring functions.

The implementation of strict regulations in industrial safety and in road traffic has reduced the number of casualties resulting from industrial and road accidents. From 1970 to 1982, the incidence of all accidents, including accidents at home, fell from 10,018 (5.9 in 10,000 population) to 6,425 (3.8 in 10,000 population) despite considerable growth in the number of cars. The rate of occupational accidents per 1,000 employees went down from 41 in 1970 to 16 in 1983 (Staatliche Zentralverwaltung 1984).

Newly registered persons with occupationally generated diseases also decreased between 1977 and 1983 by 30 percent, from 12,063 to 8,510. This downward trend is particularly apparent for diseases caused by exposure to chemicals. The one exception to this trend is diseases cause by germs and parasites contracted in tropical regions.

Care for the Elderly

Apart from children and the disabled, special attention is attached to social care for the elderly. The main stress is on their integration into the community. To this end, good medical care and cultural options are provided. Senior citizens stay in contact with their former enterprises, health facilities, and social organizations like the Nationale Front (a pool in which all political organizations work together) and the *Volkssolidaritat* (an organization which arranges cultural and social care for the elderly).

Several hundred blocks of flats have been designed to meet the requirements of senior citizens. These new quarters have improved the living conditions for more than 21,000 elderly people. There are 1,350 state-run old people's and nursing homes which provide facilities for 128,200 old people, 79,720 (62 percent) of which can live in nursing homes (Institute für Sozialhygiene 1983).

Prescription Drugs

In 1982 there were 1,975 pharmacies in the GDR with a staff of 18,840. The state-run wholesale trade in medicines and medical equipment runs ten depots with 62 dispatch stores. All drugs prescribed by a physician are available free of charge to the patient.

Health Personnel

In 1983, in a total national workforce of 10.7 million, 385,000 were employed in the health service and 138,300 in social care facilities affiliated with the Ministry of Health. This includes child care and old-age and nursing homes.

Table 5
Number of Physicians and Dentists

	PHYSICIANS			DENTISTS		
	total number	per 10,000 popul.	citizens per doctor	total number	per 10,000 popul.	citizens per dentist
1949	13,222	7.0	1,429	7,100	3.8	2,661
1955	13,755	7.7	1,296	7,259	4.1	2,457
1960	14,555	8.5	1,181	6,361	3.7	2,702
1965	19,528	11.5	872	6,207	3.6	2,743
1970	27,255	16.0	626	7,349	4.3	2,391
1975	31,810	18.9	530	7,968	4.7	2,115
1980	33,894	20.3	494	9.709	5,8	1,724
1985	37,943	22.8	439	11,757	7.1	1,416

The total number of 524,100 employees in health and social care make up 5 percent of the GDR workforce. Of these employees, 85 percent are women.

Great efforts have been spent over the last 40 years to increase the number of physicians and dentists (see Table 5). To this end, three independent medical academies (Dresden, Erfurt, and Magdeburg) were founded in 1954. At these academies and at six universities (Berlin, Greifswald, Halle, Jena, Leipzig, and Rostock), 2,000 physicians and dentists are trained annually.

In 1983 the GDR had 36,181 physicians—a ratio of one physician to each 462 citizens—and 10,903 dentists—one dentist to each 1,532 people.

Financing

The GDR, as a socialist society, guarantees the social security of its citizenry in case of illness, disability, or maternity. This guarantee is implemented through a substantial subsidy (approximately 50 percent of the total cost) provided by the state to the state-administered sick fund system.

Since 1956 a homogeneous insurance system comprised of two branches of insurance has existed. The budgets of these two insurances are merged into that of the state. The two insurances are essentially identical with regard to services;

the difference lies in the eligibility group: shop-floor workers and other employees in one group, and farmers, craftsmen, and others in the other. The sick funds' direct revenues come from a system of employee and employer payments. Employees pay 10 percent of their gross monthly wage; employers pay a second 10 percent of their employees' wages. The combined total of both fees, however, is capped at a maximum of 60 marks per employee (or 10 percent of an employee's first 600 marks of income)—a ceiling which has prevailed for some decades. To allow comparison, the average monthly income of an industrial employee was 1,100 marks in 1983. The remainder of the sick fund's revenues are provided through the subsidy payment from the state budget.

For instance, in 1983, the largest insurance scheme—that for industrial and office workers—received fee revenues of 14.5 billion marks. In contrast to this, its expenditures amounted to 26 billion marks, with roughly 12 billion marks spent for medical care and sickness benefits alone. The difference (11.5 billion marks) was paid from the state budget (Staatliche Zentralverwaltung 1983).

Taken overall, the GDR spent 5.5 percent of its gross domestic product for health and social care (retirement pensions excluded), although additional resources are provided by industrial enterprises for in-house health and social care.

Medical Scientific Societies

Medical scientific societies were founded in the GDR to promote scientific progress, translate new findings into practice faster, extend national and international exchange of experience, improve professional upgrading, and develop cooperation and contacts between colleges.

These societies are arranged under six umbrella societies:

- GDR Society for Experimental Medicine
- GDR Society for Clinical Medicine
- GDR Society for Hygiene
- GDR Society for Stomatology
- Pharmaceutical Society of the GDR
- GDR Society for Military Medicine.

Affiliated to these umbrella societies are 66 branch societies such as the Biochemical Society, the Society of Surgery, the Society for General and Community Hygiene, the Society for Children's Dentistry, and over 350 sections, chapters, and groups, and more than 120 regional organizations. At the end of 1982, the medical scientific societies of the GDR had a membership of almost 60,000.

In addition to these scientific societies, there is one union for all health workers (*Gewerkschaft Gesundheitswesen*). Wages are negotiated between this union and the government.

Development Trends

Further improvement of medical and social care continued to be a priority in GDR social policies over the 1986–1990 5-year-plan period. The main emphasis will be laid on extension of preventive health care; improvement of primary health care, particularly in big cities and industrialized conurban areas; extension of health facilities in industry; establishment of new dental treatment centers; improvement of special treatment such as traumatology, orthopedics, urology, pediatrics, and vascular surgery. Other items of primary importance are care for mother and child, for the elderly, and for the disabled. According to plan, the ratio of physicians to the population is to be raised to 1 physician for fewer than 400 people and the ratio of dentists to 1 dentist for fewer than 1,200 people.

References

Institute für Sozialhygiene und Organisation des Gesundheitsschutzes "Maxim Zetkin" Berlin. 1983 and 1985. *Das Gesundheitswesen der Deutschen Demokratischen Republik 1983 und 1985*. Vols. 18 and 20. Berlin: Ministry of Health.

Staatliche Zentralverwaltung für Statistik. 1984 and 1986. *Statistisches Jahrbuch 1984 und 1986 der Deutschen Demokratischen Republic*. Vols. 29 and 31. Berlin: Staatsverlag der DDR.

Winter, K. 1980. *Das Gesundheitswesen in der Deutschen Demokratischen Republik. Bilanz nach 30 Jahren*. 2. Revised ed. Berlin: Verlag Volk und Gesund.

GREAT BRITAIN

Stephen Harrison

The Demographic and Epidemiological Context

The total population of Great Britain has grown continuously since the early nineteenth century, but the rate of growth has declined markedly during the present century. The population doubled between 1801 and 1850 and again between 1851 and 1901, but grew by only 32 percent between 1901 and 1951; from 1951 to 2000, it is projected that an increase of a further 16 percent will have taken place. The 1982 population was just over 54 million, with an estimated 4.5 percent increase by 2000 (CSO 1983). This is largely the result of two factors. First, a marked improvement in total expectation of life has occurred during the present century. Life expectancy at birth has improved from under 50 years to over 70 years (76 for females) during this period. The improvement in life expectancy for adults has, however, been much more modest and in 1980 remained at its 1950 figures of 77 for men aged 65 years; for women of the same age it improved only slightly, from 80 to over 81 years. When expectation of life at specific ages is examined in detail it can be seen that most of the improvement is a result of the increased likelihood of survival by infants. This is confirmed by examination of infant (i.e., under one year) and perinatal (i.e., under one month) mortality rates, both of which have fallen considerably, not only since 1900 but in recent years also. The infant mortality rate for 1981 was just over 12 per 1,000 live births, and the perinatal mortality rate just over 13 per 1,000 total births, both having fallen from over 30 per 1,000 in 1949 (DHSS 1982).

The second underlying trend has been the fall in the crude birth rate. This fell steadily from 1900 until the postwar "baby boom" from 1947–1948 and a secondary boom from 1955–1964; the rate then fell again rapidly to a 1977 low of 62 percent of the 1964 peak. Since then the rate has fluctuated, and, in 1981, it stood at 12.9 per 1,000 population (CSO 1983). It is difficult to forecast whether the rate will rise in the immediate future. As can be seen, the fall in birth rate has been more than offset by the improvement in life expectancy.

In addition to fostering this net increase in population, these trends have resulted in an aging population in both absolute and relative terms. Thus, while only 4 percent of the 1901 and 11 percent of the 1951 population were 65 or more years of age, the proportion had risen to 14 percent by 1981, where it will remain until beyond the end of this century. The absolute numbers of those over age 64, but especially of those over 74 (and even over 84), have also increased rapidly (CSO 1983). The over-74 age group, which will peak at about 3.5 million in 1991, is especially important in terms of health-care finance, since it necessitates about five times the per capita expenditure of the mean for the total population, a differential which has been widening recently (DHSS 1983). The over-64 age group accounts for some 40 percent of all expenditures on health and personal social services, and it is reckoned that the effect of demographic changes alone has been to increase demand for health care by over 0.5 percent each year (DHSS 1981). The size of the tax base for supporting increases in demand for health care is also important; the proportion of the total population that is of working age has remained constant throughout the present century, but recent high levels of unemployment (doubling in five years to reach 11.3 percent in 1981) reduce the tax base while necessitating high levels of public expenditure on social policies generally.

Turning to epidemiological factors, it can be send that, with falling death rates and rising life expectancy, has come a shift in the pattern of causes of death. Much of the improvement in the former has been brought about by a reduction of mortality from infectious disease, leaving the so-called diseases of affluence as the major causes of death. In 1981 the major causes of death were ischemic heart disease (27 percent of all deaths), followed by malignant neoplasms (22.5 percent) and cerebrovascular disease (12 percent). Accidents (2.5 percent of the total) are the major cause of death between the ages of 1 and 40 years.

Patterns of morbidity are much more difficult to specify due to problems of definition and data collection. The pattern of hospital discharge diagnoses mirrors the pattern of mortality described above; cancer, heart and hypertensive disease, circulatory disease, respiratory disease, and digestive diseases are (excluding pregnancy) the major groups at rates of between about 45 and 85 discharges per 10,000 population. Not surprisingly, the pattern of consultation of general practitioners (i.e., primary care physicians) is rather different, with much greater prominence of disease of the nervous system, skin and musculoskeletal system, and (for women) both the genitourinary system and mental illness. Respiratory disease seems, however, to be the most common reason to consult general practitioners; over one-quarter of both the male and female populations consult for this reason each year. Finally, diseases of the respiratory and circulatory systems are by far the largest cause of sickness certified for the purpose of receipt of state welfare benefits, though these figures count only incapacity of at least three days' duration (OHE 1977). None of the above data covers undiagnosed disease, and it needs to be noted that the incidence of self-defined illness (OPCS 1982) and of certified incapacity to work has increased over the last decade, perhaps an indication of rising expectations (OHE 1977).

Finally, the above epidemiological profile needs to be qualified by reference to three kinds of inequality in distribution. First, there are inequalities of gender; women make greater use of health-care facilities (which may or may not reflect a difference in morbidity), but they have greater life expectancy than do men. Second, there are substantial geographical variations in mortality and morbidity, which, within England at least, tend to correlate inversely with the extent of health service resources and the frequency of their utilization. Thus, male standardized mortality ratios for 1977 varied between 113 for northwest England and 89 for eastern England. Mortality in Wales and Scotland is higher than in England even though health service resources are greater there. Third, there are major differences in the health experiences of different social classes, which may be exemplified by differences in mortality. Although the absolute mortality experience of all social classes has improved throughout the present century, the gap between the higher and lower classes has widened. Thus, in England and Wales, the standardized mortality ratio for males in professional occupations fell from 82 in the 1920s to 77 in the 1970s, whereas the equivalent figure for unskilled occupations rose from 125 to 137 in the same period (Royal Commission 1979).

Government and Politics in Great Britain

Although Great Britain is a unitary state (comprising England, Wales, and Scotland), it has a long tradition of national, regional, and local differences in administration. Separate central government departments exist for Wales and Scotland; these have responsibility for some policy areas (including health) which, in England, are the responsibility of functionally organized departments, such as the Department of Health and Social Security (DHSS). In addition to the organs of central government, elected local authorities exist throughout the country; arrangements differ somewhat between England, Wales, and Scotland, and within England, between metropolitan and other areas. These are all multipurpose authorities, funded partly by local property taxes and partly by central government grants, whose functions include education (except universities), road transportation, environmental health, and personal social services. In addition, there exist a number of single-purpose public authorities whose members are not elected: as discussed in more detail later, health authorities fall into this category (Hanson and Walles 1981).

In terms of both national and local politics, Britain has usually been characterized as a two-party sytem in the sense that, although a number of parties exist, effective competition for government at any one time has been confined to two major parties, though this may currently be undergoing change. In terms of political culture, Britain has been relatively homogeneous. Although there is considerable religious and ethnic diversity (partly due to immigration patterns in both the distant and recent past), these diversions have so far been incorporated into existing political cleavages, although the last decade has seen some activity by nationalist parties in Wales and Scotland. As a number of political scientists have observed (Peters et al. 1977), the conjunction of government by competitive elites and a homogeneous political culture tends to produce a particular style of public policy, one of which is termed "self-regulating." In other words, interest groups are often organized at the national level and are recognized by governments as involved in the policy-making process: In some cases, this process has gone so far as to leave particular interest groups to be self-regulating.

In the British health sector, this policy style is particularly highly developed. Its most formal manifestation is the arrangement whereby professional licensure is largely centrally controlled by the professions themselves. Physicians have been required to be licensed to practice since the Medical Act of 1858; this created what is now called the General Medical Council (GMC) whose tasks are to recognize qualifications for registration, to maintain a register of medical practitioners, and to administer a disciplinary code. The GMC's membership is heavily dominated by physicians, over half of whom are elected by the profession, with others nominated by the medical schools and medical corporations (Watkin 1975). These medical corporations (Royal Colleges, etc.) also have a substantial influence on postgraduate posts and trainees. Moreover, the doctors, often but not exclusively through the British Medical Association (BMA), are involved in a wide range of joint committees with government, and indeed there is a DHSS career structure for doctors which parallels the normal administrative one (Harrison 1981).

The same policy approach is evident with regard to other health-care professions. Midwives were first required to be state certified in 1905, and nurses registered since 1919. Recent legislative changes have reorganized the various registration bodies into a United Kingdom Central Council for Nursing, Midwifery, and Health Visiting, together with boards for each of the four constituent nations. Membership of these bodies consists largely of nurses.

Historically, a number of occupations have grown as offshoots from medicine and nursing. The duties of these professions "supplementary to medicine" involve specific diagnostic or treatment procedures, and the medical profession has therefore been as concerned to control them as has the state. Prior to the inception of the NHS, a nonstatutory form of registration existed via the BMA. It was not until 1960 that legislation required state registration for the occupations of physiotherapy, occupational therapy, remedial gymnastics, chiropody, radiography, orthoptics, dietetics, and medical laboratory technology. A two-tier system of control consists of a board for each of the eight professions, responsible for registering practitioners and recognizing qualifications and schools, and a Council for Professions Supplementary to Medicine which supervises the boards. Each board has a constitutional majority of members elected by the particular profession. The extent to which these professions are self-regulating is shown by the fact that each of the first six boards listed above recognizes for state registration only the qualification issued by the relevant professional association, which functions also as a trade union involved in pay bargaining. There is thus substantial control over the intake of students, the content of training, and the numbers trained (Harrison 1981). The medical profession is heavily represented on the council.

The above description of licensure arrangements demonstrates the extent to which health-care-producer interest groups are embedded in the standing arrangements of government. As commentators such as Richardson and Jordan (1979) have noted, however, British governments have been generally willing to acknowledge the involvement of interest groups in ad hoc issues; in the field of health care, as the following account shows, this approach has been evident.

The Creation of the NHS

A considerable variety of types of health-care institution existed prior to 1948, when, as is detailed below, the NHS was formally created (see Watkin 1975 and 1977, Klein 1983). The most prestigious institutions were the voluntary hospitals, so called because of their extensive support from charitable sources. The oldest had their origins in medieval monastic foundations, but many were the results of private charity in the eighteenth century and others of public subscription as memorials to World War I. These institutions provided hospital care for which a charge was made if the patient had the means to pay; they often in addition offered contributory schemes by which working people could be indemnified against subsequent charges. By the 1930s, many voluntary hospitals were in financial difficulties. Voluntary hospitals were administered by boards of (unpaid and mainly lay) governors who employed an administrator and a nursing and domestic staff. Consultant medical staff (specialists) gave their services on an honorary basis, though the association with such an institution, especially one connected with a university medical school, offered status and reputation which could enhance earnings from private practice.

Other hospitals were provided by local government authorities, funded partly from local taxation, though along with many other local government activities, increasingly assisted by central government grants. Many of these hospitals provided care for the elderly and chronically sick, having developed from recommendations made in 1834 and 1909 that these categories should not be housed in the same institutions as the able-bodied poor. In addition, local authorities had been required by legislation in 1867 and 1868 to provide separate facilities for tuberculosis, smallpox, mental illness, and fevers. After 1929, local authorities were permitted to provide general hospital facilities, though the permissive nature of this legislation led to substantial variation. Local authority hospitals were often managed by a medical superintendent. Public health had been the responsibility of local government since the legislation of 1848; by the

1930s, this function was normally headed by a medical officer of health, who also managed other local authority health services, such as home nursing and midwifery which had originally been provided by voluntary agencies. A school medical service had existed since 1907.

Finally, primary medical care was provided by general medical practitioners (GPs). Prior to 1911 their services were purchased for cash, although it was possible to insure against the cost through "friendly societies," and some local communities formed associations either to pool the risk of paying fees or even to employ a physician. In 1911, a scheme of national insurance was introduced providing, in addition to other welfare benefits, free access to GP services and drugs which they might prescribe: This covered about half the population. GPs were not salaried employees, but they continued to be independent contractors and were remunerated through local insurance committees on the basis of an annual capitation fee.

The considerable development of health-care institutions and services, which took place from the mid-nineteenth century to the mid-twentieth, and the increasing involvement of the state (a Ministry of Health had been established in 1919) did not always reflect altruistic reasons. The creation of local government hospitals originated in a nineteenth-century attempt to reduce public expenditure by discriminating between the deserving poor (i.e., the sick) and the undeserving poor; the school health service was introduced in response to a high level of medical rejections of volunteers for the British Army in the Boer War; and the 1911 National Insurance Act was modelled on a German scheme designed as a balance against political upheaval.

After World War I, however, there began a long period of pressure for a more rational and comprehensive health service. In the interwar period, more than half a dozen reports were produced by a range of bodies with different ideological perspectives. The BMA, the Socialist Medical Association, the Labour Party, the official Dawson Committee, and an independent foundation all agreed that a comprehensive service was required, though there was considerable disagreement over whether such an arrangement would be financed through insurance or taxation, and whether doctors should be treated as salaried employees.

The outbreak of World War II did nothing to interrupt the process of planning for a comprehensive service. Indeed, the temporary wartime funding and management of hospitals in the form of the Emergency Medical Service served as a demonstration that more integrated arrangements were practicable. Wartime discussion mirrored the prewar pattern with widespread agreement that a comprehensive service was required, yet considerable disagreement about who should run it, how it should be funded, and how doctors should be paid. In response to the much publicized Beveridge Report of 1942, successive (Conservative) ministers of health in the wartime Coalition Government prepared plans which were widely criticized by the medical profession. The first postwar general election produced a Labour Government with a large majority, committed to a welfare state, including a comprehensive national health service. The National Health Service Act was enacted in 1946, effective from 1948.

The formal objective of the resulting NHS was (and remains) "to secure improvement in the . . . health of the people." Its organization made separate arrangements for hospitals, community services, and primary medical and dental care, thus becoming known as the "tripartite structure." Most hospitals were taken into public ownership and arranged into administrative regions. Each English region contained at least one medical undergraduate teaching hospital or group of hospitals, whose board of governors was responsible to the Minister of Health. Other groups of hospitals in a region were managed by hospital management committees (boards of management in Scotland), which were responsible for regional hospital boards which were, in turn, responsible to the minister. The various boards and management committees were nonelected lay bodies upon which a number of doctors could and did serve, though formally in an expert rather than representative capacity. Hospital staff, including doctors, were salaried employees, and the day-to-day management of groups of hospitals was usually vested in an administrator, the Secretary. Individual hospitals were usually managed by an administrator and a matron, who was in charge of nursing and hospital support services. In some former, local authority, single-specialty hospitals, a medical superintendent was retained. Hospital consultants (specialists) were salaried, but, except in teaching hospitals, they became regional hospital board employees, effectively insulated from hospital management committees.

Local authorities remained responsible, through a health committee chosen from among their elected membership, for community services such as home nursing and midwifery, health visiting, ambulance services, and public health. The Medical Office of Health was normally the chief officer with functional specialists in charge of the various services reporting to him. In the area of primary medical and dental care, the strong desire of practitioners to remain independent led to their being self-employed but in contact with the NHS via bodies called executive councils. These councils replaced the old insurance committees and administered claims for remuneration for GPs and dentists: doctors continued the 1911 arrangements for capitation fees, and dentists later were paid a fee per item of service. Similar arrangements were adopted for opticians and pharmacists outside hospitals.

All services were available to the entire population, though hospital treatment, except in emergencies, could be obtained only by referral from a GP. Services were free at the time of use and financed from general taxation. Patients could, if they wished, elect to be treated privately, and for this a proportion of private beds in NHS hospitals was designated. Consultant medical staff could elect to work for the NHS on a part-time basis and to use their remaining time in private practice. Private patients were required to pay the ostensibly full cost of their hospital stay as well as the physician's fee. GPs were also allowed to practice privately, though few did so to any substantial degree.

Early experience with the NHS was that it seemed to be expensive. Initial estimates of the cost had been based on extrapolation of prewar expenditures, and supplementary finance had to be provided in the first several years of its existence. In time, the Guillebaud Report of 1956 was to show that, apart from being the manifestation of a large backlog of demand for spectacles and dentures, the apparent excess cost was largely due to inflation. However, by this time, not only had both Labour and (after 1951) Conservative governments introduced small but significant patient charges (initially for dentures and spectacles, but later for dental treatment and for prescriptions), but also the fallacy underlying the Beveridge Report's arguments for an NHS as an economic investment had become clear. It is now a commonplace that the total morbidity and mortality that can be reduced by medical intervention is not fixed, but rather that the demand for health care is potentially infinite. In Klein's (1983) phrase, though, the 1950s were mainly a period of consolidation with relatively little change.

By the 1960s, a number of important changes were beginning to occur. These are perhaps best summarized as four overlapping trends for the period from 1962 to 1982: professionalism, managerialism, trade unionism, and consumerism.

The NHS from 1962 to 1982

Professionalism

The NHS is, of course, dominated by professionals in the everyday sense of that term: almost 50 percent of its employees would thus describe themselves. There has been considerable academic dispute (Johnson 1972) over how useful it is to view professionals as they view themselves (as altruistic experts who invoke the assistance of the state in order to protect the public from charlatans), rather than as monopolists of knowledge and practice who use their monopoly to achieve social and economic dominance over nonprofessionals. These divergent views, however, both reflect three key notions: autonomy, individualism, and specialist knowledge.

The notion of autonomy is archetypal in the clinical freedom of the NHS consultant or GP to treat his or her patients by whatever means he or she chooses within the available resources. This freedom has been recognized by governments since the earliest state involvement as a third party in the doctor-patient relationship, and it is reflected in legal and ethical views of the physician's prime responsibility to his or her own patients, irrespective of other considerations. The operational implication of this freedom is the open-ended budget of the GP, quasiownership of hospital beds by consultants, and ultimately the fact that the total pattern of health care is little more than the aggregate of individual clinical decisions about admission, discharge, prescription, diagnosis, and treatment. Haywood and Alaszewski (1980) have shown that, despite government policies of redistributing resources away from the acute medicine, additional resources had not only been allocated to this sector, but had been used to diagnose and treat an existing number of patients even more intensively than before. The steady expansion of health-care resources throughout the 1960s and early 1970s presented no challenge to this autonomy which was buttressed by the professional self-regulation already described and by the independent status of GPs and consultants.

The notion of individualism from the point of view of the professional is subsumed in the above discussion, but a further aspect of individualism is the attitude of the health professional toward the notion of ill health. This attitude is essentially a view of illness as pathology of the individual, susceptible to alleviation or cure by medical treatment of the individual. Although there now exists a substantial radical literature which argues that such a model is misleading because it places insufficient emphasis upon societal and environmental factors as determinants of ill health (McKeown 1976), the individualistic model remains the basis of most professional treatment. The emphasis of the 1960s and 1970s was, in practical if not always in rhetorical terms, upon curative medicine.

Finally, the degree of occupational specialization of health services workers has increased considerably. In medicine, the number of officially recognized specialties has more than doubled since 1949 (DHSS 1982), and the activities of the Royal Colleges as described earlier have intensified in accordance with this. At an informal level, there is increased subspecialization within specialties and increasing reluctance for doctors to provide out-of-hours cover outside their own specialty. Increased specialization has also occurred in other categories of staff. In nursing, the existing degree of specialization into patient care groups was completed by a steady shedding by qualified nurses of "nonnursing duties." An early shedding of responsibility for instrument and dressing sterilization in the 1950s was followed by the elimination of domestic work in the 1960s and ward-level clerical work in the 1970s (Watkin 1977). Among other health-care professions, increasing specialization can be typified by the increasing division of labor (accompanied by increasingly specialized education) of pathology laboratory workers between biochemistry, histopathology, and hematology. One consequence of this trend has been the creation and expansion of a series of subordinate occupations, such as nursing auxiliaries and physiotherapy aids, to carry out the lowest level tasks rejected by each profession.

Managerialism

The concept of managerialism summarizes the attempt to introduce a range of practices and analytic techniques normally associated with commercial organizations, aiming at greater efficiency in and greater control of health services. Its history in the NHS began with the Hospital Plan of 1962, which aimed to replace a substantial proportion of building stock (which was largely old and in poor repair) with district general hospitals of from 600 to 800 beds serving a population of from approximately 100,000 to 150,000. The planning and commissioning of these began to require both the employment of additional administrative doctors at the regional level, and the formal involvement in management of hospital consultants. The latter need was the subject of the series of "Cogwheel" Reports from 1967, which recommended the creation of a two-tier committee for each speciality electing representatives to a medical executive committee for each hospital or group of hospitals. These recommendations were, however, adapted as widely as they were adopted.

Health service administrators increasingly came to see themselves as managers and to specialize as well. During the period from the 1960s to the early 1970s, the management division of labor became more specialized with the emergence of the so-called functional management of support services such as laundry, catering, and domestic work (partly as a result of the shedding of duties by other groups of staff, especially nurses). Over the same period, the subdivision of the administrative function proceeded with the emergence of finance, supplies, personnel, and, occasionally, planning as de facto specializations not recognized in official grading structures. Simultaneously, there was a steady increase in the average size of hospitals and therefore also of both concentrations of workers and the opportunity of further managerial and professional specialization. The same trend was evident in nursing, where reports of 1966 and 1968 recommended hierarchical management for both hospital and community nurses. The 1970s saw these principles extended to some of the professions supplementary to medicine.

The late 1960s also saw the introduction of quantitative techniques of management such as time study and methods study, initially in response to a need to raise the pay of hospital manual workers through incentive payment schemes during a period when other forms of increase were effectively precluded by government pay policy.

The 1974 Reorganization. The NHS reorganization of 1974 can be seen as a rationalization of the trends of professionalism and managerialism, as well as a response to the major problem brought about by these trends: the problem of integration or coordination of increasingly specialized and fragmented services. The lack of coordination resulting from the tripartite structure and from the semi-independence of clinicians had been the subject of comment in various reports from 1956 onward, and various solutions were offered. Serious government interest in a reorganization was engaged from about 1968, especially after the integration of government health and other social welfare responsibilities into the new DHSS. A series of consultative documents was produced by different ministers and different governments, culminating in a decision to reorganize the service to coincide with a reorganization of local government. The actual reorganization was presided over by a Labour Government, although most of the arrangements had been made by its Conservative predecessor.

The form of organization adopted in England in 1974 was to retain the regional "tier" from the former structure (renamed regional health authorities, or RHAs) and to create below it area health authorities to take on the function of the former hospital management committees, boards of governors, and local authority health committees. The geographical boundaries of the area authorities coincided with those of local authorities, who remained responsible for environmental health and personal social services, and with whom statutory joint consultative committees were created. About two-thirds of the areas thus created were considered to be too large for the operational management of health services and were therefore subdivided into from two to six administrative districts, each nominally focused upon a district general hospital. The RHAs and area statutory authorities were basically nonelected lay bodies, though membership contained both physicians and nurses as well as representatives from the relevant local government authority. Health authority members were unpaid, except for chairmen who received part-time salaries. Authorities at each level were advised by committees of physicians and nurses. It was not thought possible to integrate fully primary medical and dental services, and the former executive councils were replaced by family practitioner committees with a partial responsibility to area authorities. GPs, dentists, pharmacists, and opticians remained self-employed and remunerated as before.

The funding arrangements for the service remained unchanged, though from 1978 geographical distribution of funds, previously based on historical patterns, was increasingly achieved by the use of the so-called RAWP formula, whose principal components are population served, standardized mortality ratios, and service utilization rates.

Structures of occupations were left largely unchanged; the 1974 organization remained functional and therefore still susceptible to coordination problems. Such problems were to be solved by three means. First, a planning system, rational-comprehensive in nature, was introduced (from 1976) as a means of attempting to translate perceived health-care needs into priorities and action. Second, great stress was laid upon detailed definitions of the roles and relationships expected of the various organizational actors (Jaques 1978). Third, and perhaps most significant, consensus decision making by multidisciplinary management teams was introduced. Teams at regional and area levels comprised the full-time chief officers: administrator, nurse, medical officer, and treasurer, with the addition of a works officer to the regional team. At the district level (and in those areas not subdivided into districts), the district management team (DMT) consisted of full-time administrator, nurse, community physician (combining public health, epidemiological, and paramedical management responsibilities), and finance officer, with the addition of two part-time clinicians (one consultant and one GP) elected as representative of their respective colleagues. A common feature of all these teams was that decisions were to be made by consensus, that is, with the agreement of each member. Issues that could not be resolved in this way were to pass to the authority for resolution. There was no direct authority relationship between officers in a particular discipline at regional, area, or district levels; the relationship was to be one of monitoring, that is, of seeking information and advising. Both area and district teams were responsible to the area authority (Harrison 1982). Scotland and Wales were also reorganized, though with some differences in structure.

The 1974 structure can be seen as a way of trying to satisfy demands for both managerialism and professionalism. It created an organization largely characterized by nonauthority relationships. Managers themselves benefited in terms of status, gradings, and salaries, both from the reorganization itself and from preceding trends. Professionals other than doctors benefited from their own arrangements into managerial hierarchies. As Klein (1983) has argued, these arrangements, however, satisfied no one and attracted a good deal of criticism due to their complexity, though lack of perceived success can be associated with a number of social, political, and economic changes that occurred in the early years of the reorganized system's operation. These included a marked reduction in growth money available for the NHS, a turbulent period of industrial relations (see below), the beginnings of an apparent breakdown of the party political consensus about the service, and increasingly critical social and academic attitudes toward the professions and large organizations. In these lay the roots of a further reorganization and the present structure of the NHS.

The 1982 Reorganization. In 1976 a Royal Commission had begun to consider "in the interest both of the patients and of those who work in the National Health Service the best use and management of . . . financial and manpower resources . . . " (Royal Commission 1979). Like the earlier Guillebaud Report, the Report of the Royal Commission, which was published in 1979, was supportive of the NHS and its overall achievement. The majority of the report's recommendations were for low-key change, though it did suggest that the Secretary of State's direct responsibility for the whole of the service be attenuated to strategic issues and the detailed responsibility be devolved to regional health authorities. It also concluded that the 1974 structure contained one surplus tier of management.

By the date of publication of the report, a new Conservative Government had been elected. In December 1979, it published a consultative document, "Patients First," in response to the Royal Commission. This led to a further reorganization of the NHS in 1982. The major change on this occasion was the abolition of area health authorities and their replacement by statutory district health authorities (DHAs), based largely upon the boundaries of the 1974 districts. There was therefore no longer a one-to-one correspondence between health authorities and the local government authorities responsible for social services and environmental health. Similarly, there was no longer a one-to-one correspondence between health authorities and FPCs, the latter having retained their 1974 boundaries. Other changes included a simplification of the planning system and the professional advisory machinery.

Although DMTs and consensus decision making were retained, the above changes can be seen as deemphasizing comprehensiveness and integration. Another change gave greater priority to what might be seen as their corollary—managerial decentralization. Below district level, management units were created, each managed by a senior administrator, a nurse, and a clinician, though they did not formally constitute a consensus team. Chief officers at district level were urged to delegate as much as possible to these units, consisting of one or more hospitals, community services, or a mixture of the two.

Again, there were differences in the changes made in Wales and Scotland,

and, again, it was subsequently felt that the changes were inadequate. The 1982 reorganization was not to be the last.

Trade Unionism

Levels of trade union membership as a proportion of all workers (union density) are fairly high in Britain in comparison with most countries. In the NHS, the recognition of unions was established at the creation of the service, and a national system of bargaining for pay and conditions was established. In 1949 some 42 percent of NHS workers were unionized compared with 45 percent in industry as a whole and 70 percent in the public sector. Density in the NHS actually fell until the mid-1960s when it rose sharply and rapidly to 76 percent in 1978, compared with a figure of 53 percent for all industries (Bain and Price 1980). More then 40 different unions are officially recognized for different staff groups, although the two largest (so far as NHS membership is concerned), the Confederation of Health Service Employees and the National Union of Public Employees, recruit across many different categories of staff and together account for some 60 percent of all NHS trade unionists. Some quite small organizations have a high proportion of specialist groups in membership, and, as already noted, a number of professional associations such as the BMA, the Royal College of Nursing, and the Chartered Society of Physiotherapy also perform trade union functions.

A number of reasons for this membership increase may be adduced, but perhaps the three strongest are the introduction of the ''check-off'' of subscriptions from pay; the competitive union recruitment in an area of the public sector which was, as has been seen, relatively underorganized; and the effect of the trend of managerialism. The latter has fallen upon unskilled NHS workers rather than upon the professional groups, and the late 1960s marked for many such employees the end of a paternalistic approach by their superiors. At the same time, the introduction of payment-by-results systems, necessarily negotiated at the local level, gave credibility to local (branch) union officers. Thus, in addition to growing union membership, the 1970s saw increasingly local union activity in terms of organizing activity, negotiations, and consultation with management.

Prior to 1972, industrial action such as strikes or slowdowns was a rarity in the NHS, and many pay disputes were settled by arbitration. In 1972–1973, however, a major dispute, involving both strikes and other forms of coercive action, occurred as hospital manual workers pursued a national pay claim: Some 289,000 person-days of work were lost (Royal Commission, 1979). Although this action was relatively unsuccessful from the workers' points of view, it broke an effective taboo against industrial action in the NHS, for since then virtually every NHS staff group (including physicians) has been involved in coercive action in either local or national disputes. The complexity and interdependence of health service organization make it particularly susceptible to disruption by strategically placed occupational groups, though it has been rare for any such action to be taken without provision for continuing emergency coverage.

The effect of these changes has not been entirely clear. There is a danger of confusing activity, of which there has been a great deal, with outcome. While there is little doubt that union activity has restricted some areas of management decision making, it is debatable whether many of the disputes, especially those involving ancillary workers, have been economically successful (Sethi and Dimmock 1981).

Consumerism

The final trend that underlies changes in the British health system during the 1960s and 1970s can be termed consumerism, since it represents an increased level of activity by and on behalf of health-care consumers. It has three distinct strands all of which, notwithstanding the very high level of opinion poll support for the NHS, can be seen as expressing dissatisfaction.

First, the period saw a growth of the private health sector. Although, as has been noted, the arrangements for the inception of the NHS provided for a number of NHS hospital beds to be used by part-time consultant medical staff, the number of these beds (as well as the number of doctors practicing privately in addition to their NHS work) fell from the mid-1950s onward. The creation of the NHS had left a large number of nursing home beds in private hands, and the number of these beds remained static. At the same time, however, there was a steady increase in the proportion of the population which chose, in addition to access to NHS services, to be covered by private health insurance. The number covered by such insurance, mainly for acute medical care, rose from about 600,000 in 1955 to 4.2 million in 1982 (Lee Donaldson Associates 1984). It is not therefore surprising that the number of private acute hospital beds began to grow, presumably partly in response to this demand; by 1980, there were some 4,500 such beds. The majority of those subscribing to such insurance schemes did so through group schemes (often employment based), and they are likely to be of higher socioeconomic status seeking to circumvent the NHS's system of rationing by queuing. It is also likely, therefore, that the premiums paid are well below what would be actuarially fair for the whole population. This trend is widely seen as having social and political significance beyond that suggested by its size.

Second, the period from 1960 has seen a growth in the number of consumer pressure groups operating in the health field. There is a wide range of such groups, some of which (such as the Abortion Law Reform Association) are political pressure groups and some of which (such as Age Concern or MIND) also provide voluntary services to clients. It should be noted that almost all of these groups are concerned with a relatively narrow client group, and they often have their origins in campaigns against specific dissatisfactions. Thus, the National Association for the Welfare of Children in Hospital began as a campaign to extend hospital visiting hours. A number of these groups have become incorporated into the policy process to the extent of receiving substantial financial support from DHSS.

Third, certain health institutions were developed explicitly as consumer safeguards, often in response to scandals involving theft from or violence toward inmates of long-stay mental illness or mentally handicapped hospitals. Examples include the Health Advisory Service and the Development Team for the Mentally Handicapped, which carry out multidisciplinary visits to long-stay institutions, making reports to DHSS and the health authority. In addition, the scope of the Parliamentary Commissioner for Administration (the Ombudsman) was extended to include nonclinical health issues. Perhaps the most highly developed form of institutionalized consumerism is represented by the creation (as part of the 1974 NHS reorganization) of community health councils (CHCs). A CHC was created for each district, with a membership of between 18 and 30 persons drawn from voluntary organizations with an interest in the health field, from the matching local government authority, and from nomination by the regional health authority. CHCs have a small, full-time staff, and they are entitled to send a representative to speak at health authority meetings, to be consulted about health plans, and to delay hospital closures and major service changes by requiring their referral to the Secretary of State.

The NHS: 1983 to Date

The current NHS remains tax financed (with about 2.5 percent of income from prescription, dental, and optical charges), and, with the exception of these charges, services are free at the point of delivery to the entire population. Expenditure currently represents just under 6 percent of the gross domestic product, compared with just under 4 percent in 1949. In volume terms, the service has grown by over 200 percent since its inception (OHE 1977), and currently employs slightly in excess of one million full-time equivalent staff and independent practitioners in Great Britain. Nursing and midwifery staff account for almost 45 percent of this total (CSO 1983). The service is highly labor intensive; about 75 percent of current expenditure goes for direct labor costs, and about 75 percent of the staff is female (Royal Commission 1979). A total of 440,000 beds are provided, and some 6.8 million inpatients and 20.1 million outpatients are treated per annum (CSO 1983). During the 1980s, the number of patients treated has increased more quickly than the volume of resources (DHSS 1983), reversing the trend during the 1970s when additional resources went into the more intensive diagnosis and treatment of the same number of patients (Haywood and Alaszewski 1980). Two major changes relating to management have occurred recently.

First, a number of further changes in formal organization have resulted from the Report of the Griffiths Inquiry into NHS Management, published in 1983 and accepted by the government in 1984 (NHS Management Inquiry 1983; for a critical review see Barnard and Harrison 1984). The inquiry team, which consisted largely of businessmen, proposed a health services supervisory board to take national strategic decisions about NHS objectives, a full-time NHS management board to take over all existing NHS management responsibilities within the DHSS, and the identification (from any discipline, or from outside the NHS) of general managers at regional, district, and unit levels of organization, which supersede consensus decision making. In addition, the partial responsibility of FPCs to DHAs is severed; the former became independent statutory authorities in 1985. Figure 1 attempts to characterize the organization structure of the NHS in 1985; differences in Scotland and Wales will remain, though the general manager innovation will apply in both.

Second, there has been growing concern with the monitoring of health authority performance, and a series of government initiatives have been concerned with this. Thus a number of regions have created management advisory services to monitor the quality of management of health services by the districts within the region. Other examples of such initiatives include the detachment of senior officers to perform ad hoc scrutinies of expenditure on particular items, the use of commercial auditing firms (rather than the DHSS) to examine accounts, the establishment of an inquiry team to identify surplus land and property for disposal, and the development of indicators by which health authority performance might be defined (Long and Harrison 1985). Perhaps most important among these initiatives are the regional review process and management budgeting. The former of these is an annual review of RHAs by the Secretary of State, of DHAs by RHAs, and of units by DHAs, at which performance is reviewed in relation to established priorities and plans. The latter includes various budgeting experiments which seek to establish a financial base for the monitoring of management performance.

One common feature of this latest set of changes is that they appear to originate almost entirely within the government, unlike earlier reorganizations, for which at least some impetus came from within the NHS. On the face of it, these changes are explained by the political ideology of the present Conservative Government. However, a major difficulty in assessing the role of politicians in the development of the NHS is that there has been little evidence that ideological differences have in the past led to substantially different treatment of the service by different political parties when in government. Rather, there has been for the most part a substantial consensus, with little attempt to reverse the policies introduced by earlier governments. Thus notwithstanding rhetoric to the contrary, prescription charges have remained through successive governments, as have the tax-based rather than insurance-based funding and the health policies articulating an intention to give increasing priority to services for the elderly, mentally ill, and mentally handicapped. The process of the 1974 reorganization was initiated by a Labour Government, designed in detail by a Conservative Government, and implemented by another Labour Government.

All this suggests that ideology frequently operates as a post facto rationalization of political decisions and that it may occasionally create rather perverse policy outcomes. Attempts by the Labour Government from 1975 onward to phase out

Figure 1
Organizational Structure of English NHS, 1987

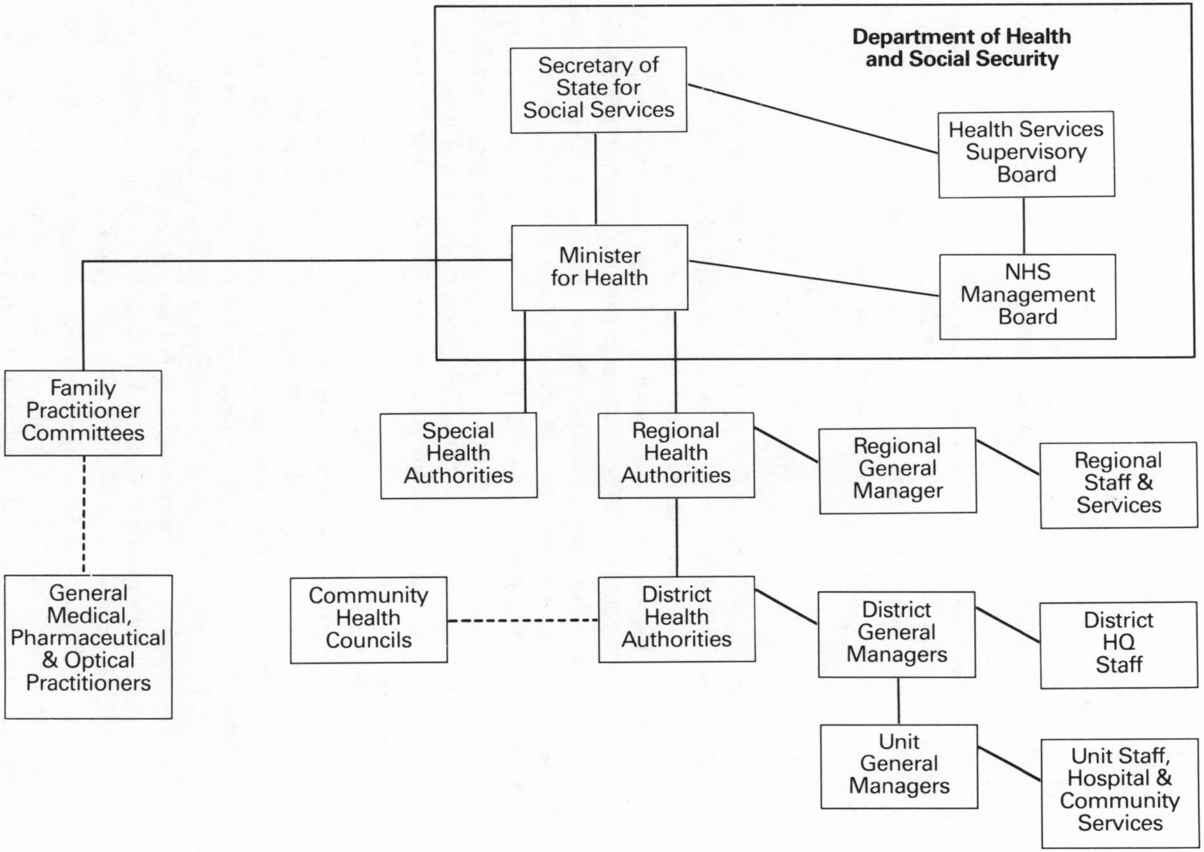

private beds from the NHS under trade union pressure served to encourage the growth of the private acute sector to its present figure of some 6,500 beds (Klein 1983). Attempts of the present government to encourage a shift of NHS hospitals' ancillary services from direct labor to outside contractors may well cost money and lower standards in the medium term. This is not to argue that ideology never drives practice, and it certainly seems likely that the form of NHS established in 1948 was to some extent the product of Labour ideology, and the full impact of the present government's conservative ideology remains to be seen. It seems clear, however, that the extent of government discretion in important components of health-care policy content has typically been somewhat limited.

One possible and perhaps more likely explanation of the recent changes in the NHS management therefore lies in the conjunction of political ideology with an economic situation that can be construed as requiring reductions in public expenditure. This possibility is further explored below.

Who Benefits?

This final section seeks to draw some conclusions about the overall performance of the NHS. Since performance is a concept which may differ with the expectations of different actors, it may be preferable to examine the points of view held by these actors.These can be stated fairly baldly: Those who work within the NHS consider it to be a satisfactory institution which is inadequately resourced; the public, though there may be specific dissatisfactions, are broadly enthusiastic in their support for it (Klein 1983). An alternative approach is for the observer to ask who seems to have benefited from the service's operation, concentrating on five major groups of actors: politicians, professionals, managers, trade unions, and consumers. This is not to suggest that these groups or their interests are completely homogeneous; what follows is no more than a brief characterization.

The NHS has served politicians well. When in government, they have claimed credit for its popularity; when in opposition, they have promised to improve it. It has been an important symbol of paternalistic government. Moreover, the service has had the very practical value of keeping health-care costs in Britain well below the level in much of the developed world. Furthermore, it has served as a device for avoiding formal decisions about rationing health care. By distributing geographically based budgets with little attempt to control the kinds of service upon which money is spent, it leaves decisions about treatment or non-treatment, provision or nonprovision, to physicians and managers, respectively. Thus, at times of economic stringency, alleged managerial failings provide a ready scapegoat (Klein 1983). It is also worth considering whether governments could actually obtain more detailed control over the NHS's activities. One explanation for the apparent long-standing political consensus is that, due to the power of clinicians to determine the pattern of service (Haywood and Alaszewski 1980), the tradition of self-regulation (Peters et al. 1977), and the existence of a nonpolitical civil service, governments are ill-equipped to procure real change themselves.

Physicians have benefited very substantially from an NHS which has relieved them of the burdens of unpaid work in voluntary hospitals, bad debts, and the necessity to work across a broad spectrum of patient groups. At the same time, they have maintained the advantages of independent practice through the doctrine of clinical freedom, the right to practice privately, and (in the case of GPs) the maintenance of self-employed status. More than one study has shown consultants to be the single most powerful group involved in the NHS (Haywood and Alaszewski 1980, Schulz and Harrison 1983). At the same time, it seems likely that the NHS funding system and methods of physician remuneration have kept doctors' earnings rather low by international comparison, although they are still high within Britain. Physicians and other health professionals have benefited from increasing job specialization in terms of both prestige and intellectual satisfaction.

Health service managers have benefited considerably in terms of earnings, gradings, and career opportunities from the trend of increasing managerialism. Moreover, the relative status of some managers (especially in nursing and building and engineering) was improved by the 1974 reorganization. Managers have also been subject to the process of increasing specialization. However, it is clear that managers are still relatively uninfluential in relation to doctors, though change is possible (Harrison, forthcoming).

The trade unions which recruit in the NHS have clearly benefited substantially from the rapid rate of which they were able to expand membership from 1966 to 1978. No doubt this trend has given unions a greater degree of control over decisions about working arrangements, and it has been the *sine qua non* of a number of industrial disputes. At the same time, however, this increased level of activity has rarely produced substantial management concessions in major disputes, and it seems less likely to do so in the future in an environment characterized by relatively high unemployment and therefore falling union membership (Barnard and Harrison 1986).

Consumers are at the same time the most important and the most difficult group of actors in respect of whom to assess benefits. The NHS ostensibly exists to serve them, yet they are much less homogeneous than other groups and are perhaps the least likely to prevail. Even where consumers have become organized through pressure groups, or represented by CHCs, their power has not matched that of producer groups (Ham 1977), and it is difficult for consumers' own views to make an impact.

It may also be helpful to consider the impact of the NHS upon consumers' health in the light of the strategy of Health for All by the Year 2000 devised by the European Regional Office of the World Health Organization (WHO 1981). This strategy has three main elements, the first of which is the promotion of healthier life-styles and environment. The NHS has devoted relatively little effort to this, perhaps not surprisingly, in view of its original conception as a means of curing the sick (Klein 1983). The second element in the WHO strategy is the reduction of preventable conditions. Although considerable improvements in the rates of mortality among children, in the incidence of communicable diseases, and in deaths from road traffic accidents have occurred, it seems that these are attributable more to such factors as better nutrition (McKeown 1976) and seat-belt legislation than to the work of the NHS.

The third element of the WHO strategy is the provision of adequate and accessible care to all. It is this respect in which the service has most obviously failed, notwithstanding the formality of free and open access to its services. Aspects of inequality in the provision and use of services and in the experience of ill health have already been discussed; the social class inequalities were the subject of a recent report (Townsend and Davidson 1983) upon which the government decided not to act. Aaron and Schwartz (1984) have recently drawn attention to the relative undersupply in Britain of such effective procedures as total hip replacement and renal dialysis. Moreover, the growth of the private sector, which has been identified above, can be taken as an indication that certain forms of service are undersupplied. Nevertheless, as Klein (1983) notes, the NHS does improve the quality of life for many who would otherwise suffer, and if the demand for health care is unlimited, it is inevitable that some demands will not be met. Given the pluralistic character of health-care arenas, it would be surprising if complete equity prevailed under either public or private financing, but there can be little doubt that an extension of the latter would reduce the degree of equity that has been achieved.

References

Aaron, H. G. and W. B. Schwartz. 1984. *The Painful Prescription*. Washington D. C.: Brookings Institution.

Bain, G. S. and R. J. Price. 1980. *Profiles of Union Growth*. Oxford: Blackwell.

Barnard, K. and S. Harrison. 1986 Labour Relations and Health Service Management. *Social Science and Medicine* 22: 11.

Barnard K. and S. Harrison. 1984. *Memorandum on the Griffiths Report*. First Report from the Social Services Committee for the Session 1983/84, House of Commons Paper 209, HMSO.

Barnard, K. A. and K. Lee, eds. 1977. *Conflicts in the National Health Service*. London: Croom Helm.

CSO. 1983. *Annual Abstract of Statistics*. HMSO.

DHSS. 1981. *On the State of the Public Health*. HMSO.

DHSS. 1982. *Health and Personal Social Services Statistics for England*. HMSO.

DHSS. 1983. *Health Care and Its Costs*. HMSO.

Ham, C. J. 1977. *Power, Patients and Pluralism*. In *Conflicts in the National Health Service*, eds. K. A. Barnard and K. Lee. London: Croom Helm.

Hanson, A. H. and M. Wallace. 1981. *Governing Britain*. London: Fontana.

Harrison, S. 1981. The Politics of Health Manpower. In *Manpower Planning in the National Health Service*, eds. A. F. Long, and G. Mercer. Farnborough: Gower.

Harrison, S. 1982. Consensus Decision Making in the National Health Service. *Journal of Management Studies* 19: 4.

Harrison, S. Forthcoming. *Shifting the Frontier?* London: Croom Helm.

Haywood, S. and A. Alaszewski. 1980. *Crisis in the Health Service*. London: Croom Helm.

Jaques, E., ed. 1978. *Health Services*. London: Heinemann.

Johnson, T. J. 1972. *Professions and Power*. London: Macmillan.

Klein, R. E. 1983. *The Politics of the National Health Service* London: Longman.

Lee Donaldson Associates. 1984. *UK Private Medical Care: Provident Scheme Statistics*. Report for DHSS.

Long, A. F. and S. Harrison, eds. 1985. *Health Services Performance*. London: Croom Helm.

McKeown, T. 1976. *The Role of Medicine*. London: Nuffield Provincial Hospital Trust.

NHS Management Inquiry. 1983. *Report*. London: DHSS.

OHE. 1977. *Compendium of Health Statistics*. London.

OPCS. 1982. *General Household Survey 1980*. London: HMSO.

Peters, B. G., J. C. Doughtie, and M. K. McCullough. 1977. Types of Democratic System and Types of Public Policy. *Comparative Politics*, April: 237–255.

Richardson, J. J. and A. G. Jordan. 1979. *Governing Under Pressure*. London: Martin Robertson.

Royal Commission on the National Health Service. 1979. *Report Cmnd 7615*. London: HMSO.

Schulz, R. and S. Harrison. 1983. *Teams and Top Managers in the National Health Service*. London: King's Fund.

Sethi, A. S. and S. J. Dimmock. 1981. *Industrial Relations and Health Services*. London: Croom Helm.

Townsend, P. and N. Davidson. 1983. *The Black Report*. London: Penguin.

Watkin, B. 1975. *Documents on Health and Social Services: 1834 to the Present Day*. London: Allen and Unwin.

Watkin, B. 1977. *The NHS: The First Phase*. London: Allen and Unwin.

WHO. 1981. *Regional Strategy for Attaining Health for All by the Year 2000*. Copenhagen: Regional Office for Europe.

HUNGARY

Iván Forgács

Health Care and Health Service

Hungary is a central European country bordered by Austria, Czechoslovakia, Romania, and the Soviet Union. Its population in 1985 was 10,657,000—5,149,000 males and 5,508,000 females. Since 1981 there has been a slight trend downward in total population, due to a decreasing birth rate as well as an increasing death rate. Of the total population, 19.3 percent lives in the capital, 36.7 percent in towns, and 44.0 percent in villages. The age distribution of the population is as follows: from 0 to 14 years, 21.8 percent, from 15 to 39 years, 35.6 percent, from 40 to 59, 24.7 percent; from 60 to 79 years, 15.7 percent; and from 80 years and more, 2.2 percent. There has been a gradual increase in the percentage of people over the age of 60 during the last 25 years.

Hungary is a socialist society, in which the preponderance of productive assets—95.8 percent—is state owned. In 1985 the gross domestic product of the country was 1033.7 billion forints, or approximately U.S. $20 billion. Administratively, the country is divided into 19 counties and the capital. Excluding the capital, there are 109 towns and 2,957 villages, each of which is considered a local municipality.

The process of industrialization over the last three decades, from a predominantly agricultural country to a moderately industrialized one, has been accompanied by numerous social and cultural changes. These changes have influenced both the distribution of manpower in different sectors of economic activity and the health status of the population. Since the most important noninfectious diseases are closely connected with life-style, and, in turn, a major factor influencing life-style is the nature of work and working conditions, the changing structure of work life has had an important effect on the health status of the population.

In 1968 a new economic policy was introduced, and the earlier extensive approach to economic development was changed to an intensive one. In agriculture and industry, an increase in efficiency has been achieved during this intensive phase, although the service sector has lagged behind. Effects of these extensive and intensive changes relevant to health care include rapid urbanization; increased geographical mobility; increasing numbers of females employed, mainly in the service sector; enhanced economic mobility between and within generations; professional redistribution among social classes; and, as a consequence of all these, changes in individual life-style.

Historical Background and Recent Health Policy

Before World War II, only 30 percent of the population belonged to a health insurance scheme. Accessibility to health service was very selective, and it depended primarily on the socioeconomic status of each individual. After World War II, a new health service strategy was adopted. The aim was to reconstruct the health-care infrastructure within the framework of a new health-care policy. The postwar development of the health service system can be divided into several distinct periods: a period of reconstruction from 1945 to 1950; the first extensive development phase from 1951 to 1965; the second extensive phase of accelerated development from 1966 to 1975; a transitional period between 1976 and 1980 in preparation for the intensive period; and the introduction of intensive development from 1981 with special emphasis on the strategy of Health for All by 2000.

During the first extensive phase, a moderate increase of health-care investment was accompanied by a rapid and significant improvement in health status. However, while mortality in both sexes and in all age groups decreased between 1950 and 1965, mortality rates increased between 1965 and 1980 for both sexes, especially for males between 35 and 59 years of age. It is paradoxical that during this period of accelerated investment in the health service, the health status of the population became worse, especially in relation to parameters concerning noninfectious diseases.

The political basis of health-care delivery was set forth in the Health Act of 1972. The main elements include free-of-charge health service, universal accessibility, equality of access to service for the entire population, priority in preventive and rehabilitative services, and community participation. The quantitative and qualitative consequences of these principles are discussed below.

Health Status of the Population

The crude birth rate increased until 1955, when it began to decrease gradually except for a jump upward between 1974 and 1977. It currently stands at 12.2 per 1,000 inhabitants. The fertility rate was 59.7 in 1960 and 50.9 in 1985 per 1,000 fertile women aged between 15 and 49 years. The stillbirth rate decreased sharply from 1950 onward and stood at 6.2 per 1,000 live births in 1985. It is worthwhile to mention that the artificial abortion rate, which was 71.5 per 1,000 in 1965, was 32.1 per 1,000 women of fertile age in 1985. The dismaturity rate (birth weight of 2500 grams or less) was 10.0 per 1,000 live births in 1985.

The infant mortality rate was 131.4 in 1938; 51.6 in 1948; 35.5 in 1960; 34.5 in 1970; 23.1 in 1980; and 20.4 in 1985 per 1,000 live births.

The crude mortality rate diminished markedly during the late 1940s and moderately between 1950 and 1965; however, there was a sharp increase between 1965 and 1985. In this later period, the mortality rate began to increase from 25 years in men and from 35 years in women, and it remained higher up to 59 years in both sexes.

In 1982 the age specific mortality rates of men were 2.16 in the age group 15–34; 10.99 in the age group 35–59; 47.60 in the age group 60–74; and 141.91 in the age group from 75 and up per 1,000 men in the corresponding age group. According to the same age grouping, the respective figures in women were 0.69, 4.97, 26.85, and 110.25, respectively, per 1,000 women. In the same year, the cause-specific mortality rates were hypertensive and cardiac diseases, 376.4; malignant tumors, 263.9; cerebrovascular disease, 222.6; generalized arteriosclerosis, 96.8; accidents, 68.4; suicides, 43.5; and infectious diseases, 2.4 per 100,000 inhabitants.

The life expectancy at birth increased between 1950 and 1970 in both sexes. From 1973 there has been a slight decrease in men and a moderate increase in women. In 1985, the life expectancy at birth was 73.6 years for women and 65.6 years for men.

Structure and Management of the Health Service

Institutions providing preventive and curative services are operated both by the Ministry of Health (university clinics, national institutes, sanatoriums) and by various levels of local councils (local, village, municipal, and county councils). However, institutions run by the councils are also supervised by the Ministry of Health and by the National Institutes on the basis of uniform, professional guidelines.

The Health Act of 1972 stipulates that every patient should have ready access to adequate, high-quality preventive and curative care irrespective of place of residence. This requirement could be fulfilled only if all health delivery institutions in the country belonged to a single homogeneous system, in which the tasks of the subsystems are well defined and the various levels cooperate to establish a system of progressive health-care delivery. Because health care in Hungary is available as a citizen's right, the state is responsible for the provision of full-scale health care for the entire population free of charge. Since good geographical distribution of primary medical facilities had already been achieved, the specialization of services was speeded up under the 1972 law. By 1985, more than 75 percent of all working doctors had specialist qualifications. At the same time, specialization of paramedical personnel (nurses, assistants, etc.) has now reached a fairly advanced stage as well. Simultaneously, organizational measures were implemented to allow for a better distribution of specialized professionals within the health-care delivery system.

Primary health care, the basis of the Hungarian health service, comprises the following services: district physician (general practitioner); district pediatrician; school health service; occupational health service; maternity and infant care (including family planning, genetic counseling, and so on); district dental service; ambulance service; certain outpatient departments that accept patients without referral; basic services including public hygiene, environment, labor, food and nutrition, as well as epidemiology; and health education.

Primary health care has been fully organized, including district physicians, district pediatricians, and occupational services in factories and other places of production. The average of 1 general practitioner (GP) per 2,400 population does not fully reflect the true rate of primary care delivery, however, since a segment of the population also receives treatment from physicians in factories and district pediatricians in towns.

Since 1951 occupational health care has been a state responsibility. Today, every enterprise employing more than 500 workers has an industrial physician. During the past twenty years, the number of occupational health service hours has increased by a factor of 2.5.

District pediatric services take place in towns, cities, and major settlements. At the village level, the district physicians are assisted in maternity and infant care activities by maternal and child health (MCH) nurses in the Primary Health Care (PHC) team and by mobile specialist services staffed with obstetricians and pediatricians.

The school health service, composed of a doctor and an MCH nurse, provides school health care to 2,000 to 3,000 adolescent school children from fourteen to eighteen years of age to ensure continuous care through regular screenings.

The dental services in 781 districts provide dental care to the inhabitants of villages or smaller communities. In towns and cities, this service is performed by the dental departments of the polyclinics. Preventive care for children is a priority area for dentistry. There is an average of 1 dentist per 3,800 inhabitants.

The ambulance service is a national organization under the direct supervision of the Ministry of Health. There are 66 ambulance stations and 1,823 ambulance vehicles in the country. All ambulances are linked by continuous radiotelephone contact with one another and with the national headquarters. The ambulance service has a double task: saving lives and transporting patients. Special paramedical units often begin emergency treatment on the spot when it is indicated.

Hospital-based inpatient and outpatient services provide the conditions of most doctor-patient encounters. There is, however, a compulsory referral system in

Hungary. If the primary level is unable to treat a patient, the patient must be referred to polyclinics staffed by specialists. Generally, such polyclinics are located in towns and cities as integrated parts of municipal hospitals. On an average, a municipal hospital is responsible for the out- and inpatient care of from 110,000 to 120,000 people.

Cases requiring complex diagnostic or therapeutic treatment are treated in large county hospitals where most of the medical disciplines are represented and sophisticated medical equipment is available. These county hospitals typically have a complement of from 1,000 to 2,000 beds. If necessary, municipal hospitals can transfer their patients to county hospitals. Of course, the county hospitals also handle routine cases in their catchment area. They provide services for an average of from 400,000 to 600,000 people.

In certain specialized areas of medicine, where the incidence and prevalence of diseases is rather low (neurosurgery, cardiac surgery, vascular surgery, transplantations), highly specialized hospitals function as regional or national centers. It is compulsory to refer patients with indicated conditions to such institutions. The responsibility of the regional centers generally extends to two or three counties with approximately one to two million in population. When necessary, the patient may be sent to this level directly from the primary sphere, bypassing intermediate levels. At present, seven regional centers are operating in the country.

This progressive form of health system organization is both professionally and economically efficient, making possible the effective deployment of highly specialized staff and of sophisticated equipment, while, at the same time, ensuring patients the best possible care. These national institutes also guarantee that modern techniques will permeate every discipline and speciality, and simultaneously provide the Ministry of Health with the professional information required to make decisions on future organizational development.

This approach to health-care organization is facilitated by the relatively short distances inside Hungary, by its well-organized mass transportation systems, and by the availability of ambulances and emergency aircraft. (It is worth noting that there is practically no point in the country farther than 25 kilometers away from a hospital.)

At night and on holidays, patients are handled by regular duty services organized all over the country, both at the primary and at the inpatient levels. This is in addition to the ambulance service.

Sanitary services and epidemiological prevention are supervised by the National Institute of Hygiene, but there are sanitary and epidemiology stations in every county, with well-equipped laboratories performing microbiological, water, air, and soil tests and investigations; offering laboratory monitoring of production technologies and biological and chemical safety of food production and marketing; and providing protection against radioactive materials. These institutions conduct necessary epidemiological investigations, including screenings, and organize vaccination campaigns. In towns, local services fulfill basic public health–epidemiological tasks. The structure and administrative operation of the health service is shown in Figure 1.

Function of Health Service

Compliance with the basic principles of Hungarian health policy has several consequences relevant to the health manpower projections. The fact that services are free at the point of delivery promotes a higher case load, especially at the primary level. Accessibility requires a good geographic distribution of the available health manpower. In Hungary since the mid-1970s, integrated and outpatient systems have existed at town, county, regional, and country levels. From town to country level, the diagnostic and therapeutic facilities increase progressively. This progressive increase demands a higher degree of manpower specialization. The priority of prevention, e.g., mass screening and vaccination, is also a factor which increases manpower needs.

Primary Health Care

The number of GPs increased by 20 percent between 1950 and 1965 and by another 20 percent between 1965 and 1980. The number of GPs in 1985 was 4,416. The geographical redistribution is seen from the following: The GP per population ratio in 1950 was 1:2,400 in Budapest and 1:3,400 in the provinces; in 1980, the ratios in Budapest and in the provinces were the same. The case load of the GPs in 1965 was 47 million per year, and about 4 million home visits were made. About 5 percent of the patients were referred to outpatient clinics, and 0.5 percent were sent to a hospital. In 1985 the case load diminished to 38 million; the number of home visits increased to 4,444,000; about 5.5 percent of the patients were referred to outpatient clinics and 0.4 percent to inpatient clinics. These figures show that, on an average, every Hungarian adult citizen consulted his or her family physician 4.5 times a year. On the other hand, in 95 percent of the cases, it was not necessary to refer patients to a higher level of care. Also, in 1985, the number of primary health-care nurses was 4,595 and they made 5,965,106 home visits. There is an increasing number of long-term care patients at the primary health-care level. In 1970, 721,000 were registered compared to 1,252,492 patients in 1985. The number of primary health-care pediatricians increased from 395 to 1,227 between 1965 and 1985, while the case load increased from 2,200,000 to 8,313,730, and 43 percent of the home visits were of a purely preventive nature.

The overall case load of primary health-care dentists in 1985 was 10,855,000, showing a slightly decreasing trend. The number of extractions decreased by 10 percent compared to 1981. On the contrary, in child dentistry, the case load increased by 14.6 percent.

Figure 1
Health Care in Hungary

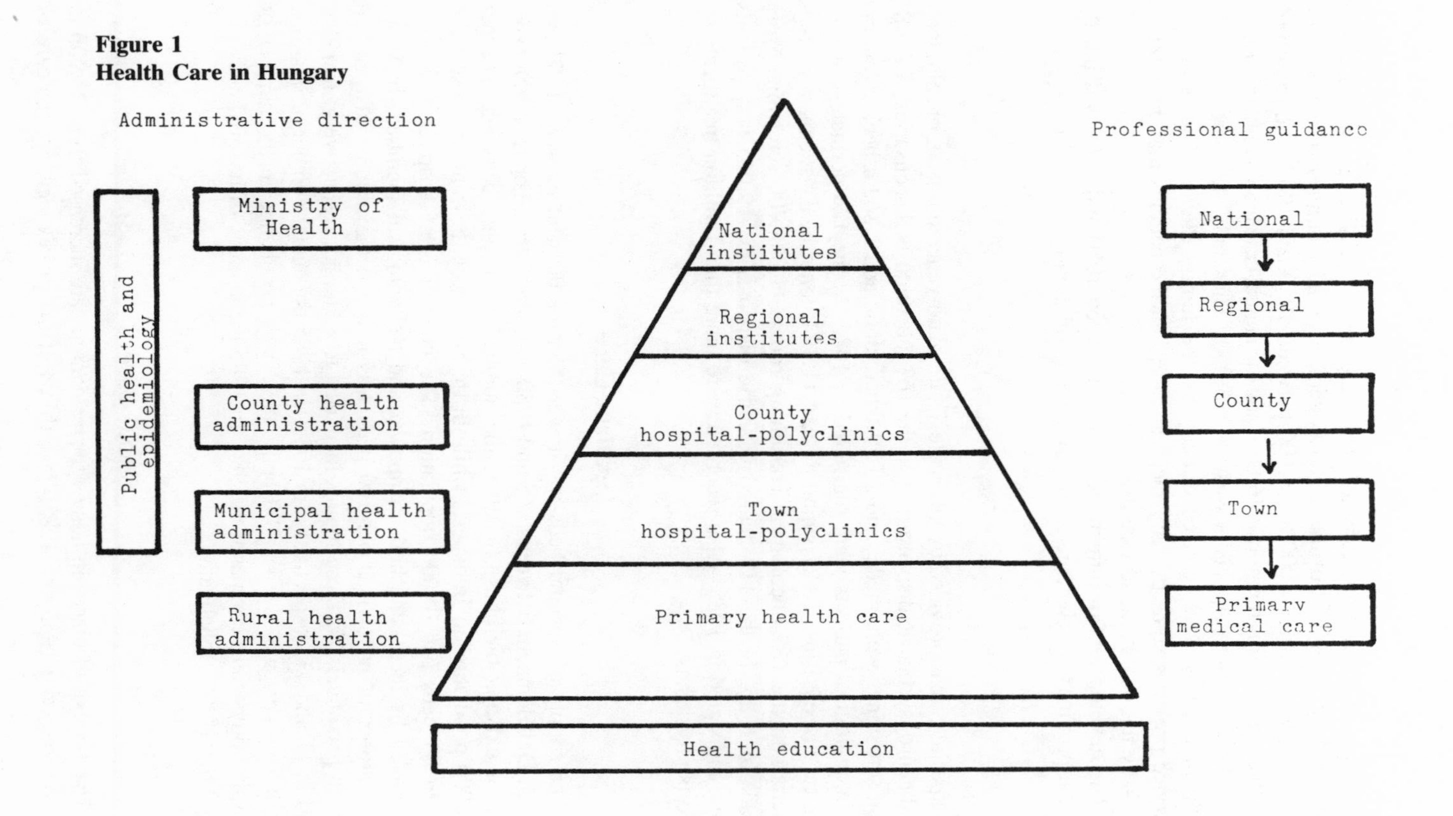

Outpatient Care

During the years from 1950 to 1975, outpatient specialist care was the most rapidly developing part of the health system. The daily number of consultation hours increased from 7,000 to 26,000 between 1950 and 1965, and to 44,000 in 1980. In 1985 this figure was 46,000, and the annual case load without dentistry and clinical laboratory visits was 38,716,000. Thus only 6.3 percent of the outpatient cases were referred directly by the family doctor. The outpatient service provides some primary medical care, and the patients may be referred back by the outpatient service itself.

The development of outpatient services between 1950 and 1965 was mostly in the provinces to compensate for the maldistribution of hospital beds.

Dispensary Care

Special care is provided by tuberculosis, dermato-venereological, oncological, and neuropsychiatric dispensaries. In the 163 tuberculosis dispensaries, 5.8 million screenings were made, and 2,059 tuberculotic and 1,862 aspecific (tumor) pulmonological patients were registered in 1985. In the 124 dermato-venereological dispensaries, 1,627 syphilitic and 11,194 gonorrheal patients were registered. In the 165 oncological consulting rooms, 1,005,700 screenings were made in 1985. In the 113 neuropsychiatric dispensaries, 19,065 new patients were registered in 1985. Also recorded were more than 1 million treatments by sports physicians.

Inpatient Care

The supply of hospital beds was lower than the demand between 1950 and 1965. Development between 1965 and 1980 was concentrated on more intensive use of existing facilities. In 1985, the number of hospital beds was 148 per 10,000 population in Budapest, while in the provinces these figures rose from 46 to 83 beds per 10,000 population. The conditions of hospital care were improved by increasing both manpower and technological facilities. In 1950, the number of physicians per 100 beds was five and the number of qualified health personnel, 17; these figures increased to 8 and 33, respectively, in 1965, and to 11 and 33, respectively, in 1980. In 1985 the actual number of qualified health workers was 51 per 100 beds; there was no change in the number of hospital physicians compared to 1980. In 1985 the average of hospital beds was 96.2 per 10,000 inhabitants.

Social Care

The number of places in homes for residential care increased from 23,000 to 37,706 between 1965 and 1985. Two-thirds of the places were for the care of elderly persons. The places in day-care homes for the elderly numbered 30,183 in 1985. The number of elderly participants in home care service was 27,608 in 1985. The number of professional social workers in these fields was 3,078; 20,450 voluntary social workers assisted at the community level. Approximately 50,000 of those 70 years or older received some kind of social care in 1985. The demand is still rising. Taking into account that the demographic changes show a significant increase in the proportion of the elderly population for the year 2000, the social care of this group will become an increasingly essential part of the health-care system.

Health Economy

In 1965, the total health expenditure consumed 3.5 percent of the national income; in 1985, this proportion had risen to 4.5 percent.

The approximate distribution of the total health budget was as follows: inpatient care, 49.0 percent; outpatient care, 8.9 percent; primary health care, 7.8 percent; mother, child, and youth care, 12.3 percent; public health and epidemiology, 3.3 percent; university clinics, 8.5 percent; and postgraduate medical school, 0.1 percent. Of the total expenditure on wages, the proportion spent on the inpatient sector was 40 percent and on the outpatient staff, 60 percent. The overall proportion of wages in the financial budget for the health sector was 44 percent.

Health Manpower

About 20 percent of the population lives in Budapest; more than 30 percent of the physicians work there. The average number of active physicians per 10,000 population is 58 in Budapest, 40 in the country towns, and 8 in the villages. The highly specialized institutions with national and regional tasks are situated mainly in Budapest. Among inpatient facilities in the university clinics, there are 23 doctors per 100 beds; in hospital clinics, there are 9–10 physicians per 100 beds. In intensive care wards and rehabilitation wards there are 58 and 1 physicians, respectively, per 100 beds. The numbers of working health personnel in 1985 included the following: physicians, 29,524; hospital nurses, 30,371; infant nurses, 16,121; MCH nurses, 5,168; PHC nurses, 4,747; midwives, 2,564; public health personnel, 2,394; pharmacists, 4,566; and other middle-level health personnel, 60,000.

Training of Doctors and Pharmacists

In 1951, the medical faculties detached themselves from the science universities and were transferred to the direct authority of the Ministry of Health. At present, there are four medical schools with faculties of medicine, stomatology, and pharmacy, and one postgraduate school of medicine.

The first three years of general medical training offer a broad theoretical curriculum. Upon this is built the second three-year cycle, the clinical training that aims at training "basic doctors" familiar with the fundamental social medical theory and practice. In the first two years, stomatology students study the same curriculum as the medical students, and, during the next three-year preclinical-clinical cycle, the aim is to train dentists capable of working independently in their own field.

Pharmacists are trained at only two medical schools. In the course of training, biological and medical knowledge has come to assume increasing importance.

Specialist training and continuing education are carried out at the Postgraduate School of Medicine, which has university status.

The Postgraduate School of Medicine organizes and runs regular as well as special training courses. Its principal aims are to train specialists, to keep expert knowledge up to date, and to teach new methods in various specialities.

College-Level Education and Training

A Health College was organized as a faculty of the Postgraduate School of Medicine in 1974. The college trains health professionals to work under professional medical guidance with relative independence. The training is provided for MCH nurses, physiotherapists, dieticians and public health–epidemiology inspectors: nurse teachers, chief nursing officers (matrons), and ambulance officers.

Regular and compulsory postgraduate training for the college graduates is the responsibility of the Health College faculty itself.

Intermediate-Level Training

Intermediate-level health professionals are trained in two types of schools: health speciality secondary schools and health speciality schools. The two types of school provide almost uniform basic training. The graduates receive certificates entitling them to work as basic nurses. Beyond this basic education, a nurse can pursue post-basic training in 34 different specialities.

Looking Toward Health Care in the Year 2000

By the end of the century, the aging of the population will exercise a major influence on the structure of disease and, particularly, the use of the health institutes. The projected population decrease of about 400,000 persons will be mostly in the younger age groups; the number of those above 60 years of age will grow by approximately 200,000. This trend will increase morbidity and, consequently, the load upon the specialized services of health institutes.

The health status of the older age groups will also increase the need for social care. Needs in these areas can be effectively met by a united network of preventive-curative and social institutes. However, it is not forseen that these institutes will take over the role of families and individuals in the care of the elderly.

The health field exercises a direct influence on the level of national income by protecting and renewing manpower. The strategy for the protection of manpower must be organized in a more complex way since the process of changes in the structure of the national economy and the increased number of career choices foreseen will probably produce a rapidly changing life-style. These changes can occasionally overburden the individual.

The continuation of the process of urbanization will exercise a persistent influence on the mode of life. The influence of general environmental and occupational factors will grow, and only effective environmental protection will stop diseases caused by a deterioration in the quality of water and air and by an increase in soil pollution and noise. Changes in the mode of life in the next decades (resulting from the economic, technical, and environmental changes) will lead to a need for improvements in life and health habits (e.g., leisure time, balanced nourishment). This can be realized by devising more effective methods of, and a comprehensive social basis for, health education. The stage of development of the national infrastructure—educational and cultural provisions, construction of homes—becomes an increasingly important factor in shaping the health status of the population.

The importance of scientific and technical development in health care and medical research will continue to grow. Basic research will be profitable only in the framework of multinational cooperation. The importance of complex programs (combining prevention, cure, and rehabilitation) will increase, especially in the following fields: cardiovascular diseases; cancer; maternal care, perinatal intensive care; accident; suicide; physical, mental, and social problems of the aged; problems of social policy; environmental protection; and organization of health services.

During the next twenty years, the prevention, treatment, and long-term care of noncommunicable diseases will be very important, with special regard to cardiovascular diseases, accidents, tumors, and mental diseases. It will be necessary to devise long-term special programs and detailed short-term programs to treat these diseases successfully. The number of new cases also will increase due to greater screening and the early detection of cases. This will slightly increase the number of so-called first appearances of first doctor-patient interactions while the care of detected cases will result in dynamic growth in the use of regular services. A reasonable level of utilization will be possible only through efforts to develop definitive care at the primary health-care level.

The proportion of hospitalization will grow slightly while the average duration of stay can be shortened by more intensive examinations and by widening the variety of treatments available on an outpatient basis. To compensate for the increased use of hospitals, there is also a need to plan out more intensively the possibilities for primary health care, screening and care, and social care.

Public health services can fulfill their tasks of protection against environmental hazards by developing laboratory facilities for the diagnosis of diseases caused by harmful chemical substances and medicines and by physical factors, such as vibration, noise, and radiation.

There will be an increase in the number of cases where first aid and transportation to a health institute will have decisive influence on the course of an illness. Thus it is essential to secure an accessible, efficient emergency service outside normal working hours and during weekends.

Care must be organized for the main groups of diseases and for special age groups. Though it cannot be extended to cover the whole population by 2000, this kind of activity must form the basis of the work of the primary health-care teams. The number of persons who need medical and social care at the same time will increase in the future. Thus it is important to create a model for home nursing and social care within the framework of a primary health-care team.

Screenings must be gradually extended, with special attention given to high-risk groups. These examinations must be performed with standardized methods and optimal periodicity. The treatment of detected cases should be the task of primary health care.

During the projected period, the role and importance of primary health care within the framework of health services will continue to grow. The optimal composition of the primary health-care team and its relations to second- and third-level care must be better worked out.

In the field of maternal, infant, and child protection, perinatal mortality can be further decreased. For this purpose, the care of pregnant women and infant protection must be improved, and child health must be optimized by better coordination of district and school health.

In the field of inpatient care, there is no need to raise the total number of beds, but it is necessary to adjust the proportion of acute/chronic beds. In the area of medical rehabilitation, the inpatient services of cardiological, locomotor, and mental rehabilitation must be provided within the framework of existing hospital facilities together with their outpatient sections.

References

Forgács, I. 1984. Strategies and Technics for the Implementation of Health Manpower and Other Projections: The Care of Hungary. *World Health Statistics Quarterly 37*: 256–80.

Forgács, I. 1985. *Egészségügy* [*Health care*]. Budapest: Kossuth Publ., pp. 1–103.

Forgács, I. 1986. Work and Health in Hungary. *World Health Organization* (WHO), October. Pp. 23–24.

Forgács, I. 1986. Health and Health Care in Hungary: A country report. *WHO*, Geneva. Pp. 1–72 (in manuscript).

Forgács, I. and M. Kökény. 1987. Towards a New Health Policy in Hungary. *Health Policy* 8, No. 2.

Kökény, M., I. Gyárfás, P. Makara, J. Kishegyi. 1986. The Role of Health Promotion in Preventive Policy against Cardiovascular Diseases. *Health Promotion* 1: 85–92. Oxford: University Press.

Kökény, M., ed. 1987. *Promoting Health in Hungary*. Budapest: Central Statistical Office, pp. 1–57.

Statistical Yearbook (Statisztikai évkonyv). 1986. Budapest: Central Statistical Office.

Yearbook. 1986. Budapest: Ministry of Health.

ISRAEL

Shlomo Barnoon and
Joseph S. Pliskin

The state of Israel came into being in 1948 following a decision by the United Nations General Assembly. Prior to this date, the country had been ruled by the Turkish Ottoman Empire until the end of World War I, at which time the League of Nations gave the British government a mandate to rule and organize the part of the country that was named Palestine.

The Jewish population had increased rapidly from 56,000 in 1918 to 650,000 in 1948. After the establishment of the independent state and the passage of the Law of Return (by which every Jew who wished to become a citizen of the new state automatically received citizenship), the Jewish population grew at a rapid pace. It reached 1.6 million in 1955 and 3.4 million in 1982. At the same time, the non-Jewish population increased from 156,000 in 1948 to about 700,000 in 1982. (These figures do not include the non-Jewish population in the West Bank and Gaza Strip regions.)

The surface area of the State of Israel is 21,500 square kilometers. The southern region of the country is a semiarid land comprising almost 70 percent of the total area but less than 15 percent of the population. Forty-five percent of the population is concentrated in the central region of the state which comprises less than 10 percent of the total area. The state is situated on the shore of the Mediteranean Sea, and it has a subtropical climate.

Health Status of the Population

The health status of the population in Israel has improved considerably since 1948. The general health picture resembles other industrial countries with a declining birth rate and increased longevity, an increasing proportion of elderly people, less incidence of infectious diseases but more chronic diseases. The main causes of death are from cardiovascular diseases, cancer, and accidents. Tables 1,2, and 3 present data on the evolution in infant mortality, life expectancy, and the leading causes of death, respectively, between the years 1950 and 1982.

Historical Development

Health services in Israel provide a classic example of the problematics of pluralism. The system of health-care delivery consists of two different types of organizations: the governmental Ministry of Health and the various sick funds (*Kupot Holim*), which are similar in nature to Health Maintenance Organizations (HMOs) in the United States. Until the end of World War I, health care to the Jewish population was provided mainly through charitable organizations. The first sick fund was founded in 1912 by an organization of agricultural workers and had 150 members. In 1920, with the formation of the *Histadrut* (the General Federation of Hebrew Workers in Israel), the sick funds of the two major parties in the *Histadrut* merged to become the *Kupat Holim Klalit* (General Sick Fund). This fund, which was strongly associated with the labor movement, initiated a political process which is primarily responsible for today's pluralistic system.

Due to political antagonism between various factions of society during the pre-state era, two other sick funds were established to serve nonlabor-aligned segments of the population. In 1931 farm workers not belonging to any of the socialist parties organized themselves under the sponsorship of *Hadassah* to establish the Amamit Sick Fund. The National Sick Fund (NSF) was established in 1933 to serve ''nationalist workers'' who were associated with the revisionist party. In 1936 the General Zionist Party established its own Central Sick Fund of the General Zionists. The latter was merged with the Amamit Sick Fund to form the United Sick Fund. Waves of immigration in the mid-1930s brought large numbers of physicians from Europe who had difficulty integrating themselves into the health-care system. One group formed the Maccabi Sick Fund in 1941 as a joint venture of private practitioners to capture part of the market that was by then accustomed to the sick fund concept. The Israeli Medical Association established two regional sick funds: in Tel-Aviv in 1942 and in Haifa in 1950. These two were merged in 1962 to form the Assaf Sick Fund, which was merged with the Maccabi Sick Fund in 1975.

This close association between the sick funds and the political parties in the country explains the great dependence of today's health policy decisions on the political framework of the State of Israel. While health policy is always in some degree dependent on political processes, in Israel this dependency is magnified manifold.

Upon the establishment of the State of Israel in 1948, the various sick funds provided health care to the majority of the population, The newly formed government assigned the responsibilities for planning, supervising, and coordinating health-care services to the Ministry of Health. The massive numbers of immigrants in the early 1950s found the sick funds unprepared and unwilling to provide

Table 1
Infant Mortality Rates (per 1000 Live Births)

	1950	1960	1970	1980	1982
Total	N.A	31.3	24.2	15.1	13.9
Jews	46.2	27.0	18.9	12.1	11.6
Non-Jews	N.A	48.0	37.3	24.4	21.0

Table 2
Life Expectancy at Birth

		1950	1960	1971	1980	1982
Total	males	N.A	N.A	70.1	72.1	72.5
	females	N.A	N.A	73.4	75.7	75.8
Jews	males	67.2	70.6	70.6	72.5	72.8
	females	70.1	73.1	73.8	76.2	76.2
Non-Jews	males	N.A	N.A	68.7	70.0	70.8
	females	N.A	N.A	72.8	73.4	73.3

Table 3
Leading Causes of Death (per 100,000 Population)

	1950-54	1960-64	1970-74	1980
Cardiovascular diseases	201.4	252.1	249.1	252.7
Malignant neoplasms	85.3	106.2	131.4	136.1
Cerebrovascular	63.5	67.5	100.0	76.5
Infectious diseases	46.9	12.5	5.1	12.0
Accidents	N.A	N.A	35.4	22.9
Others	248.9	149.9	215	206.9
Total	646.0	588.2	(1) 736.0	(1) 707.1

(1). Excluding war casualties in 1967 and 1973.

them with services. As a result, the Ministry of Health took charge of the provision of various services to the mainly homeless and poor immigrants, and became directly involved in health-care delivery. Today, the ministry controls more than half of the available beds in general, and long-stay hospitals and most of the family health centers that mainly provide preventive services.

Organization of Services in the Country

The policy of Israeli governments has been to promote welfare mechanisms for the benefit of society. Health services have been regarded as a basic right of the population and as an obligation of society to its members. The existence of the various sick funds provided a reasonable mechanism of delivery based on a prepaid system subsidized by the government. There has been an ongoing debate on the various forms of a national health insurance act that would augment or replace the existing system.

Currently, approximately 95 percent of the population is covered by the network of sick funds. Every household pays a monthly membership fee, which is supplemented by employer contributions. This membership entitles every individual to comprehensive health care including virtually unlimited outpatient, inpatient, and rehabilitative services, medications at nominal fees, and heavily subsidized medical equipment. Most dental services are not covered but are provided by private practitioners or for a fee by clinics of the sick fund.

The health services sector in Israel employs over 60,000 people which accounts for close to 6 percent of the labor force. Total estimated expenditure on health remained basically steady at about 5.5 percent of the gross national product from 1962 to 1972, increased to 7.7 percent in 1979, and declined due to budgetary cuts to about 7 percent in 1982.

The two main providers of care are the Ministry of Health and the General Sick Fund (GSF). The ministry controls and operates 48 percent of general acute beds and about 41 percent of long-term (psychiatric, geriatric, and rehabilitative) beds. It provides most of the preventive care including maternal, infant, school, and some adult services, as well as all public health oriented services. The GSF provides services to approximately 75 percent of the population. It owns and operates a network of outpatient clinics, pharmacies, hospitals, laboratories, and other diagnostic and therapeutic facilities. It is the only sick fund that owns and operates hospitals, and it accounts for about 31 percent of general acute beds and 9 percent of long-term beds.

The other sick funds cover about 20 percent of the population. They provide outpatient services directly through their own clinics or through private clinics via financial agreements. Similarly, they reimburse hospitals directly for inpatient care provided to their members.

In addition to the government and GSF hospitals, there are public (nonprofit) hospitals, which account for 19 percent of general acute beds and 27 percent of long-term beds, and private hospitals, which account for only 3 percent of the general acute beds but for 31 percent of long-term beds. Table 4 presents the distribution of beds by ownership.

The following are the main components of the Israeli health-care system:

1. Government ministries and organizations
2. Social Security
3. Local (municipal and rural) government authorities
4. Voluntary health insurance agencies (the sick funds)
5. Voluntary associations for general and geriatric hospitalization
6. Voluntary organizations.

Table 4
Hospital Beds by Owner (1982)

Ownership	Total	General acute	Psychiatric	Long term
Government	11980	5680	4087	2213
GSF	4865	3615	526	724
Public	4460	2252	271	1937
Private	5942	329	3408	2205
Total	27247	11876	8292	7079

In an attempt to achieve efficiency and continuity in hospital care, the country was divided into six regions. Each region has been assigned one tertiary care hospital and a number of secondary care hospitals according to their availability. Patients in each region are referred to hospitals in their region, and to other regions only when a service is not available and only upon special authorization.

The routine flow of patients through the system is described in Figure 1. Patients usually go first to a primary care clinic, either public or private. The public primary clinics include family physicians, pediatricians, and occasionally various specialists. Most of these clinics have pharmacies or at least a small medications room on the premises and are capable of dispensing most of the drugs prescribed by the clinic physicians. Provisions are made to reimburse patients for drugs purchased in private pharmacies whenever they are not available through regular channels.

Organizationally, both for the Ministry of Health and the GSF, there are two managerial entities responsible for the delivery of care. The first is responsible for ambulatory primary and specialty clinics which are grouped geographically under separate managements. They are responsible for all manpower, supplies, buildings, and diagnostic and therapeutic facilities in their respective regions. The second managerial entity is responsible for the delivery of inpatient care. The hospitals operate emergency facilities which serve simultaneously as triage centers and channels for admission to the hospitals. The outpatient clinics are also under the responsibility of the hospital managements. This total organizational separation between ambulatory and inpatient services causes many inef-

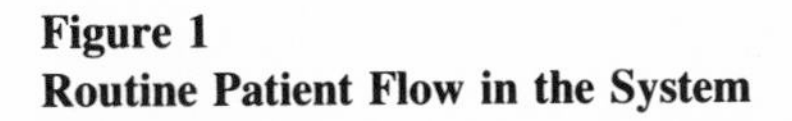
Figure 1
Routine Patient Flow in the System

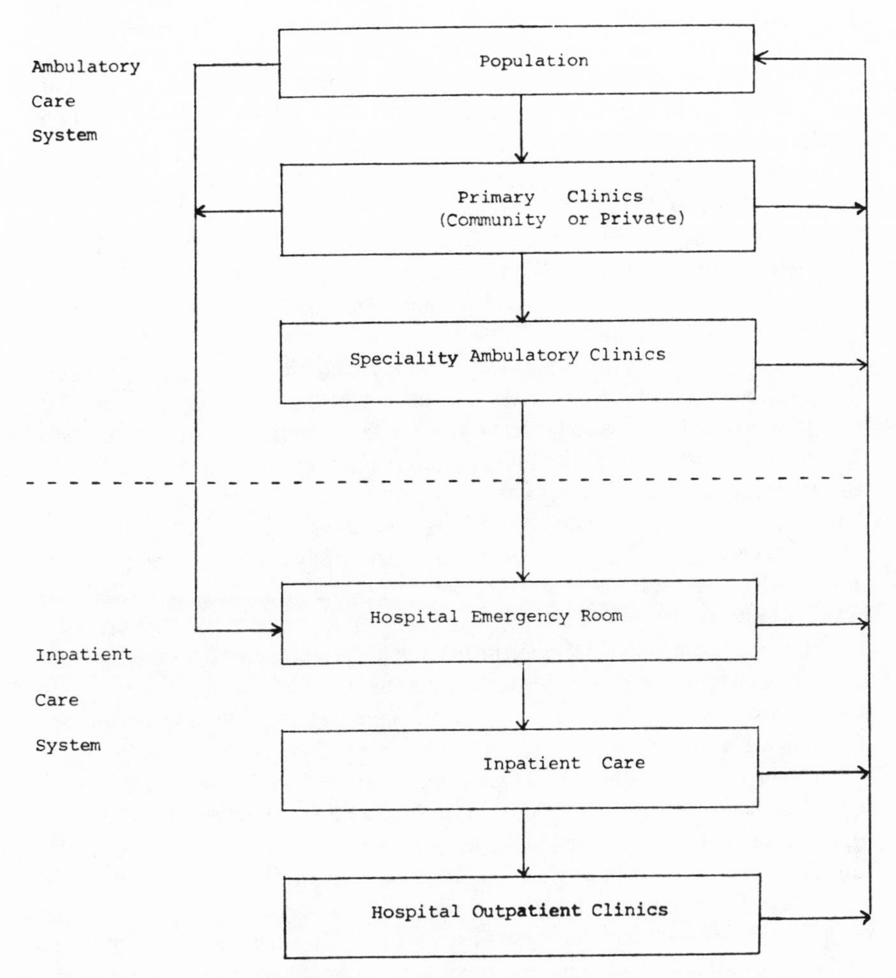

ficiencies due to duplications of laboratories, personnel, equipment, supplies, and so on. Physicians, nurses, and other health workers who provide services in one setting, e.g., ambulatory care, do not, as a rule, provide care in hospitals and vice versa.

A major component of the Israeli health-care system is the medical corps of the Israeli Defense Forces. It provides all services to enlisted and reserve personnel through a network of primary care infirmaries, specialty clinics, field hospitals, and contractual arrangements with some of the civilian hospitals. During periods of war, the military medical corps assumes total responsibility for managing all of the hospitals in the country.

Medical Education and Personnel

The Israel health-care system includes four medical schools which rely upon a network of teaching hospitals and which require six years of training plus a year of internship (like the European system). There are also training facilities for nurses and other health professionals. In addition, there are two schools of dentistry, a school of pharmacology, a school of public health, and programs for health-care management,

Health professionals are organized in professional unions which are primarily responsible for negotiating wages, salary, and working conditions. The Medical Association is further responsible for setting standards, for conducting tests for the various medical specialities, and for recommending graduates for licensure by the Ministry of Health.

More than 50 percent of the physicians in the country have earned their medical degrees in schools outside of Israel. About half of those are people who were born in Israel and went to other countries for their medical training; the others are new immigrants. The multiplicity of training backgrounds has frequently had a poor effect on the quality of care.

Most physicians are salaried employees who work either in a hospital or in the primary ambulatory setting. A small number of physicians and most dentists engage solely in private practice. Some of the full-time salaried physicians engage in private practice as well, causing continuous public controversy. Currently, only the Hadassah Medical Center in Jerusalem formally enables its senior salaried physicians to see private patients within the hospital. Most private practice services are paid by patients out of pocket. Some services are covered by capitation agreements.

In recent years, registered nurses have begun receiving academic degrees along with their professional training in four-year programs. Most registered nurses, however, are still being trained in nonacademic, three-year professional schools. They may specialize in one of four fields: public health, surgery, midwifery, or psychiatry. Some nurses who are working in rural settlements serve as nurse practitioners although they have not been certified. This has been brought about by the scarcity of physicians in these areas. In addition, there are one-year training programs for practical nurses who help overcome the chronic shortage of registered nurses. The system also employs the usual array of health professionals including laboratory and X-ray technicians, dieticians, social workers, pharmacists, psychologists, physiotherapists, and others.

Health System Finances

The sick funds are financed approximately two-thirds through membership fees and employer contributions and one-third by the government. All hospitalizations are reimbursed by the sick funds to the hospitals. Reimbursements are negotiated on a cost basis for each provider and financing source separately,

Table 5
National Expenditure on Health by Source (in Percent of Total in 1982)

Source	Percent
Government	44.0
National Insurance Institute	3.9
Local authorities	3.6
Voluntary sick funds	32.2
Private sector	14.6
Others	1.7
Total	100

usually on a per diem calculation. Even within the GSF, which operates its own hospitals, hospitalization cost for its members is covered through internal transfer of funds from the ambulatory regional offices to the hospital. Though it owns hospitals, the GSF purchases more than 50 percent of total hospitalization days for its members from governmental and public facilities.

Most physicians in the ambulatory setting are salaried, and a small number work in private clinics under capitation arrangements with the sick funds. Only in private practice is a fee-for-service arrangement available. The sick funds do not reimburse physicians or patients for private care unless the patient was referred to such care. For all practical purposes, there are no financial barriers for entry into the system by patients. Except for symbolic fees for medications, there are no out-of-pocket expenses to sick fund members. The Ministry of Welfare pays the GSF membership fees for all registered welfare recipients.

Table 5 presents a percentage breakdown of the national expenditure on health. Table 6 presents the distribution of health expenditures by type of service.

Problems of the System

The Ministry of Health operates a network of services including hospitals, family health centers, and community programs. As such, it places itself in direct competition with other providers in the country, especially the GSF. This competition may cause interference in the orderly flow of funds and resources from the ministry to the other providers. It also affects policy decisions which favor ministry operation to those of other providers. Because the ministry has the authority to allocate governmental funds, it has a built-in conflict of interest that some critics find unethical. Certainly, this situation produces less than optimal performance in the delivery system as a whole. It is very difficult for the Ministry of Health to effectively discharge its responsibility for planning, coordinating,

Table 6
Distribution of Health Expenditures by Type of Service (in Percentages of Total)

Hospitalization	44.0
Drugs	6.3
Primary care	19.5
Mental care	4.4
Long term care	3.1
Dental care	6.5
Capital investment/ facility construction	8.0
Others	8.2
Total	100

and supervising services, when it is also one of several competitive agencies involved in the direct provision of care.

For many years, the system has been struggling with ways to resolve problems arising from the fragmentation of care. Fragmentation presents itself in many forms. First, the multiplicity of providers which are based on rival political groups leads to competition that is not health related and results in vast duplication of services, personnel, facilities, and equipment. These organizations do not compete in the usual sense of the market, but rather under political pressures and prestige considerations which do not result necessarily in an advantage to the patients. Further fragmentation exists administratively within the GSF, by the separation of responsibilities between hospital management and the regional ambulatory care management. This managerial dichotomy created a duplicate system of facilities within a small area. Both the ambulatory system and the hospitals operate laboratories, radiology units, and pharmacies. Similarly, there is duplication in all managerial functions, e.g., accounting, personnel management, warehousing, and so on. In addition to the duplication of resources and facilities, there is duplication in the use of services. Laboratory and other diagnostic procedures completed within the ambulatory care system are frequently repeated whenever the patient is referred to the hospital.

The total separation between the ambulatory and the inpatient systems results in two levels of quality of care in the country. The hospital has been an attractive employment center for most graduating Israeli physicians, both in terms of specialization opportunities and prestige. This resulted in the hospital systems' employing the higher quality, better trained physicians while the community primary care system has ended up with many immigrant physicians of varying professional standards, some of whom were rejected by the hospitals. In addition, the community primary care clinics have been forced to hire and employ a high proportion of retired physicians. In general, community physicians in Israel, including specialists, are not involved in hospital care, which contributes to the discontinuity between hospital and primary care.

Despite the relatively high ratio of physicians to population, there are regions in the country which suffer from acute shortages of physicians and hospital beds. These regions are usually populated by groups of mid-to-lower income levels, and the poor distribution of medical personnel becomes an issue of social discrimination in addition to the obvious diminution of health services. There is an increasing tendency among the non-Jewish population to enroll in the sick funds. There is equal access to all members of the sick funds to all services.

An extensive effort has been invested in the formation of a totally accessible primary care system. The lack of financial barriers, the convenient walking-distance location of neighborhood clinics, the convenient working hours of the clinics, the presence of pharmacies on the premises—all have contributed to high-utilization rates of these services. It is now believed that the system is being overused and even abused because of the lack of barriers. There are currently a number of attempts to introduce various types of minimal barriers to limit the number of unnecessary visits. Copayments have been introduced by one sick fund for primary care services and have shown to be effective. Currently, other sick funds are considering the introduction of similar measures.

Future Trends

The problems of the Israel health-care system have been stated and reiterated by a number of national commissions. Several suggestions for the reorganization of the system have been designed, and two major plans have been discussed and debated in the *Knesset* (the Israeli house of representatives) for possible legislation. These proposed plans did not pass the legislative process because both were politically loaded and included many aspects not directly related to health care.

Currently, attempts are being made to further decentralize the system, both by the Ministry of Health and by the GSF. To achieve this end, the country was divided into regions. Four of these regions have been designated by the Ministry of Health as experimental service regions. A joint regional health management group, established in each region, is responsible for all health services for the population within the respective region. The lack of total collaboration by all providers has been the major stumbling block to the success of this experiment.

Another experiment has been in effect for the past ten years in the Negev, the southern region of the country. In this experiment, the establishment of a new medical school gave the impetus for an attempt to merge all health services with medical education. The dean of the University Health Sciences Center is at the same time the regional director of health services. A joint management group is coordinating the operations of the various provider organizations in the region. This effort has been relatively more successful than other experiments mainly because of the good intentions of local personnel despite the rivalry between the parent organizations on the national level.

The Ministry of Health in determined to continue its efforts to change the voluntary nature of health insurance in the country into a compulsory national health insurance act. The argument is that the government's share in financing health services is continuously growing. It was 33 percent in 1969, and it reached 56 percent of the national expenditure in 1982. The ministry believes that the voluntary part, as indicated by the share of personal and employer contributions, is shrinking, and the public share is increasing. Therefore, the ministry has proposed that the entire system should be financed by the treasury.

There is a general belief in the country that ''Health for All'' has been virtually achieved because an overwhelming majority of the population has ready access to comprehensive health-care services.

References

Adrian, A. 1981. Health Care in Israel: Political and Administrative Aspects. *International Political Science Review* 2: 43–56.

Barnoon, S. 1976a. Cost Containment: A Goal of Health Planning. In *Policies for the Containment of Health Care Costs and Expenditures*. Washington, D.C.: Department of HEW (NIH).

Barnoon, S. 1976b. Process or Outcome Measures for Cost Containment of Health Care. In *Policies for the Containment of Health Care Costs and Expenditures*. Washington, D.C.: Department of HEW (NIH).

Ben-Sira, Z. and R. Duchin. 1981. *Ambulatory Medical Services in Israel: Utilization Patterns and Image*. Jerusalem: The Institute of Applied Social Research.

Doron, H. and A. Ron. 1974. The Organizational Structure of Kupat Holim Services According to Regionalization and Integration. In *Kupat Holim Year Book* 3: 9–23.

Ellencweig, A. Y. 1983. The New Israeli Health Care Reform: An Analysis of a National Need. *J. of Health Politics Policy and Law* 8: 366–86.

Greenberg, D. S. 1983. Health Care in Israel. *New England J. Med.* 309: 681–84.

Grushka, T. 1968. *Health Services in Israel*. Jerusalem: Ministry of Health.

Halevi, H. 1980. *The Bumpy Road to National Health Insurance: The Case of Israel*. Jerusalem: Joint Israel Brookdale Institute of Gerontology.

Halevi, H. S. and P. Ever-Hadani. 1979. Health Expenditure under Multiple-Priority Pressures. *Israel J. Medical Sciences* 15: 43–54.

Margolis, E. 1977. National Health Planning and the ''Medical Model'': The Case of Isarel. *Soc. Sci. and Med.* 11: 181–86.

Palley, H. A., Y. Yishai, and P. Ever-Hadani. 1983. Pluralist Social Constraints on the Development of a Health Care System: The Case of Israel. *Inquiry* 20: 65–75.

Pizam A. and I. Meiri. 1974. The Management of Health Care Organization—Medical vs. Administrative Orientations: The Case of Kupat Holim. *Medical Care* 12: 682–92.

Statistical Abstracts of Israel, no. 34. 1983. Jerusalem: Central Bureau of Statistics.

Yishai, Y. 1979. Autopsy in Israel: Political Pressures and Medical Policy. *Ethics in Science and Medicine* 6: 11–20.

JAPAN

William E. Steslicke

The story of Japan's emergence as an advanced industrial nation is quite complex. Historians typically concentrate upon the economic developments that have contributed to contemporary Japan's high status in the international community and emphasize the role of the state in fostering economic growth. The fact that private industry continues to accept the legitimacy of state intervention is generally regarded as a key ingredient of Japan's economic success and one of the lessons to be learned from the story of Japan's late but rapid industrialization (Johnson 1982).

Although it has attracted less attention, the marked improvement in the health status of the Japanese people since the end of World War II is another success story that similarly calls attention to the role of the state. Of course, economic factors have an important bearing on health status, and it should not be surprising that the Japanese people enjoy a level of general well-being commensurate with their economic prosperity. However, the dynamics of state intervention in the organization, financing, and delivery of both public and private health services during the past century and the continuing acceptance of the legitimacy of state intervention are factors that have also affected contemporary health status. Given the rapid aging of Japanese society and the leveling off of economic growth, an especially heavy burden has been placed upon state agencies to respond to the changing economic and demographic circumstances and to provide appropriate resources and guidance (OECD 1972, Steslicke 1982a). What the state does or does not do in the future will have profound impact on the future health and welfare of the Japanese people.

Health Status in Contemporary Japan

According to Article 25 of the Japanese Constitution of 1947: "All people shall have the right to maintain the minimum standards of wholesome and cultured living.'' Article 25 also declares: ''In all spheres of life, the State shall use its endeavors for the promotion and extension of social welfare and security, and of public health.'' For two decades following its adoption, the constitutional mandate to promote and extend social welfare was not given high priority by public policymakers. Japan was regarded as a ''welfare laggard'' both at home and abroad. Instead of welfare, Japanese political leaders emphasized economic growth and social stability. ''Production first'' was the basis for state intervention in all spheres of life (Bennett and Levine 1976). By the early 1970s, however, the combination of high economic growth and increased pressure from the citizenry for a bigger share in the benefits of prosperity forced national policymakers to place ''promotion and extension of social welfare and security, and of public health'' on their agenda.

Indicative of the changing priorities was the *Basic Economic and Social Plan 1973–1977* approved by the cabinet in 1973 and subtitled, ''Toward a Vigorous Welfare Society.'' It declared:

> As a result of Japan's rapid economic growth to date, major improvements have been possible in income and consumption levels, full-employment has been approached, and progress has been made in such basic life fields as education and medicine. Still, there are major problems remaining, such as the anxieties of the aged and the handicapped and the lag in housing supply, and even greater efforts are being called for in a wide range of fields, including education and medical care, as the people's expectations become more diversified and more sophisticated to create a new situation. While the necessary policies are to be forcefully instituted with the establishment of a stable and comfortable life for all people as one of the top priorities for the future, ambitious attempts are also to be made to expand social security, to improve housing and the living environment, to diffuse the five-day workweek thus ensuring more free time, to improve education, to raise worker welfare standards, to promote consumer protection, and to institute other basic measures (Economic Planning Agency 1973).

Indeed, there were ''ambitious attempts'' to implement the social policy goals set forth in the 1973 plan and, by the end of the decade, Article 25's prescription was being filled. ''Production first'' was not replaced as the basis for state intervention; however, the welfare gap (*fukushi gappu*) was bridged. ''Growth Japan'' and ''Welfare Japan'' were brought closer together than at any other time in modern Japanese history. With regard to health status, not only had minimum standards been firmly established, but also the Japanese people had access to high-quality personal and public health services that were quite affordable (Macrae 1984). As they entered the 1980s, the Japanese people could take pride in their accomplishments in both health and welfare as well as in the economic sector (JICWELS 1983).

Objective measurement and international comparison of health status are, of course, quite crude. In terms of the most commonly accepted indicators, the Japanese people appear to be among the healthiest in the world. For example, the estimated life expectancy at birth for males has increased from 23.9 years in 1945 and 59.57 in 1950 to 73.32 in 1980; for females, from 37.5 years in 1945 and 62.97 in 1950 to 78.83 in 1980 (JICWELS 1983, 1). These figures are the highest in the world. Life expectancy at age 60 of 18.27 years for males and 21.96 years for females in 1980 may also be the highest in the world. As might be expected, available statistics indicate a dramatic improvement in the infant mortality rate during the twentieth century (Table 1). In 1900, the infant mortality rate was 155.0 per 1,000 births. By 1950, it had dropped to 60.1 (still quite high internationally), but, by 1980, it had dropped to 7.5 and to 6.6 in 1982—once again, among the best. As measured by these three indicators, therefore, the Japanese state of health is excellent, and various subjective assessments tend to agree. Moreover, all available evidence suggests that the Japanese people place a high priority on health status and that they have come to expect access to high-quality personal and public health services as one of the amenities of daily life in an advanced industrial society (Economic Planning Agency 1981).

Although one of two persons born in 1980 could expect to live to age 80, 722,792 deaths were also recorded. As indicated in Table 1, the flunctuation in the death rate per 1,000 persons after World War II from 14.6 in 1947 to 6.0 in 1982 in noteworthy. Although the fluctuations in the death rate from 7.6 to 6.2 per 1,000 persons between 1960 and 1980 was slight, the age distribution changed markedly. In 1955, of 690,000 deaths, 17.3 percent were fourteen years of age or below. In 1980, the ratio dropped to 2.9 percent and a corresponding decrease in the mortality rate for those aged 15 to 64 years from 38.6 percent to 27.5 percent was also recorded. By 1980, 69.6 percent of the deaths recorded were for persons 65 years or older, as compared with 44.1 percent in 1955 (JICWELS 1983, 2). The changing age distribution reflects the demographic changes in contemporary Japan as well as the sharp decrease in infant mortality and in tuberculosis-related deaths in the age group from 15 to 64.

For the first half of the century, pneumonia-bronchitis, gastroenteritis, and tuberculosis were the leading causes of death but, in keeping with the level of economic development, the so-called advanced country diseases have come to predominate. Cerebrovascular diseases were the leading cause of death beginning in 1960 and continued as the second leading cause of death in 1981 when cancer emerged as the leading killer. However, heart diseases, the third leading cause of death since 1960, have been on the rise, as has cirrhosis of the liver, which has increased by 81.6 percent over the same period and is now the eighth leading cause of death with a rate of 14.2 deaths per 100,000 persons in 1980.

Table 2 compares the leading causes of death in Japan in 1980 with recent figures from the United States, the United Kingdom, France, and West Germany. Interestingly, Japan compares quite favorably with those nations in terms of motor vehicle and other accidental deaths. The accident death rate has declined from 42.5 to 24.7 per 100,000 persons between 1970 and 1982 in spite of the spectacular increase in automobiles in recent times. Although the suicide rate in Japan of 17.7 per 100,000 persons in 1980 remains relatively high internationally,

Table 1
Trends in Vital Statistics, 1900–1982

Year	Live Births	Deaths	Natural Increase	Infant Mortality	Neonatal Deaths	Natural Stillbirths	Artificial Stillbirths	Perinatal Deaths
	(Per 1,000 Population)			(Per 1,000 Births)		(Per 1,000 Deliveries)		(Per 1,000 Live Births)
1900	32.4	20.8	11.6	155.0	79.0	–	–	–
1910	34.8	21.6	13.2	161.2	74.1	–	–	–
1920	36.2	25.4	10.8	165.7	69.0	–	–	–
1930	32.4	18.2	14.2	124.1	49.9	–	–	–
1940	29.4	16.5	12.9	90.0	38.7	–	–	–
1947	34.3	14.6	19.7	76.7	31.4	–	–	–
1950	28.1	10.9	17.2	60.1	27.4	41.7	43.2	46.6
1960	17.2	7.6	9.6	30.7	17.0	52.3	48.1	41.4
1970	18.8	6.9	11.8	13.1	8.7	40.6	24.7	11.7
1980	13.6	6.2	7.3	7.5	4.9	28.8	18.0	21.7
1981	13.0	6.1	6.9	7.1	4.7	28.8	20.5	10.8
1982	12.8	6.0	6.6	6.6	4.2	27.7	21.3	10.1

Source: Ministry of Health and Welfare, *Health and Welfare Services in Japan*, 1984, p. 72.

Table 2
Leading Causes of Death in Five Industrial Nations

Countries / Causes of death	Japan (1980)	U.S.A. (1977)	U.K. (1977)	France (1976)	West Germany (1978)
Total causes	622.0 [a]	877.9	1,172.5	1,051.6	1,179.3
Heart disease	106.3	327.2	379.1	200.2	335.1
Cancer	139.2	178.7	254.9	225.4	252.9
Cerebrovascular disease	139.7	84.1	149.3	141.0	166.0
Cirrhosis of the liver	14.2	14.3	3.7	32.9	27.6
Motor vehicle accidents	10.1	22.9	11.9	23.3	23.1
Other accidents	15.0	24.8	17.4	48.6	26.1
Suicides	17.7	13.3	8.0	15.8	22.2

[a]Number of deaths per 100,000 persons.
Source: Economic Planning Agency, Government of Japan, *In Search of a Good Quality of Life: Annual Report on National Life*, 1981, p. 107.

it is down from 21.6 per 100,000 persons in 1960 and postwar high of 25.7 in 1958 (Economic Planning Agency 1981, 109).

As might be expected from this brief review of mainly mortality-related data, statistics pertaining to morbidity rates and medical care utilization also reflect Japan's stage of economic development. The most important source of data is the annual National Health Survey *(Kohumin Kenkŏ Chŏsa)* conducted since 1953 by the Ministry of Health and Welfare *(Kŏseishŏ)*. In 1980, approximately 54,000 individuals from 16,000 households were interviewed between September 15 and 17 in order to estimate the extent of injury, disease, and use of medical services for the population as a whole. For present purposes, four general findings from the 1980 survey are relevant (Ministry of Health and Welfare 1981).

First, of the total number of households included in the sample, 25.9 percent reported one or more injured or diseased members (up from 25.8 percent in 1979), and 10 percent of those individuals interviewed reported personal injury or disease (also 10 percent in 1979). Given the morbidity or prevalence rate, estimated at 110.4 per 1,000 persons, it seems that one in every 9.1 Japanese was injured or ill in 1980. This figure has remained relatively stable for the past several years (Ministry of Health and Welfare 1981). Diseases of the circulatory system had the highest rate at 36.6 per 1,000 persons. Within that category, the rate of hypertensive disease was 24.1 per 1,000 persons. Diseases of the respiratory system (15.5) and diseases of the digestive system (14.4) were the next two highest disease categories reported.

Second, in terms of age bracket, the morbidity rate of 87.4 per 1,000 persons in the category from 0 to 4 years of age tapers off to a low of 30.2 in the category from 15 to 24 years of age, and then gradually rises to 437.3 in the 75 years of age and older bracket. Persons under 35 years of age reported the highest rate of diseases of the respiratory system; those between 35 and 44, digestive disorders; and persons 45 and above, diseases of the circulatory system. The overall morbidity rate was higher for females (117.8) than for males (102.6), and it was higher in large cities (121.7) than in smaller communities where morbidity rates ranged from 112.0 to 103.4.

Third, though seven of ten persons reported themselves in good health, only 1.3 percent indicated that they had received no medical treatment during the year of the survey. Of those receiving some sort of treatment, 87.5 percent went to hospitals or clinics, 8.8 percent purchased drugs at pharmacies, and 1.4 percent relied on massage, acupuncture, moxibustion, or Judo corrective exercises. Of the total, over 40 percent reported taking at least one type of medication in the month before the survey.

Fourth, the majority of those included in the 1980 survey (61.9 percent) reported that they had not been confined to bed during the survey year and 30.5 percent reported bed stays of from one to ten days. Needless to say, the older age groups reported more and longer bed stays, but the majority of individuals in all age categories, including those 75 years and older, reported no bed stays. The health-care needs and demands of Japan's rapidly aging population will be discussed in greater detail later.

Personal Health Services in Japan

Personal health services, or medical care, refers to the organization, financing, and delivery of diagnostic, curative, rehabilitative, and preventive services to individuals. In 1981, more personal health services were utilized than ever before, and the increasing incidence and prevalence of "advanced country illness" described above suggest that demand for services will continue to grow, particularly with respect to the middle-aged and elderly segment of the population. The system is pluralistic and incorporates traditional and modern components (Ohnuki-Tierney 1984, Broida 1980).

Kanpŏ, a traditional Japanese medicine of Chinese origin, has undergone extensive transformation since its introduction into Japan during the sixth century, and its basic treatment methods currently include plant and animal medicine, acupuncture, and moxibustion. At the time of the Meiji Restoration in 1868, *kanpŏ* practitioners outnumbered practitioners of the western style medicine that had been developing for roughly 200 years by at least five to one. However, the Meiji political leaders were determined to foster development of western science and technology in Japan and took steps in the 1870s that led to the official establishment of what is termed "biomedicine" (or sometimes, "cosmopolitan medicine") based on the European—mainly German—tradition. Although the several hundred *kanpŏ* practitioners in contemporary Japan have enjoyed a revival in demand for their services, biomedicine is firmly established as the dominant system. The fact that *kanpŏ* persists in contemporary Japan is significant. As pointed out by Ohnuki-Tierney,

> Perhaps the basic reason *kanpŏ* has not only survived oppression but has actually gained strength is that throughout its long history in Japan, the basic premises and principles of *kanpŏ*, as revealed by its diagnosis and treatment methods, have always been very close to the views held by most Japanese. To the Japanese public, *kanpŏ* does not appear as a distinct or alien system of medicine, but rather as an integral part of their own health maintenance practices. (1984, 91–92).

Ohnuki-Tierney also notes:

> *Kanpŏ* obviously is not a folk medicine. Despite its roots in the folk perception of health and illness, it has become a highly developed medical system effectively contributing to the health maintenance of the Japanese. It offers an effective alternative to biomedicine, since the two systems are almost ideally complementary; the weakness of one is the strength of the other. (1984, 122)

Kanpŏ and other alternatives are available in contemporary Japan, but most of the biomedically based services that constitute the mainstream are quite similar to those found in other advanced industrial societies. In 1981, more Japanese than ever before availed themselves of such services at the rate of 7,266 per 100,000 persons. As determined by the annual patient survey conducted by the Ministry of Health and Welfare on July 15 of that year, one in every 13.8 persons was receiving some type of medical care. A brief description of the mainstream providers, institutions, and financing mechanisms follows.

Providers of Personal Health Services

Since the official establishment of biomedicine in the 1870s, provision of medical services has been restricted to individuals and organizations designated by the state. This state-supported monopoly of medical practice is administered and enforced by government officials at the national and prefectural levels (Steslicke 1972). Currently, duly licensed physicians, dentists, pharmacists, nurses, public health nurses, midwives, physical therapists, and occupational therapists provide medical services according to national statutory guidelines in a division of labor that is physician dominated.

In 1981, there were 162,882 physicians, 56,841 dentists, 120,444 pharmacists,

18,633 public health nurses, 27,048 midwives, 548,534 nurses and assistant nurses, 3,045 physical therapists, and 1,089 occupational therapists (JICWELS 1983, 5). Although the physician and dentist ratio to population grew steadily as a result of national policy during the 1970s (there were 80 medical schools with an annual enrollment of 8,360 students in 1981), there remains a serious maldistribution with the public health services, and remote areas of the country are in short supply. Nurses, midwives, and especially public health nurses are also in short supply, and this is regarded as a serious problem calling for appropriate state intervention during the 1980s.

With respect to physicians in contemporary Japan, three points are important. First, as indicated in Table 3, in the annual survey conducted by the Ministry of Health and Welfare in 1980, only 1,633 physicians engaged in clinical practice reported their specialty as general practice; the remaining majority identified themselves with one of 29 other specialties. However, such specialties are self-reported, and there is no nationally recognized system of specialty training and registration. Second, physicians often advertise multiple specialties but most are actually engaged in general practice in both clinics and hospitals. Of the 1980 total physician population of 156,235, 148,815, or 93.3 percent were engaged in clinical practice, and, of that number, 65,114, or 41.7 percent were owners of hospitals or clinics. This means that, in 1980, 83,701 physicians in clinical practice, or 53.6 percent of the total, were salaried employees. Moreover, 24,879 (15.9 percent of the total physician population) were employed in medical school hospitals. Historically, private, solo, fee-for-service practice has been the dominant mode but, at present, the majority of Japanese physicians are salaried employees in both public and private hospitals and clinics. Third, Japanese physicians enjoy a relatively high socioeconomic status, but there is a growing sense of disenchantment with the medical mystique among health-care professionals and laypersons alike. As a result, physician power and influence at both individual and collective levels is being challenged by patients and public policymakers. Even the Japan Medical Association, which still has the greater majority of physicians as paying members at national and regional levels, finds itself in competition in the health policy arena with numerous other groups and individuals who refuse to accept that "doctor knows best" in the allocation of scarce resources (Steslicke 1982a).

Personal Health Services Organization

The Medical Service Law of July 30, 1948, as amended, provides a statutory basis for organization and delivery of personal health services throughout Japan. The law distinguishes between hospitals and clinics as the two basic units of organization by number of beds. Hospitals have twenty or more beds and clinics have nineteen or fewer. A general hospital is a facility of 100 or more beds that also meets certain other specifications. Hospitals and clinics must be managed by a physician regardless of ownership.

Table 3
Physicians by Speciality and Major Activity, 1980

		Major Professional Activity					
		Patient Care			Other Professional Activity		
Specialty	Total Physicians	Patient Care Total	Office-Based Practice	Hospital-Based Practice (Full-Time)	Teaching or Research Other Than Clinical Medicine	Administration and Public Health	Others
Total physicians	156,235	148,815	70,395	78,422	3,664	2,099	1,657
Internal medicine		24,571	6,827	17,744			
Respiratory		467	19	448			
Gastroenterology		946	123	823			
Cardiovascular disease		968	35	933			
Pediatrics		7,342	2,475	4,867			
Psychiatry		1,349	60	1,289			
Neurology		203	22	181			
Neurology (internal medicine)		463	9	454			
General surgery		10,406	563	9,843			
Orthopedics		5,418	781	4,637			
Plastic surgery		280	12	268			
Beauty surgery		11	8	3			
Brain-neurological surgery		2,025	11	2,014			
Respiratory surgery		92	—	92			
Cardiovascular surgery		347	—	347			
Pediatric surgery		236	33	203			
Obstetric-gynecology		8,422	3,697	4,725			
Obstetrics		28	4	24			
Gynecology		240	112	128			

Table 3 (continued)

Specialty	Total Physicians	Major Professional Activity: Patient Care			Other Professional Activity		
		Patient Care Total	Office-Based Practice	Hospital-Based Practice (Full-Time)	Teaching or Research Other Than Clinical Medicine	Administration and Public Health	Others
Total physicians	156,235	148,815	70,395	78,422	3,664	2,099	1,657
Ophthalmology		6,182	3,887	2,295			
Otorhinolaryngology		4,767	2,936	1,831			
Broncho-oesophagus		15	—	15			
Dermatology		2,460	869	1,591			
Urology		1,909	79	1,830			
Venereal diseases		8	6	2			
Anal		125	86	39			
X-ray therapy		125	6	119			
Radiology		1,508	43	1,465			
Anesthesia		1,645	15	1,630			
General practice		1,633	1,447	186			
Internal medicine and related specialties		33,493	23,906	9,587			
General surgery and related specialties		10,412	6,591	3,821			
Internal medicine and surgical specialties		19,375	15,567	3,808			
X-ray Therapy and Radiology		9	4	5			
Others		1,014	91	923			
Unknown		321	69	252			

Source: Masami Hashimoto, "Health Services in Japan," *Institute of Public Health*, pp. 365–66.

In 1980, there were 9,005 hospitals and 77,611 clinics (28,956 with and 48,655 without beds). Of the total number of hospitals, 8,003 qualified as general hospitals, 977 as mental hospitals, 39 as tuberculosis hospitals, 16 as leprosy hospitals, and 20 as infectious disease hospitals. There were 1,319,406 hospital beds in 1980 and 287,000 clinic beds giving Japan a bed-to-population ratio of 13.7:1,000 persons. A review of the statistics related to distribution of hospitals by type of ownership and the number of hospitals by specific type of control, number of beds, and average size indicates that there is a substantial public sector involvement in the delivery of personal health services. Indeed, public hospitals are of high quality and, historically, have been in the forefront in technical development. They command considerable respect in contemporary Japan. Nevertheless, the bulk of personal health services are delivered through the private sector (about 79 percent of all hospitals and 60 percent of all hospital beds, plus more than 90 percent of Japan's 77,000 clinics are privately owned and operated). Hospitals and clinics, both public and private, are highly competitive and offer very similar services. Since there are really no acute care hospitals as such and few special long-term care facilities, acute, chronic, short-term, inpatient, and outpatient care tends to be delivered in the same institutions—for young and old alike—with a resulting average length of stay in hospitals of 38.3 days in 1980. Most Japanese hospitals have not adopted an open-staff system. Thus, hospitals and clinics try to offer ''all-in-one'' medical services in order to keep patients (Ichijo and Kiikuni 1982). There are other peculiar features of health-care organization and delivery in Japan too numerous to mention here; however, Ohnuki-Tierney calls attention to one cultural twist in Japanese hospitalization worth noting:

> . . . the patient role in Japan reinforces individual identity, as well as each patient's identity as a social persona. This is indeed ironic, since Japanese culture is not known for its emphasis on the individual. In Japan, where one must usually wear a uniform from kindergarten all the way through high school, and formerly through the university, hospital patients use their own nightwear. The use of personal nightwear may seem trivial. However, its symbolic significance in the retention of the patient's individual identity becomes clear with increased understanding of the patient role in the Japanese medical system. Nightwear is one of the most welcome gifts to a patient, chosen especially by those who know the patient well. Attractive nightwear is thought to cheer the patient. The patient must change this clothing often, since it gets soiled, or symbolically polluted, by the sick body more quickly than usual. Extra nightclothes ease the work for the family, which usually is in charge of laundering them, and also make the patient presentable to visitors. (1984; 194–95)

Financing Personal Health Services

In describing the financing of personal health services in Japan, it is important to remember that cultural nuances can have an important bearing on costs and incentives that are not readily apparent. Perhaps the single most important feature of Japan's approach to personal health services is the system of comprehensive, universal, compulsory health insurance that has covered virtually the entire population since 1961. Based on the Health Insurance Law of 1922, the first of its kind in Asia, the system has grown incrementally to include other employment-based schemes for seamen, day laborers, teachers, and government workers. Individuals not covered by one of the employment-based schemes are entitled to coverage under the National Health Insurance Law of 1958, which requires that every city, town, or village in Japan offer health insurance to its residents and collect a special tax from those covered. Insurees are expected to share the costs of benefits with the appropriate community insurer and the national treasury.

The major features of the health insurance system are outlined in Table 4. It is unnecessary to go into the details of the various plans here except to note that there is a marked disparity in the level of benefits and cost-sharing between employment-based and community-based plans. Within the former category, members of society-managed plans tend to be much better off than members of government-managed schemes, many of which are chronically in the red (National Federation of Health Insurance Societies 1984). It is a complex system that reflects the politics of labor-management relations and the dual economy of modern Japan rather than the ideals of health-care planners for a more rational, efficient, and unified system. Although there have been numerous changes over the years, efforts to reform the system more fundamentally have been frustrated by the veto power exercised by the Japan Medical Association and other influential professional, labor, and management groups (Steslicke 1982b).

From the standpoint of the individual citizen, the health insurance system offers relatively free access to personal health services on an inpatient as well as on an outpatient basis and assurances that illness will not led to financial disaster. From the standpoint of the provider, the system guarantees that fees for service will be paid and that consumers will be encouraged to enter the market for services quite freely. Even though they benefit from the way it has operated in the past, providers tend to be highly critical of many aspects of the system. They particularly demand increased payments under the unit-point system and a loosening of the many restrictions on treatment practices in the national fee schedules. Still, neither providers nor consumers are as troubled as insurers and payers have been with the rise in overall medical expenditures during the past decade.

In Japan, as in the United States and in various other advanced industrial nations, cost containment has become a major concern. The situation is less urgent in Japan than in the United States, but it is being taken very seriously. By 1980, the rapid growth of medical care costs reached 12,000,000 yen, an estimated 5.01 percent of the GNP and 6.18 percent of the national income (JICWELS 1983, 10). It was of small comfort to concerned Japanese that their figures remained relatively lower since they realized that certain hidden costs were not revealed by their accounting system. For example, the traditional Japanese practice of gift giving is followed by many patients in dealing with physicians, and the resulting transfer of cash or merchandise over and above the prescribed insurance fee for service may increase overall medical expenditures by as much as 15 percent. As indicated in one recent Japanese assessment:

> During the period of high economic growth it was possible for the expanding economy to absorb the increase in medical care costs and they were not a matter of concern. However, following the oil shock, and even when the economy reverted to stable growth, medical care costs continued to rise at a faster pace than economic growth. (JICWELS 1983, 10)

In brief, it is not simply the rapid increase in medical costs but also the changing economic and demographic circumstances that have put cost containment on the national agenda.

How is the burden of medical costs distributed in contemporary Japan? According to one Health and Welfare Ministry estimate, in 1980 the national treasury's share was 30.5 percent of total medical care costs, and local governments contributed 2.9 percent of the total. Employer contributions of 23.8 percent and insuree contributions of 30.7 percent meant that 54.5 percent of total medical care costs were covered through the health insurance system, and 88.2 percent of the total by combined state and insurance system contribution. Thus, the direct patient share was ll.8 percent of the total (a share that has steadily declined from 20.6 percent in 1965 to 12.9 percent in 1975 to 10.8 percent in 1981) (JICWELS 1983, 10). Whether or not a redistribution of the burden is desirable or even possible is highly controversial, but increased patient cost-sharing is being supported in business and government circles. The principle has been incorporated into recent health insurance legislation of 1983 and 1984 despite fierce resistance. Rationalization of medical care costs in the 1980s has precipitated a struggle between various forces in Japanese society, and the strategy of state intervention developed during the happier days of high economic growth is changing accordingly.

Public Health Administration and Services

The form, content, and degree of state involvement in the organization, delivery, and financing of personal and public health services in modern Japan have changed over time more or less in keeping with the emphasis on economic and industrial development and on catching up with the advanced western nations. Since the early 1870s, government officials at national and regional levels have played an important role in health policy development and administration, and the line between public and private was not clearly drawn. At the national level, the Ministry of Health and Welfare (MHW) has exercised major responsibility for health administration since its establishment in 1938, but its jurisdiction is by no means exclusive. It shares responsibility with a number of other governmental agencies.

Table 4
Outline of Health Insurance, 1983

Scheme			Insured Persons	Insurer
Employee's Insurance	Health Insurance	Government-managed Health Insurance	Employees at places of work where health insurance societies are not established (small and medium size enterprises)	State
		Society-managed Health Insurance	Employees at places of work where health insurance societies are established	Health Insurance Societies 1,703
	Seamen's Insurance		Seamen (on designated vessels)	State
	Day Labourers' Health Insurance		Day Labourers { Employed on day-to-day basis, for fixed time less than 2 months, etc.	State
	Mutual Aid Association Insurance	National Public Service MAAs	National public service employees	25 MAAs
		Local Public Service MAAs	Local public service employees	54 MAAs
		Public Corporation Employees MAAs	Employees of Japan National Railway, the Salt and Tobacco Monopoly, and Nippon Telephone and Telegraph	3 MAAs
		Private School Teachers and Employees MAA	Private School teachers and employees	1 MAA
Community Health Insurance	National Health Insurance		Those not covered by employees' insurance (agricultural workers, self-employed, construction workers, doctors, employees at small scale places of work)	Cities, Towns, Villages 3,272 National Health Insurance Associations 169

Insurance Benefits				Financial Resources	
Medical Care Benefits			Cash Benefits	Insurance Contribution	State Subsidy
Medical Benefits	Dependants Medical Expenses	High-Cost Medical Care			
100% some cost-sharing	In-patient 80% Out-patient 70%	Note: Patient cost-sharing ¥51,000 For low income persons, excess of ¥15,000	Injury and Sickness Allowance Maternity Allowance Childbirth Expenses	8.5% special benefits contribution — 1% (November, 1981)	16.4% of benefit costs
100% (as above)	In-patient 80% Out-patient 70% supplementary benefits exist		As above supplementary benefits exist	7.947% (average for all societies, 1980)	¥1,500 million as benefit cost assistance (1982)
100% (as above)	In-patient 80% Out-patient 70%	As above	As above	8.2% (April, 1982)	¥2,700 million as benefit cost assistance (1982)
100% (as above)	70%	Cost-sharing of ¥39,000	As above	Special Grade 1 — ¥20 per day Grades 1~8 — ¥60~¥660 per day	35% of benefit costs plus ¥600 million fixed sum (1982)
100% (as above)	In-patient 80% Out-patient 70%	As for Health Insurance	As above (supplementary benefits exist)	6.05 ~ 11.85% (April, 1981)	None
70% (both head of household and members) (benefit rate can be raised)		Cost-sharing ¥51,000; ¥39,000 for low income persons	Midwifery Expenses · Funeral Expenses Nursing Allowance (optional)		45% of medical care costs plus temporary grant for financial adjustment 25 ~ 40% of medical care costs plus temporary adjustment assistance grant

Source: JICWELS, *Trends and Policies of Health Services in Japan: Rationalizing Medical Care Costs*, p. 24.

In broad functional terms, Japanese national health administration is usually divided into three main categories: general health administration, school health administration, and industrial health administration. Environmental protection should probably be added as a fourth functional category. In each of these areas, state intervention has led to the emergence of a complex administrative apparatus that is likely to grow in the 1980s in spite of the ''administrative reform'' policies embraced by recent governments.

Overall responsibility for environmental protection is assigned to the Environmental Agency, headed by a director-general with the rank of minister of state. Established in 1971, the agency is divided into a number of bureaus and departments that employed over 900 officials in 1981. Ancillary bodies include the Central Council for Environmental Pollution Control and the National Institute for Environmental Studies. As a result of the flurry of legislative activity in the late 1960s and early 1970s, the agency administers a relatively complete set of environmental laws, the cornerstone of which is the Basic Law for Environmental Pollution Control of 1967 as amended (Reich 1983). According to Article 4 of the Basic Law,

> The State has the responsibility to establish fundamental and comprehensive policies for environmental control and to implement them, in view of the fact that it has the duty to protect the people's health and conserve the living environment.

State responsibility is made even more explicit in Articles 10 and 17, which relate to emission control, control of land use and installation of facilities, establishment of surveillance and monitoring systems, dissemination of knowledge and information, and similar matters. The law also requires submission of an annual report and an implementation statement to the National Diet.

State involvement in industrial or occupational health and safety has also become quite extensive in the postwar period. At the national level, the Ministry of Labor has been assigned primary responsibility for implementing the relevant sections of the Labor Standards Law, the Workmen's Accident Compensation Insurance Law, the Industrial Safety and Health Law, the Working Environment Monitoring Law, the Pneumoconiosis Law, and other rules and regulations dealing with detection, prevention, compensation, and research related to work and health. Since 1960, there has been a steady decrease in work-related injuries for which the ministry's five-year Industrial Injury Prevention Programs can claim some credit. During the 1980, the degree of state commitment to maintain or improve occupational safety and health will be put to the test, and the special requirements of middle-aged and older workers will be of great concern.

At the other end of the age scale and life cycle, state involvement in school health activities has also increased in the postwar period, and the Ministry of Education, Science and Culture has become the main national administrative agent, with the ministry's Physical Education Bureau bearing major responsibility. The ministry is also involved through the Medical Education Division of its Higher Education Bureau (Sakuma 1978).

With the environmental, industrial, and school health exceptions noted, general health administration is centered in the MHW. Established as a result of pressure from the Japanese military leadership shortly before World War II and reorganized under the aegis of the Supreme Commander for the Allied Powers during the occupation of Japan, the MHW was organized into nine bureaus, two departments, and one separate agency as of 1980. It was also responsible for 19.1 percent of the total national budget in 1980. Basically, the MHW is involved in four types of programs: public health and medical care; social welfare and public aid; social insurance; and education, research, and information gathering.

Of the total number of national laws under the jurisdiction of the MHW, well over 100 deal with public health and medical care. According to one audit, 9 deal with disease prevention, 25 with environmental health, 11 with general public health administration and health statistics, 14 with medical care organization and personnel, and 9 with pharmaceutical affairs. Not included here are the various social and health insurance laws. The MHW oversees the administrative and programmatic activities of perfectural, city, town, and village governments related to personal and public health services as well as the extensive system of health centers. It also plays an important role in health planning at the national and regional levels. Though part of a complex and overlapping system of organization and programs, the MHW is the most visible and concrete manifestation of the Japanese state in contemporary health administration.

In summary, the Japanese state was engaged in the following basic activities related to health care at the beginning of the 1980s: development of plans, programs, and policies; regulation of services and providers; provision of services; financing and subsidization of services and providers; research, education, and information gathering; and integration and coordination of health and medical affairs with other state activities and priorities. It is not possible to describe how these health-related state activities are organized at the prefectural and local levels in detail. However, a brief look at Japan's health center network will provide a basic understanding of public health services delivery in the postwar era.

The contemporary health center network is based on the Health Center Law of 1947, a complete revision of the 1937 statute that established the prewar network through which public health services were delivered throughout Japan. At present, Japan is divided into 47 prefectures, which are further subdivided into cities, towns, and villages. The 1947 law requires all prefectures and 30 larger municipal governments to establish and maintain health centers on the basis of 1 per 100,000 persons. In 1980, the actual rate was 1 per 136,000 persons, and a total of 855 health centers were in operation—655 prefectural, 144 municipal, and 53 Tokyo Metropolitan. Of these, 275 were classified as urban, 98 as urban-rural, 320 as rural, 128 as L (a small population in a large area), and 34 as S (an area of less than 30,000 population).

The legally prescribed functions of the health centers are as follows: (1) control of communicable diseases including preventive vaccination; (2) prevention of tuberculosis by mass medical examinations, detailed examinations, and medical aid; (3) control of venereal diseases; (4) control of other diseases, e.g., trachoma parasitic diseases, and degenerative diseases; (5) promotion of mental health; (6) maternal and child health (health guidance for pregnant women, nursing mothers, and babies and infants, medical guidance for handicapped children, mothers' classes, and so on); (7) consultation on eugenic protection; (8) dental hygiene; (9) improvement of nutrition; (10) food, milk, and meat sanitation; (11) rabies prevention; (12) maintenance of environmental sanitation (houses, hotels, public bathhouses, entertainment facilities such as theaters, laundries, barbershops, beauty parlors, garbage and waste disposal, water supply, sewage disposal, and graveyards); (13) matters related to environmental pollution; (14) medical affairs; (15) public health nurse activities such as home visits and health education; (16) medical social work; (17) public health laboratory service; (18) maintenance of health and vital statistics; and (19) public health education (Ministry of Health and Welfare 1981). Of course, the performance of these legally prescribed functions varies, and it is affected by personnel shortages and funding priorities. However, the health center record is, in most respects, impressive.

According to one leading Japanese authority,

> During the first decade after the war—when urbanization and industrialization were hardly noticeable due to the destruction of the war, and health activity of cities, towns, and villages was very weak—health centers contributed remarkably to the improvement of community health, especially in communicable disease control, maternal and child health, nutrition, tuberculosis control, food and sanitary inspection, public health nursing, health education, and so on. Afterwards, however, particularly since the 1960s, the country underwent drastic socioeconomic changes, and there have been notable shifts in community health and demands due to the changes of disease patterns and different modes of living of the people. (Hashimoto 1984, 356–57)

Thus, revision of the public health services delivery system in keeping with changing economic and demographic circumstances is also on the national health policy agenda during the 1980s, and bold efforts are under way to coordinate and integrate both state and privately supported public health, personal health, and welfare services and programs. The developing health and medical services system for the elderly is generally regarded as the first step in that direction.

Health and Medical Services for the Elderly

As a relative latecomer in the industrialization process, Japan has had a number of advantages in the international marketplace. Among them is the fact that, during the period of recovery and high economic growth in the 1960s and 1970s, Japan has had a young population and a healthy work force, as well as a comparatively small dependent elderly population. By 1980, the proportion of Japan's

Table 5
Trends in National Medical Care Costs for the Elderly, 1973–1982

(Units: ¥100,000,000, %)

Year	National Medical Care Costs	Rate of Increase	Medical Care Costs for the Elderly	Rate of Increase	Ratio of Medical Care Costs for the Elderly per National Medical Care Costs
1973	39,496	–	4,289	–	10.8
1974	53,786	36.2	6,652	55.1	12.4
1975	64,779	20.4	8,666	30.3	13.4
1976	76,684	18.4	10,780	24.4	14.1
1977	85,685	11.7	12,872	19.4	15.0
1978	100,042	16.8	15,948	23.9	15.9
1979	109,510	9.5	18,503	16.0	16.9
1980	119,805	9.4	21,269	14.9	17.8
1981	128,600	7.3	23,753	11.7	18.5
1982	138,800	7.9	26,903	13.3	19.4

Source: JICWELS, *Trends and Policies of Health Services in Japan: Rationalizing Medical Care Costs*, p. 19.

population 65 years and older was only 9.1 percent (compared with 11.2 percent in the United States and over 14 percent in France, Great Britain, West Germany, and Sweden). Therefore, there has been less urgency in dealing with the special problems of the elderly than elsewhere (Tominaga 1983). Unfortunately for Japan, the burden of caring for an aging and elderly population is increasing as the prospect of a population of 65 years and over of from 18 percent to 21 percent by the year 2015 lies ahead. The traditional spirit of "respect for the elderly" *(keirŏ)* is an important cultural asset, but it will be severely strained in the struggle to accommodate the needs and demands of a rapidly aging society (Steslicke 1984).

The institution of a program of virtually free personal health services for the 70 years and older population (65 years and older if bedridden) in 1973 was an expression of *keirŏ* made possible by the coming together of "Growth Japan" and "Welfare Japan," plus a "substantial commitment of political energy (Campbell 1984). The figures presented in Table 5 indicate why this remarkably generous program barely survived the 1970s. Not only did the ratio of medical care costs for the elderly soar from 10.8 percent of total national costs in 1973 to 19.4 percent in 1982, but also the burden was unevenly distributed. The national health insurance system managed by local authorities was particularly hard hit in assuming over 30 percent of the burden by 1980. While financial distress provided the most important reason for change, inappropriate utilization of personal health services and underutilization of public health services by the aging and elderly population were also seen as urgent problems by health policymakers. After several years of study and planning in both government and private health policy circles, "political energy" sufficient to enact a new Health and Medical Services for the Aged (*Rǒjin hoken-hǒ*) was finally generated in August 1982. The new system of health and medical services for the elderly depicted in Figure 1 was put into operation in 1983.

While there may be room for skepticism regarding the motives of some of the participants in the policymaking process and the extent to which the "spirit of *keirǒ*" served as a guiding light, the capacity of the Japanese state to act in a highly complex and sensitive area of economic and social life is impressive. It is too early to begin to evaluate the results, of course, but the organization and goals of the new system are also quite impressive. Writing in 1975, Steven Jonas quite accurately observed:

> The Japanese health services system is a complex one. It bears many similarities to the health care systems of the large Western capitalist countries. At the same time, as one would expect, there are significant differences as well. For the most part, as in the West, there is a rather high degree of organizational and functional separation between the preventive, treatment, and rehabilitative services. (1975, 58).

In essence, the goal of the new health and medical services system for the elderly in Japan is to integrate and coordinate prevention, treatment, and rehabilitation as well as welfare services, and thereby surpass the separation and fragmentation of services that prevail in the west. The fact that the elderly are being asked to assume some degree of cost-sharing for personal health services may not be onerous in the long run.

The Health Policy Agenda in Contemporary Japan

The major components in the delivery of personal and public health services in Japan (in spite of the separation and fragmentation noted above) are interrelated and may be thought of as a *system*. This is not to suggest that the health-care system is self-contained and fully capable of generating changes from within. On the contrary, the health-care system in Japan has proved to be highly responsive to its broader economic and political environment, and to national priorities that are determined through the political process. Setting the health policy agenda was relatively simple when national priorities called for "more of the same" as they did for roughly 20 years, beginning in the early 1960s. Accordingly, the strategy of state intervention was to balance the interests of various organized groups while also attempting to improve the general level of health. By the mid-1970s, however, "more of the same" became problematic and social policy priorities became subject to extensive reexamination. Changing economic and demographic circumstances at home and changes in the international economic order forced policymakers in Japan to intervene in the health-care system in keeping with their desire to strengthen the nation's capacity to produce goods and services competitively. "Welfare Japan" could not be al-

Figure 1
Organization of Health and Medical Services for the Elderly, 1984

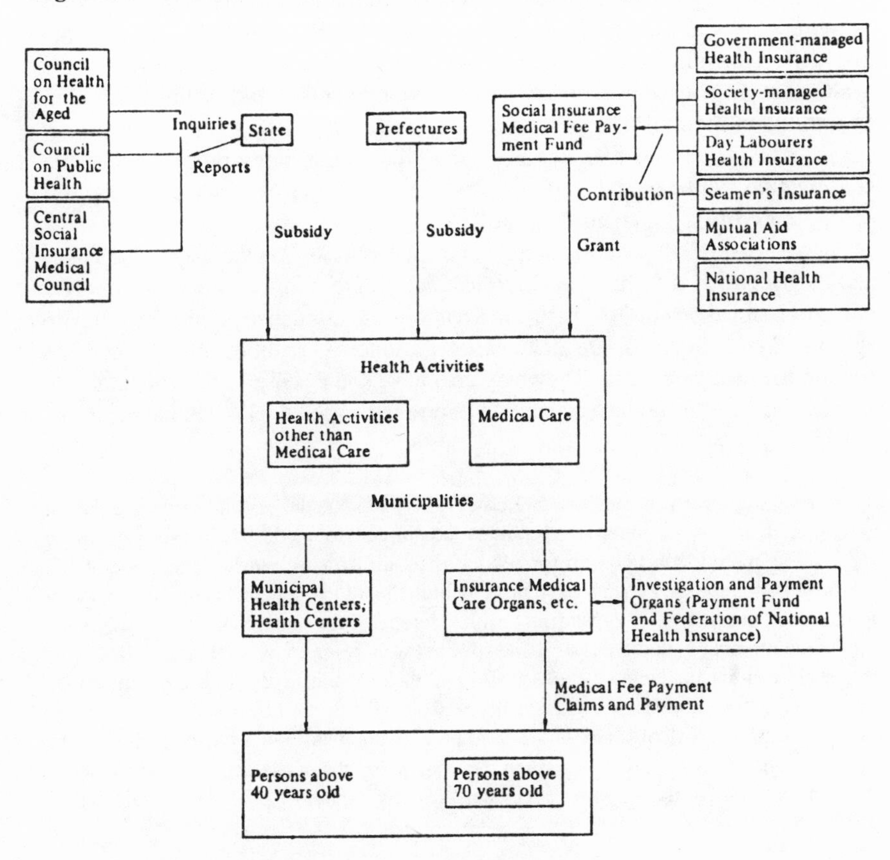

N.B. The contents of health activities other than medical care are as follows.

Issuance of Health Notebooks
Health Education
Health Consultation
Health Examination – General Health Examination – Cancer Examination
(General Examination
(Detailed Examination
(Visiting Health Examination
(Stomach Cancer
(Uterine Cancer
Therapy
Visiting Guidance

Source: Ministry of Health and Welfare, *Guide to Health and Welfare Services in Japan 1984*, p. 24.

lowed to destroy ''Growth Japan.'' Reforming the way in which personal and public health services were organized, financed, and delivered was placed on the national policy agenda in the 1980s.

What has been accomplished? Perhaps the major accomplishment of the reform effort was the enactment of the Health and Medical Services for the Aged Law in 1982. Skeptics have dismissed the changes introduced by the new legislation as more symbolic than tangible. Supporters of the new approach see it as the first step in the direction of more comprehensive and fundamental change in the health-care system with emphasis on disease prevention and health promotion as well as on high-technology curative services. They also see the new law as consistent with the self-help and beneficiary-pay ethos being propagated by the conservative political and corporate establishment—as well as a meaningful short-term cost-containment measure.

For MHW officials, ''rationalizing medical care costs'' is the major challenge, and they feel that they have made significant progress in a number of areas. As the professional agents of state intervention and guidance in the health-care system, they have a hardheaded sense of economic realities and the need to contain medical care costs. They may also have some sense of the essential role of medical care in modern Japan. As expressed in the MHW annual report of 1982:

> . . . when the problem of medical care costs is considered, the essential role of medical care should not be forgotten. Expenditure committed to medical care should not be regarded as merely consumption for service. It is difficult to translate the value of life and health into monetary terms, but quite a lot of the input into medical care is contributing to improved productivity by restoring health. Moreover, the magnitude of medical care's role in maintaining both the physical and spiritual well-being of the individual, the family and society is incalculable. . . . every effort is to be made in the future to rationalize medical care costs, but for the reasons given above it is not felt desirable to plan for the indiscriminate control of all costs. The important thing is to rigorously eliminate the injustices and improper practices within the system and the waste caused by inefficiency while at the same time investing adequately for the required medical care. (JICWELS 1983, 15).

In the effort to reach the official target for ''Health for All by the Year 2000,'' World Health Organization members should carefully examine the Japanese experience in establishing ''minimum standards of wholesome and cultured living'' and the role of the state in ''the promotion and extension of social welfare and security, and of public health'' as prescribed in Article 25 of the constitution. The interrelationship between health and economic development discussed by participants in the Alma-Ata Conference of 1978 is illustrated by the Japanese case (World Health Organization 1978). To the extent that agents of the Japanese state retain their commitment to the essential role of health and medical care during the 1980s and beyond, the Japanese people will be well served even though ''production first'' continues as the basis for economic and social policies.

References

Bennett, John W. and Solomon B. Levine. 1976. Industrialization and Social Deprivation: Welfare, Environment, and the Postindustrial Society in Japan. In *Japanese Industrialization and Its Social Consequences*, ed. Hugh Patrick, 439–92. Berkeley: University of California Press.

Broida, Joel H. 1980. Medical Technology in Japan. In *The Management of Health Care Technology in Ten Countries*, eds. D. Banta and K. Kemp, 77–91. Washington, D.C.: Congress of the United States, Office of Technology Assessment.

Campbell, John Creighton. 1984. Problems, Solutions, Non-Solutions, and Free Medical Care for the Elderly in Japan. *Pacific Affairs* 57, 1 (Spring): 53–64.

Campbell, Ruth. 1984. Nursing Homes and Long-term Care in Japan. *Pacific Affairs* 57, 1 (Spring 1984): 78–89.

Economic Planning Agency, Government of Japan. 1973. *Basic Economic and Social Plan*. 1973–1977. Ministry of Finance.

Economic Planning Agency, Government of Japan. 1981. *In Search of a Good Quality of Life: Annual Report on National Life 1981*. Ministry of Finance.

Economic Planning Agency, Government of Japan. 1982. *Quality of the Environment in Japan 1981*. Health, Welfare and Environment Problems Research Society.

Goldsmith, Seth B. 1984a. Hospitals and the Elderly in Japan. *Pacific Affairs* 57, 1 (Spring 1984): 74–77.

Goldsmith, Seth B. 1984b. *Theory Z Hospital Management: Lessons from Japan*. Rockville, Md.: Aspen Systems Corporation.

Hashimoto, Masami. 1981. National Health Administration in Japan. *Bulletin of the Institute for Public Health*, Vol 30, pp. 1–36.

Hashimoto, Masami. 1984. Health Services in Japan. In *Comparative Health Systems*, ed. Marshall W. Raffel, 335–70. University Park: Penn State Press.

Ichijo, Katsuo and Kenzo Kiikuni. 1982. Health Services in Japan. *Japan-Hospitals: The Journal of the Japan Hospital Association* 1: 3–20.

Japan International Corporation of Welfare Services (JICWELS). 1983. *Trends and Policies of Health Services in Japan: Rationalizing Medical Care Costs*. JICWELS.

Japan Institute of Labor. 1982. *Japanese Industrial Relations Series: Industrial Safety and Health*. Stanford, Calif.: Japan Institute of Labor.

Johnson, Chalmers. 1982. *MITI and the Japanese Miracle: The Growth of Industrial Policy, 1925–1975*. Stanford, Calif.: Stanford University Press.

Jonas, Steven. 1975. The District Health Center in Japan: History, Services, and Future Development. *American Journal of Public Health* 65, 1 (January): 58–62.

Lock, Margaret M. 1980. *East Asian Medicine in Urban Japan*. Berkeley: University of California Press.

Lock, Margaret M. 1984. East Asian Medicine and Health Care for the Japanese Elderly. *Pacific Affairs* 57, I (Spring): 65–73.

Macrae, Norman. 1974. Health Care International. *The Economist* 291, 7339 (April 28): 17–35.

Ministry of Health and Welfare. 1981. *Guide to Health and Welfare Services in Japan 1981*. Health and Welfare Problems Research Society. Tokyo.

Ministry of Health and Welfare. 1981. *Outline of the 1980 National Health Survey*. Tokyo: Foreign Press Center.

Ministry of Health and Welfare. 1984. *Guide to Health and Welfare Services in Japan 1984*. Tokyo: JICWELS.

National Federation of Health Insurance Societies (KEMPOREN). 1984. *Health Insurance and Health Insurance Societies in Japan 1984*. Tokyo: KEMPOREN.

Ohnuki-Tierney, Emiko. 1984. *Illness and Culture in Contemporary Japan: An Anthropological View*. New York: Cambridge University Press.

Ohtani, Fujio, ed. 1971. *One Hundred Years of Health Progress in Japan*. Tokyo: International Medical Foundation of Japan.

Organization for Economic Cooperation and Development. 1976. *Towards an Integrated Social Policy in Japan*. Paris: OECD.

Reich, Michael R. 1983. Environmental Policy and Japanese Society: Part I. Successes and Failures. *International Journal of Environmental Studies*, Vol 20, pp. 191–198.

Sakuma, Mitsuru. 1978. School Education in Japan. *Social Science and Medicine* 12, 6A (November): 551–554.

Steslicke, William E. 1972. Doctors, Patients, and Government in Modern Japan. *Asian Survey* 12, 11 (November): 913–31.

Steslicke, William E. 1982a. National Health Policy in Japan: From the "Age of Flow" to the "Age of Stocks." *Bulletin of the Institute of Public Health* 31, 1: 1–35.

Steslicke, William E. 1982b. Development of Health Insurance Policy in Japan. *Journal of Health Politics, Policy and Law* 7, 1 (Spring): 197–226.

Steslicke, William E. 1982c. Medical Care in Japan: The Political Context. *Journal of Ambulatory Care Management* 5, 4 (November): 65–77.

Steslicke, William E. 1984. An International Perspective on Health Care: Learning from Japan. *International Perspective on Health Care: Learning from Other Nations: Hearing Before the Select Committee on Aging, House of Representatives, 98 Congress, Second Session, Comm. Pub. No. 98–450*. Washington, D.C.: U. S. Government Printing Office.

Tominaga, Ken'ichi. 1983. Japan's Industrial Society at Critical Turn: Advantages Are Fading. *The Oriental Economist* (January): 32–39.

World Health Organization. 1978. *Primary Health Care: Report of the International Conference on Primary Health Care, Alma-Ata, USSR, 6–12 September 1978*. Geneva: WHO.

MOZAMBIQUE

Diana Jelley, Adrienne Epstein, and Paul Epstein

Health Profile

Mozambique, formerly one of Portugal's African colonies, gained independence in 1975 following more than a decade of armed struggle against the colonial power. The health-care system is Mozambique today reflects both the legacy of the colonial period and the experiences of the years of war, as well as the socioeconomic and political priorities of the present government.

Mozambique is a developing country in southern Africa with a population of about 12 million, of whom 800,000 live in the capital city, Maputo. The rural population, which comprises 90 percent of the total, is largely located in scattered communities without public services. The health status of Mozambique's population is similar to or even lower than that found in most Third World populations and, as such, reflects the country's low level of economic development. Fifty percent of the total population is under 15 years of age, and high infant, childhood, and maternal mortality rates contribute to an average life expectancy of approximately from 40–45 years. Detailed information relating to disease incidence and mortality rates of the total population is not available for the colonial period. Quite simply, such information was not of interest to the colonial state. Data collection was confined to the urban, European population. Since independence, considerable attention has been given to the collection of accurate data on mortality rates and disease incidence, but the paucity of resources and the scattered nature of the population limits this initiative. Such statistics as are available are presented in Tables 1 and 2.

Despite the lack of accurate data, it is clear that infectious diseases and diseases directly associated with malnutrition are the key issues in Mozambique's health profile. Recent estimates suggest that measles cause a third of the deaths of those

Table 1
Mortality Rates, 1980

	Category	Estimated Value
1.	Infant Mortality	70-100/1000 live births in Maputo 140-150/1000 live births in Mozambique
2.	Neonatal Mortality	40-50/1000 live born children
3.	Maternal Mortality	300-400 women death/100,000 live born children
4.	Birth Rate	45/1000 women 15-45 yrs

Source: Joint WHO/*UNICEF JCHP* Study, "Country Decision-Making for the Achievement of the Objective of Primary Health Care—Report from the People's Republic of Mozambique," Maputo, 1980.

under five years of age; diarrhea, pneumonia, malnutrition, and prematurity are also of principal importance. As well as being a primary cause of death among the very young, malnutrition causes anemia, blindness, skin infections, and neurological disorders. The overriding nutritional problem, however, for both children and adults is a general insufficiency of protein and calorie intake. WHO estimates, in 1980, suggested malnutrition rates in the whole country of between 25 to 30 percent. It is likely that the nutritional status of the majority of the population has considerably worsened over the last years due to the widespread disruption of agricultural production and destruction of transport systems resulting from the ongoing war with South African–backed guerrillas.

Infectious diseases also take a major toll, and the effects of many of these illnesses are much more severe in the malnourished person. Parasites such as giardia, hookworm, ascaris, and schistosomiasis are common to all ages in the Mozambican population. Gastroenteritis, anemia, or urinary tract infection is frequently the cause of debility and ill health. Airborne diseases such as tuberculosis, measles, and meningitis spread readily in the densely populated, poorly serviced, periurban areas, and the incidence of these conditions remains high although the institution of vaccination programs has helped to reduce the incidence of measles. Other widespread endemic diseases include malaria, leprosy, sleeping sickness, respiratory infections, and scabies. Outbreaks of typhoid and cholera occasionally occur (authors' personal clinical experience).

Table 2
Disease Incidences, 1980

	Condition	Prevalence
1.	Malnutrition*	25-30% of families in typical rural community. 30% of children under 12 underdeveloped with respect to weight and height.
2.	Malaria	53-5% parasite index 1976.
3.	Bilharziasis	Infection rate of 80% in children less than 12 years.
4.	Tuberculosis	200-250/100,000 people (new cases)
5.	Intestinal Parasites	(All common - no information on precise incidences)
6.	Measles	
7.	Tetanus	
8.	Diarrhoeal Diseases	
9.	Leprosy	

*Defined as an energy intake less than 1.2 times the basal metabolic rate.
Source: Joint WHO/*UNICEF JCHP* Study, "Country Decision-Making for the Achievement of the Objective of Primary Health Care–Report from the People's Republic of Mozambique," Maputo, 1980.

Dental health systems also differ from those found in developed countries. Oral tuberculosis and cancrum oris are relatively common and often require lengthy medical treatment. Dental caries are less common than in the west—one survey showed that only 28 percent of the Mozambican children have one decayed adult tooth at the age of twelve, compared to 93 percent of a similar sample in the U.K. (Hobdell 1984). However, the incidence of dental caries appears to be rising with the increased availability of refined sugar, which occurred after the country gained independence. Gingivitis occurs more commonly in Mozambique than in developing countries, possibly reflecting poorer standards of dental hygiene and nutrition.

Cardiovascular and degenerative diseases also make their contribution to mortality and morbidity, and they are predominantly seen in the urban populations who have an increased life expectancy but also a greater incidence of cigarette and alcohol consumption as well as obesity.

Historical Overview

The health-care system in Mozambique is based on both a knowledge of the principal health problems and an understanding of the major determinants of health. Health care is thus a very broad-based concept that seeks to tackle not only the end results of disease processes, but also to identify and prevent, where possible, the causes of disease.

Health care under Portuguese rule in Mozambique reflected the geographical, racial, and economic discrimination of the colonial system. There was a total bias of service provision in favor of the white urban elite, against the black rural population. Seventy percent of all the doctors worked in the capital, and all modern hospital facilities were found in the three largest cities. The few district hospitals and health centers that existed were grossly inadequate in terms of staffing, equipment, and drugs. Health care was curative; virtually no preventive activities were carried out. Health care was available not to those who needed it most but to those who could afford to pay.

During the years of the armed struggle, provision of basic health care accessible to the whole population became one of the first aims of Frelimo. Resources were very limited, but vaccination campaigns were carried out and rudimentary health posts were set up throughout the liberated areas. These served as focal points not only for treatment, but also for health education and the spread of ideas about disease prevention, the use of latrines, and so on. The experiences of the war years had illustrated the relative uselessness of high technological solutions to medical problems in the face of malnutrition and widespread infectious disease. The importance of popular participation both in treating the wounded and improving the level of health in the community was stressed. Volunteers were recruited from the local population to be taught basic first aid skills by the few available trained nurses. Minor wounds could be treated locally; major casualties were transported to Tanzanian or Zambian border hospitals. Peasants in the liberated villages distributed drugs, built health posts, and provided food for soldiers and patients. The basic principle of the involvement of the mass of the population in the organization and sustenance of health services, plus the emphasis on preventive activities, laid the groundwork for the development of Primary Health Care (PHC) as the major thrust of health policy in independent Mozambique.

Mozambique's decision to emphasize PHC as its major strategy in developing a health-care system can be clearly seen as a key aspect of its overall aim to transform the socioeconomic base of society. The development of Mozambique's health-care system is a fundamental reorientation of the total socioeconomic system to place a higher value on the needs of the less well-off. The health-care system itself is thus but one element in the intersectoral approach to improving the health status of the population.

Mozambican Health-Care System

The present health-care system in Mozambique evolved following a series of major legislative acts. The first task of the Ministry of Health was to create a national health system. Less than one month after independence, the government nationalized all health services, and private medical practice was abolished. The approach to primary health care which had been initiated during the armed struggle continued to evolve, and it was articulated as an overall policy in 1977 when the Law of the Socialization of Medicine was enacted. This law provided the legal basis for the development of PHC and the provision of health care which was free or virtually free at the point of delivery. This law also established a referral structure for the health service that is discussed below.

The Third Congress of Frelimo that took place in 1977 laid down policies for future development. The organization of a health system that benefited the whole population was made a fundamental task of Frelimo. This was to be achieved by extending the national health service to all parts of the country, giving priority to preventive medicine but not neglecting curative care, and developing a national policy to combat communicable diseases (Central Committee Report to the Third Congress, 1977).

The Fourth Congress, which took place in 1983, reviewed the progress in health-care delivery. Health service institutions had increaaed in number to such an extent that the number of people per health unit had decreased from 16,200 to 11,600. Preventive medicine had been practiced by increasing vaccination uptake, by building latrines and rubbish dumps, and by extending and improving maternal and child health services. Infant mortality in the urban centers was recorded as having dropped from 150 to 80 per 1000 live births.

The state administration system for all sectors including health is organized into eleven provinces (Maputo City has recently been given the status of province). The provinces are divided into districts, and are further subdivided into localities. The Ministry of Health is located in Maputo, and each provincial capital has its own health administration, plus district-level administrators. The immediate post-independence task of the Ministry of Health was to ascertain the numbers of health institutions still functioning, and to determine how many medical personnel remained in the country. A basic infrastructure had to be developed which took account of existing medical services and sought to weld them into a coordinated health-care system. The first national health planning meeting was held early in 1977 *(Conselho Nacional Coordinador de Saude*, or

CNCS), which involved the heads of the various directorates in the Ministry of Health plus the provincial health directors. Each directorate prepared a plan for the coming year which was discussed by the executive council, and then sent out to the provinces and districts which, in turn, held meetings to discuss the possibilities of executing the programs at each level. Revised plans were then submitted to the second biannual planning council (CNCS) for discussion and approval. The strength of this system lies in its involvement of personnel at different levels, but difficulties arise due to a scarcity of qualified, experienced cadres at the district level and the poor communication facilities. Policies have thus continued to be initiated from the center rather than the periphery; the function of the latter has largely been to approve rather than to modify directives from above.

Base Councils

An important feature of the Mozambican health system has been the establishment of base councils at all health institutions. Decision-making structures were set up within the hospitals and health centers in 1977. Workers on a ward or in a health center are elected to the council, and responsibility for various tasks such as promotion of ward hygiene, health education, and so on are allocated to the council members. Problems in the running of the ward or health center are discussed and referred if necessary to the hospital or district council. In 1979, the need to strengthen the hierarchical organization of the hospital and to reaffirm the importance of individual responsibility, particularly that of the council director, was stressed. Democratization of administrative structures could still proceed but not at the cost of workers failing to make or carry through decisions.

The Socialization of Medicine Law of 1977 established a structure for the health service. People had to go initially to a health post or health center. Only when the health center system could not cope with the problem could patients be referred to the next level of care, the district hospital, or eventually to tertiary level care at the major provincial hospitals. Table 3 shows the number of health institutions at each level of care. The delivery of PHC is principally the responsibility of the health posts and health centers. Across the country as a whole, there is a primary care unit for every 12,000 population, but some districts are still very poorly served in relation to others both between and within districts (Bell 1984).

PHC is the base level of the health service and, as such, can deal effectively with approximately 80 percent of all of the country's health problems—the remainder must be referred to higher levels of care. PHC care in Mozambique comprises the following areas:

1. Environment health measures including drinking water supply
2. School and workers' health

Table 3
Health Institutions, 1983

Description	Number	Level of Care	Appro. No. of Beds/ Unit*
Health Posts, Health Centres and Maternity Units	1069	Primary	20 Per Health Centre
Rural or District Hospitals	26	Secondary	95
Provincial Hospitals	7	Tertiary	215
Psychiatric Hospitals	4	Tertiary	280
Central Hospitals	3	Tertiary	780

*Twenty-five percent of all beds are in maternity wards.
Source: Compiled from Joint WHO/*UNICEF JCHP* Study (Maputo, 1980) and G. Walt and A. Melamed, *Mozambique—Towards a People's Health Service* (London, 1984).

3. Health education
4. Vaccination programs
5. Mother and child health and family planning
6. Control of communicable diseases
7. Basic-level curative care
8. Basic data collection.

This broad range of activities requires intersectoral planning, and this occurs in the context of national development plans in which priorities are defined for each sector in the framework of the overall aims of the ensuing five or ten years. Additionally, the political system in Mozambique readily encourages community participation in health issues. Party structures are operational from the village level upwards, and, in conjunction with the mass organizations of women and youth, workers' councils and people's assemblies provide an effective organizational base for health promotion and preventive activities. This was most clearly evidenced during the vaccination campaigns of 1976 and 1977. WHO later verified that 95 percent measles vaccination coverage had been achieved in the northern provinces despite the dispersed nature of settlement and poor transport facilities (Joint WHO/UNICEF JCHP Study 1980, 23–25). Popular participation in this context does not appear to be a function of coercion but of cooperation between the mass of the population and their political leaders.

Health Centers

The health center is the basic unit for the delivery of PHC. The role of the health center is to mobilize the people of the area to take some responsibility for their own health in terms of a range of preventive actions. Additionally, the health center must maintain close contact with the political and administrative structures in order to coordinate intersectoral activities and to receive feedback from the local population on the actions of the center (Gill and Melamed 1984). Health centers also provide basic level curative care—in the urban areas, a doctor is usually based at the health center or visits regularly. Trained nurses or medical assistants, who usually see all the patients when they first come, perform a triage function—only about 10 percent are actually seen by the health center doctor. Additional staff may run clinics for patients with tuberculosis who require long-term treatment and follow-up, and minor injuries are treated where possible to reduce the pressure on hospital accident departments. Referral to the district or provincial hospital is made in cases of serious acute illness, e.g., meningitis or tuberculosis, or in order to obtain specialist consultations or investigations. Few health centers have the facilities to perform even basic blood and urine tests. Health centers also run pre-natal and under-fives clinics. Women who, according to defined criteria, have high-risk pregnancies and severely malnourished or underdeveloped children are also referred to the hospital services. Health education activities are an important aspect of health center actions—these include explanatory sessions for pregnant women; demonstrations of weaning, food preparation, and oral rehydration mixtures; and discussions of common diseases and their mode of transmission. Environmental health activities include involving the local population in digging latrines and new wells, clearing rubbish and mosquito breeding sites, and operating vaccination campaigns in local schools and factories (Cuidados de Saude Primarios 1978).

Pharmaceutical Policy

Two further aspects of the organization of the health service may be noted. Mozambique's pharmaceutical policy has attracted international attention. This constitutes an integral part of the health service program, and in line with other initiatives, seeks to make the best possible use of available resources. During the colonial period, drug costs were borne by the patient, and for an ordinary worker a medical emergency could readily cost a month's wages. Drugs were selected for import according to their profitability, prescription was by brand name, and polypharmacy was rife. One of the first moves of the new government was to establish a drugs policy through a technical committee for therapeutics and pharmacy. The first step was to revoke import licenses for all products lacking proven therapeutic value, those with an unreasonable profit margin, and the worst examples of polypharmacy. This led to an immediate reduction of licensed products from 13,000 to 2,600. The New National Formulary, produced in 1977, eliminated outmoded or unnecessary drugs, and reduced this list to 640 items representing 408 different therapeutic substances. This list proved to be very similar to WHO's list of 200 essential drugs published the following year. A subsequent edition of the formulary lists only 355 therapeutic substances; modification and updating continues. Prescription is by generic name only, and bulk purchasing by the state pharmacy is combined with an open tender on the international market. If unit prices of acquisition are examined for 1975 to 1979, it is found that 1979 prices are up to 20 percent less than those in 1975. The price paid by the patient for drugs prescribed as outpatients has thus been considerably reduced—a sliding scale according to income is used. In making the needs of the people a priority, Mozambique has achieved a coherent and inexpensive pharmaceutical policy (Barker 1983, 780ff.).

As in many developing countries, a range of traditional medical practitioners also provides treatment to the population. This vast army of indigenous practitioners ranges from people who use spells, dances, and superstitition to those who are skilled in the use of herbs or the techniques of bone setting. The official policy has been to discourage such practices, partly because they constitute a private sector and also because of their lack of proven efficacy in many cases. In practice, however, many of these individuals continue to treat patients. This is especially true in areas where government health services are not readily accessible. In addition, a ministerial commission is studying various herbs and traditional remedies to test their therapeutic efficacy. Hence policy on this issue is not rigid; the long-term aim is to take advantage of the positive aspects of traditional medicine and to outlaw any practices that prevent individuals from seeking western medical attention.

Financing

The Mozambican health service is financed entirely by the state budget through the allocations to the Ministry of Health (Joint WHO/UNICEF JCHP Study 1980, 30–31). Along with economic and educational development, health is one of the priority sectors and as such consumes a significant proportion of national expenditure (see Table 4). In 1980 US $55.4 million was committed to the health sector representing 10.6 percent of the total state expenditure (from 2 to 2.5

Table 4
Breakdown of State Expenditure, 1979

	Sector	US Million $	Per Cent
1.	Defence	113.8	26
2.	Economic Sector	114.9	26.3
3.	Education	70.8	16.2
4.	Health	46.1	10.5
5.	Public debt, social security	49.1	11.3
6.	Central and Provincial Structures	42.2	9.7
Total		436.9	100.0%

Source: Joint WHO/*UNICEF JCHP* Study, Maputo, 1980.

percent of the GNP) and an average of US $4.50 per head per year (US $1.70 in 1975). Between 1976 and 1980, the mean annual increase of the state health budget was 8.9 percent. Further allocation is made to PHC activities via the actions financed by other sectors, such as water, sanitation, and agriculture. The expenditure on health is integrated within the National Planning Commission's ten-year plan for economic development.

Within the overall increasing expenditure on health, an attempt has been made to shift resources from the capital to the provinces and from tertiary to primary care. In 1978 the three central hospitals used up to 56 percent of the total health budget; by 1980, this had dropped to 42 percent. A breakdown of the Ministry of Health budget for 1980 shows that some 56 percent is allocated to personnel and 18 percent to pharmaceuticals as the main allocations. The share of the health units' budget allocated to primary and secondary care rose from 30 percent in 1978 to 41 percent in 1980 (Joint WHO/UNICEF JCHP Study 1980, 87). Expenditure has increased, and PHC has received a larger share of the budget, but there still remains gross inequality of resources according to geographical

Table 5
Geographical Distribution of Resources, 1979

	Maputo City	Maputo + Beira + Nampula	All 10 Prov. Capitals	All Other Distr.
% of Population	5.9	9.5	17.5	82.5
% Doctors	52.5	71.6	89.8	10.2
% All Health Workers	35.1	49.1	66.1	33.9
Population Per Health Worker	180	210	290	2,670
Population Per General Hospital Bed	385	373	420	1,512
Population Per Primary Care Unit	12,416	12,244	13,095	13,600

Source: Joint WHO/*UNICEF JCHP* Study, Maputo, 1980.

distribution (see Table 5). Today's resource allocations still reflect the colonial hierarchy—Maputo City is the most favored, followed by Nampula and Beira with central hospitals, and other provincial capitals and districts with rural hospitals. Least favored are the 70 percent of health districts that have neither health centers nor doctors. The allocation of personnel reflects the same trend with over 50 percent of the doctors and 35 percent of all the health workers based in Maputo City, which contains only 6 percent of the total population.

Health Personnel

All medical personnel are financed by the state except for the village health workers, who receive their payment from the surplus produced by the village and continue to farm themselves. Salaries are proportional to the level of training and experience, but even the best qualified Mozambican doctors do not earn more than US $8,000 per year.

The numbers and types of medical personnel working in Mazambique have changed dramatically since the colonial period. At independence over 85 percent of the country's 550 practicing doctors left, and most rural hospitals and health posts were abandoned. There was thus a demonstrable need to train health personnel at all levels. Doctors sympathetic to the aims of Frelimo were recruited from many western countries, and the socialist countries also sent specialists in many disciplines. By 1982 there were 365 doctors in Mozambique of whom 100 are Mozambican. The medical school in Maputo produces between 20 and 25 Mozambican graduates each year (according to Dr. Pamela Zinkin, Univ. of Eduardo Mondlene, Maputo, 1985). In the years since independence, the medical course has been substantially restructured. The amount of theoretical teaching in basic medical sciences has been cut, and courses on preventive medicine and community health have been introduced. More time is spent on clinical work, and students spend several periods in the rural areas carrying out epidemiological studies as well as practicing clinical medicine. Newly qualified graduates spend at least one year outside Maputo before returning to the central hospital to undergo specialist training in pediatrics, obstetrics, internal medicine, or surgery. Some Mozambican doctors go abroad for specialized training when facilities for such training do not exist within Mozambique. Allocation to speciality and place of work of Mozambican doctors is made by the Ministry of Health according to current needs, as well as attention to individual preference and aptitude.

Given the numbers of health personnel required in the post-independence period, the greatest emphasis was placed on training paramedical workers and nurses. Institutes of Health Sciences were set up in three provincial capitals, and courses were developed for nurses, midwives, medical assistants, anaesthetic technicians, and workers in preventive medicine, nursery education, pharmacy, and radiology. In addition, some dental assistants are being trained, and refresher courses for nurses and midwives have been set up. Current plans also include the training of paramedical workers in surgical techniques to enable them to carry out caesarian sections and perform some trauma surgery at district hospitals. The numbers working in the various health service sectors in 1982 are listed in Table 6. Of these workers, 30 percent are in the primary sector and 47 percent are in the tertiary sector. A separate training program was conceived for village health workers (Joint WHO/UNICEF JCHP Study 1980). The people of the village select their own candidate for the six-month training course and share the cost of supporting the health worker once the training is completed. By 1980

Table 6
Ministry of Health Personnel, 1982

Doctors	365
Medical Assistants	200
Nurses	2300
Midwives	490
Preventive Medicine	494
Other Medical Technicians	700
Dental Assistants Plus Auxiliaries	33

Source: Joint WHO/*UNICEF JCHP* Study, Maputo, 1980.

over 600 of these workers had been trained, but at least 15 percent of the villages had been unable to produce enough surplus to support the health worker.

The roles played by the various workers within the health service are largely commensurate with the length of their training. Village health workers provide simple preventive and curative care and can prescribe a small number of drugs such as chloroquin and aspirin. Medical technicians and agents with three and two years of training, respectively, are frequently in charge of health districts, and they can diagnose and treat a much wider range of conditions before referral to secondary level care.

Major Problems

This review of Mozambique's health profile and its emerging health service has sought to demonstrate the close interdependence between health and the level of development. The health status of the Mozambican population will be altered most significantly to the extent that land redistribution, increased food production, and attention to basic need provision (shelter, food, water, fuel, and so on) can be prioritized by its government. The control of some diseases, e.g., malaria and schistosomiasis, will also depnd on the development of effective vaccines backed up by vector control programs. In Mozambique, the political will to focus resources on the health needs of the majority does exist, as does a clear understanding of the major determinants of health. However, the principal problems in implementing programs derived from this knowledge are political and economic constraints.

This analysis should not be understood as minimizing recent health accomplishments in Mozambique. It has sought to implement an ambitious PHC program, and it has achieved substantial advances in the ten-year post-colonial period. Every health district in the country now has at least one medical assistant or doctor working within its area, and accessibility and availability of basic-level preventive and curative care has been greatly increased for the majority of the population. Health care is provided as a basic right, not as a privilege based on ability to pay, and the training of large numbers of health workers has meant that more care has been made available to more people.

Many problems still remain, however, in the implementation of these policies. Absolute levels of resources available for materials and personnel are an important constraint. Many difficulties have been encountered in the setting up of the organizational structure for health-care delivery and in the allocation of resources to the various sectors. Some health workers and health educators have had difficulty in making the transition from the colonial medical services and adopting the aims of the present health-care system.

A number of these problems have been highlighted in a study of PHC delivery carried out in 1981 (Jelley and Madeley 1983a, 1983b; Madeley, Jelley, and O'Keefe 1983). Although the study was limited to three health centers in Maputo and its environs, several points emerge which are likely to apply in other, less well-serviced areas of the country. A dichotomy was found to exist between the tasks ascribed to the urban health center within the framework of PHC and the feasibility of their execution given existing personnel and material resources. This was considered to derive in part from the lack of involvement of the practitioners of PHC in its organization and planning. Despite the ministerial directives concerning democratic decision making, this had not become a reality—instructions concerning changes in policy or practice were simply sent out to the health centers with minimal opportunity for discussion and reply. As a result, the Ministry of Health was receiving very little feedback concerning the actual implementation of its policies. Lack of resources at the level of primary care was preventing the health centers from carrying out more than basic curative care, and perhaps child health and prenatal programs. The broader scope of the PHC program—data gathering, outreach preventive health and vaccination programs, and environmental monitoring—could not be pursued at the present levels of funding.

In the maternal and child health clinics, a high level of technical competence was observed in the activities of weighing, measuring, and prenatal examinations carried out by the clinic nurses. The quality of care delivery was found to fall short of its specified objectives to the extent that the women and children at highest risk (e.g., obstetric problems or malnutrition) were not always given the further attention and help which their risk status would indicate. Generally, little attempt was made to determine the causes underlying the mothers' problems, and the attitude of the nurses to these women was as often punitive as supportive, discouraging them from further attendances. In addition, when the work of the health center was viewed as a whole, it became apparent that the curative and preventive services were sharply divided, e.g., children brought for curative care would not have their position on the weight for age chart checked, and basic physical illnesses were rarely identified in the preventive health clinics. Little communication or exchange of experiences was taking place between workers in the different sectors.

The Ministry of Health itself stresses the continuing problem of communicable disease control. Measles and diarrheal disease continue to take a high toll among the young, while parasitic diseases and tuberculosis are the cause of chronic ill health. Up to 90 percent of patients fail to complete antituberculosis therapy. The health service also experiences problems in the maintenance of supply of materials. This is particularly true outside the major cities, and it has been greatly exacerbated by the disruption of communication and transport networks by continuing warfare. The great success of the vaccination campaigns of 1976 and 1977 has not been followed up adequately because of the difficulties in reaching the scattered rural communities and of providing the necessary infrastructure and equipment to maintain the "cold chain" (Dick 1984, 57). In the same way, there are frequent drug shortages due to both lack of funds to finance importation and failure of the transport systems to deliver, especially to the rural areas.

The amount spent on health in Mozambique has increased dramatically over the last ten years; however, the real level of financial constraint is apparent in a comparison of the US $5.60 available per head to the US $200 per head spent annually in the United Kingdom on health care. Money spent on health is in direct competition from other vital sectors such as defense, agriculture, industry, and education, and substantial increases in the financing of any of these sectors clearly depends on economic development. In the health sector, there is a clear commitment to redirection of resources to the primary sector. However, given the overall limits on spending, this is difficult to put into practice, since the major hospitals are in the major cities, and these institutions require a high level of funding in terms of staff and materials in order to function. There is thus a limit to how much of the money currently used in the tertiary sector can be realistically diverted.

In the same way, health service personnel require a certain level of infrastructure and supplies in order to function. Moreover, these demands increase according to the level of training. Since the major health facilities are located in the urban areas, the majority of the most highly trained staff will also remain in these areas. This is clearly a danger when encouraging the increasing specialization of Mozambican doctors, as there become fewer and fewer hospitals where they can acquire and practice such skills. Specialized medicine thus remains accessible only to those who live in or can travel to the major urban centers. A further problem, which has been noted by many foreign health personnel working in Mozambique, is the persistence among some health workers of attitudes prevalent in the colonial era (Williams 1984). The desire to preserve their privileged status led some workers to continue to treat patients without respect and to ignore criticisms (Williams 1984). Work patterns in many health institutions improved as a result of the democratic structures set up in response to the party's analyses, but the process of unlearning the past and developing new patterns of work is far from complete.

Future Changes

An outstanding feature of independent Mozambique has been the determination within all sectors of government activity to examine and analyze the progress and effects of the policies being instituted. This process takes place at the district and provincial levels and culminates in the national party congresses that occurred in 1977 and 1983. The discussions leading up to and during the congresses provide the basis for the directives that will guide future policies. In the health sector, the priorities established by the Third Congress were reaffirmed. Targets for the immediate future in both preventive and curative medicine were approved by the Fourth Congress. These included increasing vaccination coverage across the country to 80 percent for antituberculosis vaccine at birth and antitetanus for school children, 70 percent for measles, and 50 percent for polio and the triple vaccine. Additionally, prenatal care was to be extended to at least 50 percent of all pregnant women. Regular medical examinations of workers in high-risk occupations were to be instituted. In terms of curative care, the emphasis was placed on increasing the numbers of health personnel and improving the accessibility of health care in the rural areas by building more health posts and by increasing inpatient and simple diagnostic facilities. All these programs were to be implemented in 1984 and 1985. Subsequent reviews will reassess the country's overall needs and priorities.

Within the context of a centrally planned economy, unplanned or uncontrolled changes still occur. Of crucial importance in this context in Mozambique are the demographic shifts that are paralleled throughout the Third World and the internal disruption that has occurred as a direct result of the guerrilla war sponsored by South Africa. (For a full account of the effects of this war see *South Africa's Undeclared War against Mozambique*, published by the Mozambique Angola Committee, 35 Wellington Street, London.)

Mozambique's birth rate is high; however, public health measures instituted to date have not yet had a great impact on infant and child mortality. As a result, population growth rates have not substantially increased. The most significant demographic trend in terms of health-care provision is the increase in urbanization. The lack of food, water, and basic commodities in the rural areas has driven many thousands to the cities in search of employment and a better food supply. The population of Maputo was estimated at 380,000 in 1974, and found to be over 800,000 in 1980 (Commusão Nacional de Plano 1982, 290). Rapid urban growth takes place on the periphery of the city and usually comprises makeshift, overcrowded housing with poor access to water, sanitation, fuel, and food supplies. Many recent migrants are unable to find work and thus increase the pressure on the incomes of relatives and friends. PHC initiatives, although initially conceived with a view to providing services to rural communities without health care, will also need to become increasingly oriented to the needs of this rapidly expanding population of urban poor.

As a final note, it is essential to relate the current problems and future perspectives for Mozambique's health-care system in the context of the ongoing war. The cessation of hostilities from Rhodesia when Zimbabwean independence was achieved was followed by a rapid escalation of activity by the South African–backed Mozambique Resistance Movement. The critical impact of these efforts has been the destruction of the rural infrastructure. The result has been starvation for many thousands, plus a massive exodus of refugees into Zimbabwe. The London newspaper, the *Times*, reported in October 1983 that over 700,000 people were suffering famine in southern Mozambique, but only 100,000 were able to reach the relief centers (O'Keefe and Munslow, March 1984). In this context, it is clear that health service provision has a minor role to play in preventing ill health when compared with the urgent need for internal political and economic stabilization.

The ambitious call of WHO for Health for All by the Year 2000 still appears a distant target for Mozambique. The social and economic priorities established in Mozambique suggest that maximum use will be made of available resources in order to drive toward this goal. A great amount has been achieved in the first decade of independence in establishing the basic tenets of PHC and in developing a coordinated national framework for their implementation. The success of WHO's initiatives, however, will not depend only on the health programs set up by individual countries. The future of Mozambique and its health service depends on the achievement of political stability and economic growth—objectives that depend as much on external constraints, such as South African and western policies, as on any Mozambican government activities.

References

Barker, Carol. 1983. The Mozambican Pharmaceutical Policy. *Lancet* January 10: 780ff.

Bell, David. 1984. Close Up on Rural Health Care. In *Mozambique—Towards a People's Health Service*, eds. Gillian Walt and Angela Melamed. London: Zed Press.

Central Committee Report to the Third Congress. 1977. London: Frelimo, Mozambique, Angola, and Guinea Information Centre. Commisaõ Nacional de Plano. 1982. *Mozambique Informação Estatística 1980/81*. Maputo.

Cuidados de Saude Primarios. 1978. Report to Alma Ata Conference from Mozambique. Geneva: WHO.

Dick, M. 1984. If You Don't Know Niassa, You Don't Know Mozambique. In *Mozambique—Towards a People's Health Service*, eds. Gill Walt and Angela Melamed. London: Zed Press.

Hobdell, Martin. 1984. The Sweet Tooth of Independence. In *Mozambique—Towards a People's Health Service*, eds. Gillian Walt and Angela Melamed. London: Zed Press.

Isaacman, Allan and Barbara Isaacman. 1983. *Mozambique—From Colonialism to Revolution, 1900–1982*. London: Gower.

Jelley, Diana and R. Madeley. 1983a. Ante-natal Care in Maputo, Mozambique. *Journal of Epidemiology and Community Health* 37, 2 (June 1983): 111–116.

———. 1983b. Preventive Health Care for Mothers and Children. *Journal of Tropical Medicine and Hygiene* 86: 229–236.

Joint WHO/UNICEF JCHP Study. 1980. Country Decision-Making for the Achievement of the Objective of Primary Health Care—Report from the People's Republic of Mozambique. Maputo (available from WHO, Geneva).

Madeley, R., D. Jelley, and P. O'Keefe. 1983. The Advent of Primary Health Care in Maputo, Mozambique. *Ambio* XII, 6: 322–25.

Munslow, Barry. 1983. *Mozambique: The Revolution and its Origins*. London: Longman.

O'Keefe, P. and Barry Munslow. March 1984. "Drought, Floods and Destabilization in Mozambique." An Earthscan Feature. London *Times*.

Walt, Gillian, and Angela Melamed, eds. 1984. *Mozambique—Towards a People's Health Service*. London: Zed Press.

Williams, R. 1984. The Ebb and Flow of Democratization. In *Mozambique—Towards a People's Health Service*, eds. Gillian Walt and Angela Melamed. London: Zed Press.

NETHERLANDS

Adrian A. de Roo

Introduction

In 1983 the Netherlands had 14.4 million inhabitants and a labor force of 6 million, of whom 13.5 percent were unemployed. While nearly 29 percent of the population was younger than 20 years of age, 14 percent was 65 years of age or older. Approximately 560,000 inhabitants (4 percent) had foreign nationalities, with Turks (155,000) and Moroccans (101,000) forming the two largest ethnic minority groups. The Netherlands has a relatively high population density at 424 inhabitants per square kilometer, which rises to 2,221 in the large town where 3.5 million people (one-fourth of the population) lives (*Vademecum of Health Statistics* 1984).

The Dutch health-care system is characterized by a mix of profit and nonprofit elements. Provider organizations and sick funds are nonprofit private organizations, whereas the medical practice itself is a for-profit private enterprise with limited open competition (Van de Ven 1987).

Since 1814, the Netherlands has been a kingdom with a central government that delegates powers to provinces and to municipalities. Until 1974, the Dutch central government left the responsibility for the development of the health-care system to community-based initiatives. Subsequently, health providers and financiers have had to function within a tightening legislative framework.

Health-care expenditures in 1983 consumed 8.8 percent of the gross national product at market prices, a percentage that has been stable in recent years. About 85 percent of the health expenditures are paid for by sick funds, health insurance companies, and private households. The other 15 percent is paid by the government. The overall pattern of the health insurance system is such that it guarantees payment for the health care of every inhabitant of the Netherlands. Patients with compulsory insurance only in a few cases pay additional out-of-pocket charges for services. Voluntary insurance covers the costs per annum insofar as they rise above a minimum level (Van der Werff 1984).

Basic Health and Health System Statistics

In 1983 there were 170,000 live births—11.8 per 1,000 population. The infant mortality during the first year of life was 8.4 per 1,000 life births. Life expectancy at birth for girls was 79.4 and for boys 72.7 years. The main causes of death were diseases of the circulatory system, 44.9 percent; malignant neoplasms, 27.3 percent; and diseases of the respiratory system, 6.9 percent. In 1983 1,710 persons died in traffic accidents and 923 committed suicide (0.10 per 1,000 population). In 1982 4.7 induced abortions per 1,000 women (between the ages of 15 and 44 and living in the Netherlands) were performed in specialized clinics. There were 13.0 consultations of a general practitioner and 7.0 of a specialist per 100 population in 1983. There were 8.1 contacts with dentists per 100 inhabitants (*Vademecum of Health Statistics 1984*).

Inpatient short-term care was offered in 1983 in 177 general and 48 specialized hospitals, which had a total of 69,583 beds (4.8 per 1,000 population). Nearly one-third of the hospitals have between 400 and 1,000 beds; 28 percent have fewer than 200 beds. There were 98 nursing positions per 100 occupied beds. The admission to general hospitals was 8.4 per 100, and surgical procedures were performed on 42.0 percent of those admitted. The average length of stay was 12.5 days (*LMR Jaarboek 1984* 1986).

Long-term care was provided in 327 nursing homes—147 for somatic patients, 82 for psychogeriatric patients, and 98 for both groups. The total number of beds in these institutions was 48,108 (3.3 per 1,000 population) with 68 nursing positions per 100 occupied peds.

There were 76 psychiatric hospitals with 24,855 beds (1.7 per 1,000 population) and 55 nursing positions per 100 occupied beds. In 129 institutions for the mentally retarded, 29,915 beds were available—2.1 per 1,000 population, with 63 nursing positions per 100 occupied beds.

Ambulatory mental health care was offered by 138 institutions, which employed about 6,500 persons in early 5,000 permanent staff positions. More than 202,000 clients were helped in 1982 by these institutions. Treatment lasting less than three months was offered to 51 percent of the clients; 17 percent of them were treated for more than one year. About 13,000 persons with alcohol and 8,300 with drug problems were treated in 1982 by specialized ambulatory centers. Home care was delivered by more than 11,000 persons (on 8,400 full-time positions) employed by visiting nursing organizations. Together they had over 10 million patient contacts in 1983 (*Vademecum of Health Statistics* 1984).

In 1983 the Dutch health-care system provided employment for 5.7 percent of the labor force. There were nearly 29,000 physicians (2.01 per 1,000 population) active in the system. Among them were more than 5,600 general practitioners (0.40 per 1,000 population), 10,000 specialists (0.69 per 1,000), and about 1,500 public health physicians (0.11 per 1,000). About 4,000 physicians participated in professional training programs. There were more than 6,200 dentists (0.44 per 1,000), about 1,700 pharmacists (0.12 per 1,000), and about 1,000 midwives (0.07 per 1,000) and 9,300 physiotherapists (0.64 per 1,000 population). In 1983 Dutch universities had 1,403 medical students; there were 2,574 persons studying dentistry and 1,617 studying pharmacy.

Historical Development of the System

Up the 1960s, a basic characteristic of Dutch society was that social life was structured by groups that shared the same religious or secular worldview (Kramer 1981). This principle of social organization expressed itself in the development and structure of the health-care system. Care institutions had an overtly religious, Roman Catholic or Protestant, or secular, neutral, identity that was reflected in the selection of personnel, the name of the institution, the additional social and religious facilities offered to patients, and so on. It was quite normal for a middle-sized town to have three hospitals, three visiting nursing organizations, and three sick funds, each serving a different religious or social group.

This segmentation of the health-care system also existed on the national level. Roman Catholic hospitals were members of a national Catholic association as were Protestant hospitals and secular institutions. The same organizational triad developed on the national level for the visiting nursing services, the psychiatric hospitals, the sick funds, and so on. This type of segmentation did not, however, take place in the medical profession. The KNMG (the Royal Society for the Advancement of Health Care) has always represented the whole medical group. The same level of organizational coherence applies to other health professionals, creating a situation whereby a fragmented set of provider institutions faced a much more uniform group of health professional organizations.

In the 1960s this so-called pillar structure of Dutch society (as the segmentation has been described in sociological literature) disintegrated (Lijphart 1968). For health provider institutions, this meant that patient referrals were no longer predominantly based on one's group identity. Instead, quality criteria, personal relations between medical professionals, and so on became the decisive factors that determined the choice of a provider. In practice, this meant that the religious provider institutions lost a central component of their identity. The same happened to the other provider organizations and to the sick funds with a religious identity, as well as to their counterpart organizations on the national level.

One of the consequences of this social change was that on the local and national level, historical obstacles to collaboration disappeared. In the beginning of the 1970s, the local visiting nursing organizations fused, and between 1967 and 1981, 93 hospitals undertook some 43 mergers. In the beginning of the 1980s, the organizations for ambulatory mental care merged into less than 70 regional institutions. On the national level, existing organizations fused into new structures in which common political interest became the binding factor rather than shared worldview (Können 1984).

The governmental role in health care was minimal until 1974. It was a deliberate political choice to leave the development of the health-care system to community-based initiatives. After World War II, the government controlled the price of health services and the construction of new institutions as part of an overall policy on prices and construction. It also concerned itself with health insurance, as part of the social security legislation. In 1966, the current sick fund law (on the compulsory insurance of the dependent labor force) replaced the regulation introduced by the Germans in 1941, and in 1968 the parliament passed legislation requiring general compulsory insurance for exceptional health-care risks. But the government did not intervene in the development of the health-care system as such.

In the 1960s, however, the political climate changed toward a more active stance for the central government in the health-care system. This change reflected an overall redefinition of the government's role in the Dutch welfare state. Following three years of discussion, the parliament in 1971 passed a law that was intended to bring the expansion of hospital facilities under political control. This was the first step toward the assumption of central government responsibility for the future of the whole delivery system.

The second step was taken in 1974. In that year, the government published a comprehensive plan to bring the health-care system under central political control. In this plan, five policy goals were formulated. The first was to create a health-care system that had facilities evenly spread over the country to ensure equal access for every citizen. The second goal was to create optimal coordination of services within and between the several sectors of the system. The third goal was to rationalize the very complex pattern of health-care financing. The fourth goal was to balance the capacity of training programs for the health professions with the personnel demands of the institutions. The fifth goal was to create public participation in the decision-making processes on both institutional and political levels of the system (external democratization) (Van der Werff 1984).

These goals reflected the shortcomings of the health-care system as perceived in 1974. First, the existing pattern of health-care facilities was the result of an uncoordinated process of community-based decision making. After World War II, this had led to an unbalanced distribution of health-care institutions over the country and to an overaccentuation of inpatient care. There was no real capacity problem in the system at that time, but there were important problems to ensure continuity of care in cases in which a patient had to be referred between institutions. These problems fed the wish to create better integration of health-care activities among institutions and professionals within the system.

Second, there was growing concern about rising expenditures. The costs of health care as a percentage of the gross national product (at market prices) grew from 3.1 percent in 1953 and 5.5 percent in 1968 to 6.7 percent in 1972 (Van der Werff 1984). This created pressure for more efficiency in the system. Greater integration of health-care activities was seen as one answer; another was sought in the streamlining of the financing structure. A simpler financing structure was also believed to be an effective instrument for future cost containment. At the end of the 1960s, the first disturbances of the labor market for health personnel were observed, and this led to concerns about the capacity of the medical training programs. Additionally, the strong democratization movement of that era led to a search for instruments to enable the public to participate more directly in the governance of health-care institutions and in the preparation of policy plans.

In the 1974 plan, two new laws were announced: one to control the costs of health care and one to plan the future development of health-care prices. In 1980, the parliament passed the law on health-care charges against strong opposition of the professional groups and the provider institutions. In addition to price control, this law opened the possibility for the government to standardize the incomes of professional groups. In 1982 the law on health-care facilities was passed. This law provided the instruments necessary to create overall planning of health services on a national and a regional level.

The 1974 plan also sought to create an active governmental role in guaranteeing the quality of the caring process. This led to the preparation of a new law governing the health professions to replace the current regulation that confines health-care activities to those permitted explicitly in law. Under the new law, offered to the parliament in 1986, the title rather than the health-care activity itself will be confined to specific professional groups. This change reflects growing social recognition of alternative modes of health care.

Present System Structure

As noted before, the health provider institutions in the Netherlands were mainly established by the Roman Catholic Church, by Protestant denominations, and by secular social organizations. In 1975, 58 percent of the existing short-term hospitals had a religious background (32 percent Roman Catholic, 17 percent Protestant, and 8 percent general Christian); 30 percent were established by secular social organizations and 12 percent by the government (Können 1984).

The Dutch provider institutions, including those established by the government, are generally owned by foundations or societies. All the visiting nursing organizations, most psychiatric hospitals and institutions for the mentally deficient, and 85 percent of the short-term hospitals are in this way privately owned, as are 60 percent of the nursing homes. About 15 percent of the short-term hospitals, 40 percent of the nursing homes, and some psychiatric hospitals are owned by foundations established in most cses by the local government. In two or three cases, hospitals are run as governmental agencies. There are no institutions owned by corporations, since for-profit institutions are forbidden by law. Many psychiatric hospitals and institutions for the mentally retarded belong to multi-institutional structures. By contrast, hort-term hospitals and the visiting nursing organizations are freestanding institutions, as are most of the nursing homes.

While the health provider institutions are nonprofit, most doctors in the system work as individual entrepreneurs. General practitioners work on a fee-for-service basis for subscribers to voluntary insurance programs. They receive an annual capitation fee for patients belonging to one of the sick funds. Nearly 3,500 (58 percent) general practitioners work in a single practice, and 1,279 (23 percent) work in dual practice. Fewer than 780 (12.1 percent) work in one of the 90 group practices and 120 health centers. In a few health centers, general practitioners work on salary (*Vademecum of Health Statistics* 1984).

About 10 percent of the medical specialists work on salary basis in the short-term care hospitals, owned by the central and local government. Specialists in the psychiatric hospitals and nursing homes all work on salary. However, about 70 percent of all specialists in the Netherlands work on a fee-for-service basis, and do dentists, midwives, and physiotherapists.

After World War II, hospitals began to limit practice rights to contracted specialists who formed the institution's medical staff. In the current situation, certain subspecialists (plastic surgeons, gastroenterologists, rheumatologists, and so on) have part-time contracts with several hospitals, while most other specialists practice full time in a single hospital. In 1977, more than 90 percent of all surgeons had contracts with a single hospital, as had nearly 98 percent of all internists. By contrast, in 1978, 39 percent of the orthopedists practiced in two hospitals and 14 percent in three institutions (De Roo 1985).

In these specialist contracts, hospitals require physicians in the same specialty to develop working relationships with each other. This started a development toward group practices in the hospitals. In 1976 only 20 percent of the internists worked in a solo practice, as did 6 percent of all surgeons in 1977 and 25 percent of the orthopedists in 1978. The gradual disappearance of solo practice goes hand in hand with the concentration of outpatient activities in the hospital building. In 1976, 80 percent of all internists no longer had outpatient activities outside the hospital, while the corresponding figure for surgeons in 1977 was 83 percent (De Roo 1985).

The admitting contracts create a close structural relationship between specialists and hospitals. This relationship reflects the structural division between primary and hospital care. In the Netherlands the general practitioner is the exclusive provider of family care. A physician can be either a general practitioner or a medical specialist, but the combination of both functions is not possible. One cannot register for a specialty if one has a primary care practice. Furthermore, there are no institutional relations between hospitals and home nursing organizations. Thus hospital care, general practice, and home nursing are conducted on three separate organizational circuits, a situation which creates considerable problems in coordination and communication between the primary and hospital care sectors.

The structural relations between specialists and hospitals have consequences for institutional management as well. Admitting contracts require specialists to participate in a formal institutional group, the medical staff. By doing so, hospital management is able to communicate and negotiate with the specialists as a whole. In reverse, the medical staff strongly influences and often dominates hospital decision-making processes. The actual degree of influence depends on the extent to which the medical staff acts as a united group. The national professional organization of medical doctors does not function as a union, so it cannot support the medical staff in negotiations with hospital managers.

The influence of the medical staff also depends on the quality of hospital management. These qualities vary strongly and one recent issue has been the question of having a medical doctor as the top hospital manager. Between 1920 and 1960, the normal situation was to have a medical doctor as the general director. It is estimated that, subsequently, some 50 percent of these administrating doctors have been replaced by economists and—more recently—by professional managers. Physicians still take part in the hospital management but not any more as the leader of the team.

The influence of the medical staff on hospital decision making also depends on the role of the trustees, who represent the foundations and societies that own the institutions. There is no standard division of labor (or power) between the trustees and the directors of either hospitals or other health provider institutions in the Netherlands. In many institutions the trustees often have extended formal powers, although it is widely acknowledged that even in these cases the administrators retain actual power, largely due to their increased access to managerially necessary information. Occasionally, however, a hospital's trustees are paid parttimers who then may be very influential.

Taken together, the governance pattern of Dutch health institutions offers a complicated pattern in which trustees, directors, and medical staff interact within the limits set by the interorganizational networks the institutions participate in, the legal restrictions set by the central government, and the financial conditions negotiated with the financiers.

Costs and Financing

In 1983 the health-care expenditures were HFI 33,116 million, or 8.8 percent of the gross national product at market prices. About 65 percent was used for inpatient care, 16 percent for ambulatory care, 10 percent for pharmaceutical supplies and supplies of medical aids, 2 percent for preventive medicine, and 7 percent for administration and other activities. The income of medical doctors not on salary absorbed 10.3 percent of the total health expenditures, 5.9 percent went to medical specialists, and 4.4 percent went to general practitioners. Only 5 percent of the total health expenditures comes directly from the national (4 percent) and local (1 percent) tax revenues and 1 percent is directly financed by enterprises. The central government pays additional contributions to the several health insurance funds and by doing so ultimately pays 15 percent of all expenditures. The bulk of the money comes from private households, paid in the form of direct expenditures or fees for health insurance (*Vademecum of Health Statistics* 1984).

There are two types of health insurance in the Netherlands. These are complementary and, together, they provide coverage to the entire population. Compulsory health insurance exists for employees below a certain income level and for those who get their income from the social security funds. This insurance is offered by nonprofit sick funds. It covers primary care, hospital and psychiatric hospital care for one year, dental care, and prescriptions. Partners who do not work, children under sixteen years (under 27 years for students and the handicapped) are covered without additional payments. The premium is nearly 10 percent of the wage-earner's income and is subject to a certain maximum. It is paid on a fifty-fifty basis by the employer and the employee, hence the employee pays approximately 5 percent of wages as premium. The fee and the maximum income level are fixed annually by the national government with the advice of the Sick Fund Council.

In 1983, more than 8 million persons were covered by the compulsory insurance program. That year they paid together about 40 percent of all health-care expenditures. The other 6 million persons (self-employed people, retired workers, and employees above a certain income level) participate in voluntary insurance programs, which offer coverage of the same health risks as the compulsory insurance. They can select one of the insurance packages offered by about 80 for-profit companies and nonprofit organizations that cover together the competitive voluntary insurance market. These packages cover individual expenditures per annum in combination with their own expenditures. The central government must approve price changes for voluntary insurance (Van de Ven 1987).

Complementary of these two insurances is general compulsory insurance for coverage of visiting nursing, ambulatory mental health, hospital and psychiatric hospital care after one year, nursing home care, and other health services not covered by the two standard forms of insurance. The fee for this supplemental insurance is nearly 4 percent of earnings, again with a maximum. In the case of dependent labor, however, the employer pays the fee. Thus, in practice, an employee in the sick fund pays 5 percent of his wages while other persons pay 4 percent plus a voluntary insurance premium that can vary.

Patients with compulsory insurance in a few cases have to pay additional out-of-pocket charges for services once the fees for health insurance have been paid. For example, they pay a small amount of money for prescriptions. In 1986, the central government announced plans to extend the amount of additional charges. Persons with voluntary health insurance pay their own health expenditures to the limit defined in the contracts. There are some possibilities to vary these limits. Insurance contracts with higher limits require patients to pay more of their health costs themselves, but consequently offer lower annual premiums.

The general compulsory insurance has an income-tied copayment that must be paid for long-term inpatient care.

Health-care institutions in the Netherlands traditionally have been paid on the principle of cost reimbursement. In 1983, however, the central government introduced regulations that required short-term hospitals to operate under a fixed budgeting system (Groot 1987). One year later, the same budget approach was extended to all other provider institutions. At present, the incomes of medical specialists are outside the budgets of the institutions they work in; however, the possibility of integrating them in the near future is currently under discussion.

When fixed budgets were introduced for the first time, they were set at each institution's expenditure level of two years prior, adjusted for subsequent inflation. Every institution is required to negotiate with the local sick funds about the target level of productivity under its budget. The resulting agreements function as a basis for adaptation of the budget in the next year. If the actual productivity (in terms of admitted patients, occupied beds, etc.) is less than was agreed, the budget will be decreased. The budget can be increased if the productivity is higher than expected or if negotiations lead to decisions to expand certain services.

This approach is highly unsatisfactory for all parties, since considerable time must be invested in discussions about future changes in the allocation of money. One alternative may be to introduce regional budgets, leaving the problem of actual distribution to the institutions concerned.

Political Control of the System

Political control over the system rests on a complicated power balance between the public and the private sector. In Dutch politics the development of the health system traditionally has been considered to be the responsibility of the private sector. However, since 1974, the central government has tried to control the development of the system by regulations that restrict the policy-related decisions of both institutions and individual professionals in the private sector (Rutten 1987).

Several difficulties have, however, conspired to limit the effectiveness of the government in taking primary responsibility for the development of the system. First, the cental government has had internal difficulties in developing an integrated health policy approach. Although the Ministry of Welfare, Health, and Culture is responsible for the overall health policy, it must negotiate with the Ministry of Education concerning the academic teaching hospitals and the medical training programs. It also must deal with the Treasury as far as macro-financial policy decisions are involved. Policy decisions regarding the working conditions in the health system have to be coordinated with the Ministry of Social Affairs (Van der Werff 1984).

Second, some important policy instruments are not available to the central government. For instance, the government has no direct financial control over the system since it pays only 15 percent of the total health expenditures. Direct administrative control is similarly minimal since only a few health provider institutions function as government agencies.

Third, the process of health policy is not concentrated in the hands of the governmental bureaucracy. Dutch law requires a process of policy development that involves several nongovernmental advisory bodies in which the health field is strongly represented. Some of these bodies have implementation powers that strengthen their influence. Political tradition also requires the involvement of the provincial and local government, which, in turn, have their own health-field-dominated advisory bodies. Provincial and local governmental influence reflects the generally shared Dutch political philosophy of decentalization. The influence of the advisory bodies is political recognition of the importance of private initiative in Dutch society (Boot 1983).

Health professionals, institutions, insurers, and patients all have their own national organizations to promote their interests. The socioeconomic and scientific interests of the medical profession are promoted by the KNMG. This organization has three sections: one for medical specialists, one for family doctors, and one for physicians on salary. These sections often have opposite interests, so the KNMG often finds it difficult to function as a united group. About 65 percent of the Dutch physicians are members of the KNMG. This percentage has been declining in recent years, however, due in part to the declining effectiveness of the organization in defending the physicians' socioeconomical interests.

General hospitals, psychiatric hospitals, institutions for the mentally deficient, and nursing homes are organized on the national level in the NZR (the National Hospital Council). This Council has its own research center, the NZI (National Hospital Institute). The visiting nursing organizations are united in a national society, as are the ambulatory mental health-care organizations. The sick funds also have a national society. Nonprofit insurance organizations have their own national organization as do the for-profit companies. In addition, health insurance groups have created a joint commission. General and disease-specific patient organizations also collaborate in a national platform. A very recent development is the establishment of a national organization in which healers and patients from the alternative medicine sector collaborate.

Together with other social groups, these organizations in varying ways are represented in three of the four advisory bodies officially involved in the policy-development process on the national level. The fourth body is the Health Council, which advises the central government on scientific aspects of health care like the reintroduction of treatment of psychiatric patients with electroshock, the annual number of heart transplantations, and so on. Most advisory statements are prepared by ad hoc committees. The members are appointed by the government. They are recruited from the field for their special expertise on the subject concerned.

The advice of the Health Council is often transformed into planning proposals by the National Council for Health Care. This council advises on national health policy affairs and also functions as a forum for communication between the interest groups in the health field. This council has members that are representatives from professional groups, patient groups, employer organizations, labor unions, financiers, and the provincial and local government. Comparable councils on lower governmental levels advise the provinces and municipalities.

The Sick Fund Council provides advice to the central government on such subjects as the content of insurance coverage, the limitation of target groups for compulsory insurance, the raising of insurance fees, and so on. This council also has to approve the contractual agreements between the funds and the professional groups in the health field, and it controls the implementation of the Sick Fund Law. The council has crown members (nominated by the government) and representatives from employer organizations, labor unions, sick funds, and professional groups.

The Board of Hospital Facilities advises the central government on the planning and building of hospital facilities. In addition to this general advisory role, it prepares decisions on the allocation of licenses for specific hospitals. The board had crown members (independent persons nominated by the government) and persons representing the hospitals, the medical profession, the sick funds and insurance companies, and the provincial and local authorities.

Future Outlook

In the 1960s and 1970s, the primary political justification for bringing the health-care system under central governmental control was to make health-care services of high quality equally available to every citizen of the welfare state. However, as a result of the economic distress of the 1970s, cost containment gradually superseded the earlier policy goals. As a consequence, the new laws on charges and on health facility planning became more and more instruments for cost containment.

With regard to cost containment, the government has been successful in scaling back the rate of growth in health expenditures. The growth rate in 1977 had been 10.7 percent, which receded to 7 percent in 1982, 4.3 percent in 1983, and 3 percent in 1984. For 1985 the growth rate was 1.5 percent. Since this is less than the general inflation rate, the actual growth of health expenditures in 1985 was close to zero (*Financieël overzicht gezondheidszorg 1986* 1985).

These results partially reflect the decline of general inflation rates in the Netherlands. They also reflect the effectiveness of cost-containment measures in the inpatient sector. The introduction of budgets for health provider institutions meant a switch from output- to- input based financing that set clear limits to the expenditures. Other cost-containment measures that contributed to the declining growth rate were a forced reduction of beds (some 8,000 between 1982 and 1989, to be accomplished by changing hospital licenses) and restricted growth in the number of new health professionals (to be accomplished partially by the same method and partially by creating a new system of licenses for fee-in-service professionals). Less successful were efforts to introduce a standard income level for medical specialists. This entailed budgeting of the joint income for medical specialists, while still leaving room for individual income differences. However, since sanctions are lacking for production that leads to individual incomes above the standard, this approach has not yet been successful.

The declining growth rate has had its price in terms of increased social tensions. Hospitals complain more and more publicly about the shrinking amount of money available to them, and they try to mobilize public opinion to resist future budget cuts by arguing that they will hurt the quality of patient care. Their resistance is reinforced by the fact that in the current situation there is a growing necessity to set priorities for the treatment of patients in the face of scarce resources. Within hospitals, this leads to more and longer waiting lists for elective surgery, and also for consultation. The professional groups show growing resistance against measures designed to lower their incomes. This all, in turn, creates aggression and fustration directed at the source of these unpopular measures: the national government. As a direct outcome of this growing pressure, in 1986, the Netherlands experienced the first strike of medical specialists in its history.

Policy results in the planning of health facilities have thus far been very modest. As of 1986, the law on health-care facilities has been fully implemented on an experimental basis only in three regions. In recent years, doubts have grown about the feasibility of overall planning for health-care facilities. These doubts have developed partially from the practical difficulties experienced during the implementation of the law. Until now, the planning process has produced only minor results in terms of redistributing existing service facilities over the country or balancing the planning of new services.

These doubts also reflect the belated recognition that an effective planning process requires a complex and extended bureaucratic structure. This structure has until now been only partially developed, but it has become clear that a full-grown planning structure is a costly affair. Between 1979 and 1984, the costs for administration of the health-care system increased more than 65 percent (from 572 to 948 million guilders), while in the same period total health-care expenditure increased only 34 percent. In 1984 total costs for health care increased 3 percent, while costs for administration grew 6.2 percent. Estimates for 1986 show a 4-percent increase of administrative costs in a planned overall increase of 1.8 percent. The practical dilemma, then, is whether to put money into development of a planning structure or to use it for health care itself (*Financieël overzicht gezondheidszorg 1986* 1985).

This dilemma is becoming increasingly acute. It is politically difficult to defend lower budgets, incomes, and investments for provider institutions (against heavy resistance from the health professions, patient groups, and other stakeholders) while investing a growing amount of money in the development of a planning structure. In addition, the political climate is changing. It is becoming increasingly popular to suggest that the market mechanism is a suitable alternative to planning in reaching stated political goals. This too makes the future of the current planning approach uncertain.

Progress toward the other 1974 policy goals also has been modest. Coordination between primary and inpatient care is still considered a big problem. The government in recent years has invested substantial funds into the development of local networks between health professionals, but these networks have been paralyzed by competing interests among the participants. On a related area, the policy of external democratization has resulted in the preparation of patients' rights legislation to be presented to the parliament in 1987. This bill specifies the rights of patients, including psychiatric patients, and introduces grievance procedures to be followed in the case of complaints. The external democratization policy in some cases has resulted in changes in the composition of hospital boards; however, there has been no real breakthrough in this area.

The manpower planning issue still is unsolved. The main obstacle is the struggle over who has the right to regulate the number of new students in health training programs. While this discussion has been taking place at the national level, the professional groups who control the training programs for medical specialists have in the meantime cut down student numbers from 2,969 in 1981 to 2,374 in 1985. The intake of the medical schools, which is directly controlled by the central government, has in the same period been reduced by about 25 percent. However, these measures only take effect after a substantial time lag; in the Netherlands medical study takes six years and subsequent specialty training takes an additional five to six years. In the meantime, medical schools are producing a growing number of physicians who cannot find a position for subsequent professional training. In 1986, 1,200 of them organized into a movement for the creation of new positions inside the health-care system.

The behavior of these jobless physicians may well be decisive for future developments in the Dutch health-care system. Until now, they have sought jobs within the established pattern of the health-care system, but with less and less success. As a result, they are gradually becoming inclined to create conditions to practice outside the official system. Some of them have penetrated the alternative health-care sector, contributing to a development that moves toward a certain fusion of academic and alternative medicine. Others are involved in efforts to introduce for-profit elements in Dutch health care, using loopholes in the existing laws. Still others are participating in efforts to create new health delivery structures of the health maintenance organization type. Through their innovative behavior, these physicians will play an important role in the next years in determinating how existing problems in the health-care system will be addressed.

References

Boot, J. M. D. et al. 1983. *Structuurnota Gezondheidszorg 1984*. Utrecht: Bohn, Scheltema & Holkema.

De Roo, A. A. 1985. *De opleiding tot medisch specialist's*. Gravenzande: Van Deventer.

Financieël overzicht gezondheidszorg 1986. 1985. Den Haag: Ministerie van Welzijn, Volksgezondheid en Cultuur.

Groot, L. M. S. 1987. *Incentives for Cost-Effective Behavior: a Dutch Experience*. Health Policy 7: 175–188.

Können, E. 1984. *Ziekenhuissamenwerking, fusie en regionalisatie*. Utrecht: NZI.

Kramer, R. M. 1981. *Voluntary Agencies in the Welfare State*. Berkeley: University of California Press.

LMR Jaarboek 1984. 1986. Utrecht: Stichting Informatiecentrum voor de Gezondheidszorg.

Lijphart, A. 1968. *The Politics of Accommodation and Pluralism in the Netherlands*. Berkeley: University of California Press.

Rutten, F. H. 1987. *Market Strategies for Publicly Financed Health Care Systems*. Health Policy 7: 135–148.

Vademecum of Health Statistics of the Netherlands. 1984. Den Haag: Staatsuitgeverij.

Van de Ven, W. P. M. M. 1987. *The Key Role of Health Insurance in a Cost-Effective Health Care Market*. Health Policy 7: 253–272.

Van der Werff, A. 1984. *Health Services and Planning and Management for the Health Services in the Netherlands*. Den Haag: Ministerie van Welzijn, Volksgezondheid en Cultuur.

NIGERIA

Paul O. Chuke

Health Status

The population of Nigeria by mid–1984 was 88.1 million of which 45 percent (40,103,000) were under 15 years of age, 52 percent (46,341,360) were in the labor age-group of from 15 to 64 years, and 3 percent (2,673,540) were over 65 years of age. Females in the reproductive age group (15 to 44 years) constituted 20 percent of the population. The crude live birth rate per 1,000 population was 45, and the crude death rate per 1,000 population was 20, leaving an annual population growth rate of 2.5 percent (Kent and Haub 1984).

The infant mortality rate per 1,000 live births was 120, of which the corresponding values of urban and rural areas were 100 and 130, respectively. The adult life expectancy at birth was 49 years in 1984. There is a paucity of reliable statistics, which, coupled with the great diversity in climatic conditions and culture in the country, make it difficult to determine the most common causes of death. Statistics from Lagos, the national capital, taken as the most representative of the whole country, give the following (Williams 1971):

Disease	Percentage
Pneumonia	15.1
Gastroenteritis	10.05
Heart failure	6.03
Malaria	5.05
Hypertension	3.28

Anemia	3.08
Tetanus	2.43

The relatively low death rate from malaria is not so surprising if it is recalled that it is in the 0-to-4-year age group that malaria is most severe and accounts for 70 percent of all registered malaria deaths. Most of the anemia found in farmers is caused by hookworm infestation and in mothers and children by a combination of dietary factors and hemoglobinopathy. Apart from the latter, the majority of causes of death are infections. This is emphasized by the high rate of infection (per 100,000 population) of the top twenty major causes of morbidity from notifiable diseases (Basic Health Service Programme 1976):

Disease	**No. per 100,000**
Malaria	1,693
Dysentery, all types	338
Measles	149
Pneumonia	132
Gonorrhea	78
Whooping cough	655
Schistosomiasis, all types	47.9
Filariasis	31.7
Chicken pox	30.4
Ophthalmia neonatorum	17.0
Tuberculosis	12.5
Onchocerciasis	10.2
Infective hepatitis	8.6
Food poisoning	7.1
Trachoma	5.4
Tetanus	3.5
Syphilis	1.8
Meningitis, all types	0.8

The Evolution of the Nigerian Health-Care System

Nigeria as it is known today was created by the amalgamation of the northern and southern parts of the country in 1914. The present Gongola State, which had been functionally a part of the country since after World War I, became permanently integrated in 1960. With a population of 88.1 million (mid–1984 estimation), Nigeria has the largest population of all the African countries; every fourth African is a Nigerian. The southern border of the country is the Atlantic coastline; to the north, it borders on arid land which, farther north, merges imperceptibly with the Sahara Desert. Physically, the country has a swampy mangrove coast, followed by thick tropical forest, then from savannah to shrubland, and finally to semiarid land as one moves northward. Two important climatic influences are the southeast trade winds from the Atlantic Ocean, which bring heavy rainfall during the midyear especially to the southern parts of the country, and the dry, cool northeast trade winds in late December and early January, which blow southward from the Sahara Desert.

There are 250 ethnic groups in Nigeria, but 63 percent of the population is made up of the three major ones. Each group has it own culture, part of which invariably is its own system of traditional medicine. Before the series of events that eventually led to modern Nigeria, traditional medicine was the system of health-care delivery. Even today, it is still a force to be reckoned with, and every village has its traditional healers. They are of various types: herbalists, soothsayers, diviners, bonesetters, traditional midwives, traditional mental health therapists, and traditional surgeons. There was and still is no embracing philosophy or system; rather, each culture evolved its system in isolation. Diseases were either divine punishment for misdeeds, or they resulted from evil machinations of the enemy.

Contact and interaction with Arabic and European traders, explorers, and finally colonialists over a period dating from the second half of the fifteenth century brought about the foundation of modern medical services in Nigeria. The real roots of health care as we know it today in Nigeria is consequently exogenous in origin.

The Portuguese in 1472 were the first Europeans in Nigeria, and they were followed by the British in 1553. There is no evidence that these initial contacts resulted in any form of organized health services. This phase was followed by the era of slave trade which began with the "discovery" of America by Christopher Columbus and reached its peak in the latter half of the eighteenth century. The high mortality and morbidity from diseases, especially in the middle passage between Africa and America, led in Britain to the 1789 Act of Parliament which compelled all ships carrying slaves to have on board a licensed surgeon so as to select healthy slaves to ensure no loss of profit. Again, no evidence exists to suggest that this brought about any permanent benefit to the health of the inhabitants on land.

It was the Niger expeditions that brought about simple medical care to Nigeria. The expeditions in 1832, 1841, and 1854 followed earlier explorations on the source of course of the River Niger by Dr. Mungo Park and Richard Landar. In the last of these expeditions in 1854, Dr. Baikie markedly reduced mortality by the use of appreciable doses of quinine and opened up the hinterland to commerce.

However, while traders brought doctors with them to serve their own needs, it was the Catholic, and Protestant, including Baptist, missionaries who first established organized health care for the inhabitants in Nigeria in specific areas.

The first hospital in the country, the Sacred Heart Hospital, was built by the Catholic Mission at Abeokuta in 1895; the Church Missionary Society opened up dispensaries in Obosi (1890), Onitsha, and Ibadan (1896). Other institutions soon followed and, at Independence in 1960, the missionaries operated a remarkable proportion of the health services.

Although the missionaries established health institutions and provided health care to the population, their efforts were not coordinated nor was it their primary motive, and each mission had its own areas of influence. Health care by the missionaries was a spin-off from the real work of evangelization. It was therefore left to the government to develop nationwide health services.

Apart from Lagos, the present capital of the country, the rudiments of the government health services could be said to have started in Lokoja from the military medical service established for the troops that had been sent by the British to secure the frontier against competing European powers. By 1900, Lokoja became the headquarters under Lord Lugard, who was interested in preventive and curative medicine. Military and later civilian hospitals were established, town planning was introduced, and a building act was enacted. St. Margaret's Hospital, Calabar—the first government hospital—was built in 1889.

However, in 1902, the medical services in Gambia, Sierra Leone, Ghana, and Nigeria were merged into the West African Colonial Medical Service under the colonial office in London. In addition to the disadvantages of a centralized health care system, this resulted in the exclusion of African doctors from the Government Medical Services, an action which was regarded as retrogressive. World War I brought acute staff shortage as most of the health workers were deployed in the armies fighting in the Cameroons and East Africa. Some hospitals had to be closed. The situation was worsened by the influenza and plague epidemics of 1918 and 1924. In 1939, the Yaba Medical College, the first medical school in Nigeria, was established. Initially, it produced auxiliary health workers, the medical assistants, but subsequently it was upgraded to train assistant medical officers. Almost all of the latter went to Britain afterwards and, by joint agreement with the British Royal Colleges of Surgeons and Physicians, obtained the licentiate diplomas which converted them into full-fledged doctors. This type of institution, which trained incomplete doctors, became so unpopular that it disappeared with the establishment of the University of Ibadan and Nigeria's first conventional medical school in 1948.

World War I produced more changes. First, with the Japanese occupation of Malaya, Nigeria became an important exporter of rubber and tin, and with the new prosperity, practically every major aspect of life including health care moved forward. Second, with military campaigns in the Middle East and East Africa, West Africa including Nigeria became an important transit area for the transportation of military aircraft and, later, troops. This produced a marked increase in the military medical activities of the British and American troops stationed in West Africa. The civilian population benefited indirectly, and, after the war, some military hospitals were handed over to the civilian administration.

With increasing industrialization, health services continued to improve, and in 1952 with limited self-government for the three regions of the country, government grants-in-aid for missionary health care further enhanced this development. The latter was boosted by independence in 1960 by international aid from such agencies as WHO, UNICEF, British Technical Assistance, and American AID among others. Medical education expanded, and, by 1983, there were thirteen medical schools in Nigeria. The nineteen states of the Federation of Nigeria each has a Ministry of Health and its own health services. The central government is responsible for international and public health, specialized hospitals including university hospitals, and health policy.

Structure of the Health-Care System

Administrative Apparatus

The structure of the health services in Nigeria is based on the political divisions in the country. The Federal Ministry of Health in Lagos is responsible for international health, the collection of statistics, nationwide preventive and health education programs, and for curative care in all the university teaching hospitals in the country. It also owns and administers special hospitals (psychiatric and orthopedic hospitals). In each of the nineteen states, a state ministry headed by a Commissioner of Health is responsible for all aspects of public health in the state. It runs various general hospitals both in the rural and urban centers and in some areas where hospitals have been built by community effort, and it contributes to the joint administration of such hospitals. The smaller political divisions in the country, the local government areas, build and operate the local government dispensaries. The latter offer primary health care and receive professional supervision from the state-owned general hospitals. A National Council for Health, a body comprising the federal and state ministries of health, initiates health policy which becomes law after successfully passing through the accepted legislative processes in the country. In addition, the Nigerian Medical Council, a statutory body established by the federal government and comprising professional men from the federal and state ministries of health and representatives from the Nigerian Medical Association and of the colleges of medicine, is responsible for setting standards of health care and medical education. No medical school can operate without the prior approal of the Nigerian Medical Council. The Council keeps a register of medical and dental practitioners and could strike out any name for professional misconduct after due legal processes for which an appeal in the country's higher courts can be made.

Private Health Care. In addition to the government-operated health system, private practice is also available. Large companies operate their own health services or retain private medical practitioners for their staff and dependents. The services operated by these companies may include hospital facilities or may consist mainly of outpatient care or first aid. There is also health care by voluntary agencies which are predominantly missionary bodies. Most of the latter were of foreign origin initially but have become indeginized with independence. Only few still obtain assistance from abroad. Many receive grants-in-aid from the various governments in the country. The traditional system of health care operates not only in rural areas but also in the big cities, and it enjoys great confidence probably because it is culture bound. It is an uncoordinated system. Each practitioner operates in isolation, and the "secret" is kept within the family. Many patients invariably first consult the traditional healer and only go to the conventional hospital when the illness gets worse. Eventually, if it is a chronic illness or a potentially fatal one, they go back once again to the traditional healer.

Professional Bodies. Various professional bodies exist. The Nigerian Medical Association is a powerful body of registered medical and dental practitioners. It gives adequate support to the government in maintaining standards and has indirectly been instrumental to continued progress in the postgraduate residency programs. There are also the Pharmaceutical Society of Nigeria, the Association of Nurses and Midwives of Nigeria, and the Association of Medical Laboratory Scientists. Each of these operates in almost the same way as the Nigerian Medical Association.

Organizational Relationships

A patient has numerous options depending on where he is resident, the amount of time which he is prepared to spare, his ability to pay for services, the strength of his cultural affinity or his predilection for giving way to the cultural beliefs of relations or friends, the acuteness of his illness, his age, and possibly his level of formal education. In the rural areas, the local government dispensaries, the traditional healers, the rural hospitals, and lately private clinics form the options available. From any of these primary contacts with the health service, but least with the traditional healer, a patient could be sent to the bigger general hospitals and eventually to the university teaching hospitals should his illness demand more expertise and more sophisticated equipment.

Professional supervision of the dispensaries is conducted by the general hospitals, which often supply drugs to them as well. The outpatient clinics of the hospitals and the dispensaries are open mainly in the mornings and early afternoons on weekdays, but emergencies are accepted throughout each day in the hospitals.

Currently, more attention seems to be devoted to curative rather than preventive care. This seems to be the immediate and appropriate response to the numerous acute medical problems that are seen at health institutions every day. Every health institution operated by a government, however, has a preventive section as well. Immunization is practiced against the common childhood diseases for which vaccines are available (Bacille Calmette-Guérin—BCG, diphtheria-pertussis-tetanus, measles, polio). A revised and expanded program on immunization was launched in October 1984 in Lagos. In well-baby clinics—for which the Welesly Hospital in Ile-Ife Oyo State is a well-known pioneer—and also in prenatal and postnatal clinics, posters and health workers remind mothers of the benefits of a well-balanced diet, breast feeding, adequate waste disposal and pit latrines (where a water system is not available), potable water supply, personal cleanliness, and the wearing of shoes. Federal and state television and radio stations transmit health education programs in all major indigenous languages of the country. Intersectoral activities are best coordinated at the village level where community development programs, sometimes with the aid of the government (by a matching grants system), develop, for example, potable water supply from boreholes or build community secondary schools or community hospitals.

Long-term planning has not yet become possible. Planning has been mainly on a medium-term (five to ten years) or a short-term (annual budget exercise) basis. Both at the center and in the states, a Ministry of Economic Development and Planning coordinates planning functions with the Ministry of Finance, the cabinet office, and the relevant ministry which, for health matters, is the Ministry of Health. Programs are listed according to priority in each ministry, and each program competes for funds on this basis from the allocation for each ministry from the total projected revenue for the plan period.

The major national development plans have been 1945–1955, the First Colonial Development Plan (Decade of Development); 1956–1962, the Second Colonial Development Plan; 1962–1968, the First National Development Plan (Post-Independence Plan); 1970–1974, the Second National Development Plan; 1975–1979, the Third National Development Plan; and 1980–1984, the Fourth National Development Plan. The Decade of Development was launched immediately after World War II, and the emphasis was on health in the provision of safe drinking water and adequate sanitation in the urban areas.

The Financial Mechanisms

The major provider of health services at the federal, state, or local government levels is the government. In most cases, this service whether preventive or curative is free while, in others, a token fee is charged to the patient. In all cases, however, preschool and school children do not pay for services in government health institutions. In addition, civil servants in each state receive free medical treatment in their state hospitals. Dental care, especially when dentures are to be supplied, however, is not free.

In organizations such as big private companies or parastatal establishments, which offer limited health services or retain private medical practitioners to do so, the workers and their dependents receive free medical treatment. In some instances this is totally free; in others, a small monthly deduction from a worker's salary is added to the employer's larger contribution toward the sickness fund. In addition, members of the management staff of these companies could consult any medical practitioner of their choice at the expense of the companies. There are usually safeguards to prevent abuse.

The majority of the population who are self-employed and the bulk of whom are farmers in the rural areas have to pay for their health care, even though this payment is minimal in the heavily subsidied government or local authority health institutions.

Treatment for pulmonary tubercuosis is free in the numerous special hospitals throughout the country. The same applies to leprosy.

The Organization of Medical Personnel

In the bigger hospitals, a general outpatient department (GOPD) functions as a triage. Patients without appointment to specific specialty clinics are first seen here. Minor complaints are disposed of, and conditions needing extensive investigations or specialized care are referred to the appropriate physicians who hold clinics on specific days of the week. Accident and emergency departments, in addition, are invariably a feature of these hospitals. They receive patients 24 hours a day, and they have a small operating theater for minor surgery and a few beds for emergency treatment and observation, but, in most cases, they refer the patients for admission to the appropriate physician on emergency duty for that day. In each accident and emergency department, a separate section is developed for children. Women in labor go directly to the labor ward.

The physician's inpatient practice is developed on the traditional unit and departmental system. There are departments of internal medicine, surgery, obstetrics and gynecology, and pediatrics. Sometimes ophthalmology, otolaryngology, anesthesia, pediatrics, surgery, and others could each constitute a department or be part of general surgery. The same thing applies to internal medicine (neuroogy, dermatology, etc.) or to pediatrics and obstetrics and gynecology. The pattern seems to depend on the availability of funds and expertise. Within each department, the physicians operate in units. The unit may be for a subspeciality (e.g., chest diseases), in which case all chest physicians are grouped in the unit, or may simply be a smaller division of the department. Each unit has a head and a variable number of younger doctors from intern to senior registrar. The latter has obtained the postdoctoral diploma and is awaiting the opportunity to apply for a vacant consultant post.

The same pattern operates in big private general hospitals and mission hospitals but with fewer specialties and also fewer training doctors. In the district hospitals (government or mission) or in small private hospitals (urban or rural), one or two all-purpose medical practitioners are responsible for all major subspecialties (internal medicine, pediatrics, surgery, and obstetrics and gynecology). Limited in scope, they refer complicated problems to higher level health-care institutions, but they are nevertheless vital for emergency patients who must be treated on the spot.

Reimbursement Arrangements. Most health care in the country is provided on a fee-for-service basis. Since most government institutions are heavily subsidized and many mission hospitals receive grants-in-aid from the government, the cost to the individual patient is comparatively small. Companies that retain the services of private physicians pay a retainer on a monthly, half-yearly, or annual basis depending on mutual arrangement. In addition, the physician sends his bill to the company at the end of each month for actual medical attention given to the staff of that company during that particular month. No national health insurance health insurance scheme is yet available.

Role of Nurses and Other Professionals. Other health professionals, mainly nurses, midwives, laboratory scientists, physiotherapists, radiographers, occupational therapists, medical records officers, and social workers, play vital roles in effective health-care delivery. The nurses and midwives form the largest single group. Each group of health professionals is regulated by a separate act of government, e.g., the Medical and Dental Practitioners Act of 1963 and the Nursing and Midwifery Registration Act. Apart from the medical laboratory scientists and the midwives, the other health professionals do not seem to go into private practice on their own.

Recently, the roles of the sanitary engineers in the promotion of public health, the health planners in the development of health services, and the health economists in seeking less costly but equally effective health systems have become increasingly important.

In Nigeria, most of the health professionals are being trained in the country: doctors, dentists, nurses, midwives, physiotherapists, occupational therapists, medical laboratory scientists, and radiographers. Training at home for the Nigerian and West African postgraduate diplomas is now available but not yet mandatory.

Major Health Problems

The Third National Development Plan recognized as the major health problems in 1975: (a) a shortage of health manpower, (b) a disparity in the distribution of health facilities and institutions in the country, (c) inadequate preventive health services, and (d) poor management and utilization of health institutions. With some modification, this statement is still true. The increase in the number of medical schools to thirteen (as a result of the implementation of this plan) did reduce the doctor/population ratio from 1:22,000 in 1973 to 1:12,550 in 1980; however, the imbalance—with the preponderance in major cities—still exists. The shortages in the other groups of health workers—medical laboratory scientists and technicians, pharmacists, radiographers, and nurses—have been less dramatically reduced.

The teaching hospitals and general hospitals located in urban areas account for about 70 percent of the total number of beds available in all recorded health establishments in the country. In addition, preventive services are disproportionately developed when compared with curative services. Consequently, infectious diseases account for much of the morbidity and mortality rates. Management and utilization of health institutions need improvement. The hope that a board supervising the network of hospitals in each state would improve staff discipline and provide for better management did not materialize as inadequate manpower was assigned to it, coupled with interministerial strain.

A major problem is finance. Nigeria's health services are run predominantly on the basis of public assistance, and much of the government's allocation is used for personnel emoluments. For improved technical services, a great infusion of funds is needed. Since the average patient cannot afford this, there is need for alternative means for financing health care in the country.

Future Trends

The Third National Development Plan recognized that in spite of the progress made since 1960 in the improvement and expansion of the basic infrastructure of health services,

> the problems that still remain to be solved are so tremendous that the situation would require the application of appropriate policies and measures as well as massive physical inputs in the critical areas if the health services are to keep pace with the rapid growth of population.

The solutions proposed were increased manpower development, further development and expansion of hospital services, comprehensive health coverage of the whole country, improved disease control, efficient management and utilization of health institutions, encouragement of medical research, and improved health planning. A total amount of ₦759,928,000 was earmarked for capital health development during the plan period from 1975 to 1980. Out of this, ₦406,410,000 was for hospital programs, ₦219,175,000 was for basic health services programs, ₦70,050,000 was for training programs, and ₦64,293,000 was for the support of health programs (*Third National Development Plan 1975–80*, vol. 1, chap. 17).

The admission level in all medical schools in the country was to reach 3,000 by 1980; however, even, though this target was never reached, it had become clear by 1984 that the annual output of doctors had far exceeded the economic capacity of the country's institutions to employ them—a situation made worse by the present worldwide economic recession. Most medical schools have consequently reduced their annual enrollment. There is still a disparity in the distribution of doctors between the rural and urban centers; however, some young doctors, after the mandatory national youth corps service mostly in the rural health services (for one year immediately after internship), have volunteered to continue, but their number is comparatively small. A possible solution to this problem is the incorporation of a two-year service in rural health care as part of the postdoctoral training progam of the national postgraduate diploma.

The envisaged impact on health care by the creation, training, and deployment of a new cadre of medical personnel for the rural health services did not occur. This may be partly because the program represented an upgrading exercise rather than real creation and development of new and additional members of the health team. It is probable that, in the future, primary health-care workers will be chosen from the community and trained specifically for the health needs of that community. The large and diverse population of the country with its varying culture and socioeconomic stages of development, necessitating different approaches, has delayed rapid implementation of primary health care. A more intensive effort by the ministries of health in the various states of the federation and specific planning at this level are possible in the future. Modern health-care coverage of the population was expected to reach 40 percent in 1980 from a figure of 25 percent. The difficulties encountered seem to call for a review of the concept of health care. Use of traditional healers after the removal of the negative aspects of their practice, intensification of primary health care, and increase in the number of smaller hospitals in the rural areas are all possible. A senate committee on traditional medicine was set up in 1983. In 1984, the new government instituted a committee to study alternative medical practice in the country.

The takeover of teaching hospitals by the federal government and their increase in number to thirteen have created problems. It is possible that the number will be reduced. Medical research, especially health systems research, will assume greater importance in the future as attempts will be made to rationalize expenditure on health and to maximize the effective use of health resources.

An issue which is generating debate is the financing of health care. Public health care is greatly subsidized by government in Nigeria but, with the increasing cost of modern health care, it is becoming clear that alternative methods for economic support have to be devised. National health insurance has been proposed by various groups, notably the Nigerian Medical Association, and it is possible that this could be developed by existing insurance companies, or a totally new health insurance group could be created by a combined effort of government and private enterprise. The issue is becoming urgent as increasing socioeconomic development seems to be enhancing the percentage contributed by the private sector in the nation's total health resources.

The political will to further develop and expand health care is presently evident judging from the initial pronouncement of the new government on its disappointment that "the government health institutions had been reduced to mere consulting offices." Many state ministries of health have intensified the development and promotion of primary health care. The College of Medicine, University of Lagos, has incorporated in its curriculum one year of intensive field training in primary health care. Overall, in the spirit of social justice, the trend in Nigeria is toward Health for All by the Year 2000.

References

Adeloye, A. 1977. *Nigerian Pioneers of Modern Medicine: Selected Writings*. Ibadan: Ibadan University Press.

Basic Health Service Programme of the Federal Republic of Nigeria. 1976. Report of the Project Formulation Team, p. 10. Lagos: Federal Ministry of Health.

Dada, B. A. A. November, 1982. *Health Profile 1981/82*. Lagos: Federal Ministry of Health.

Kent, M. M. and C. Haub. 1984. *1984 World Population Data Sheet*. Washington, D. C.: Population Reference Bureau.

Schram, R. 1971. *A History of the Nigerian Health Services*. Ibadan: Ibadan University Press.

Third National Development Plan 1975–80, vol. 1. 1974. The Central Planning Office, Federal Ministry of Economic Development, Federal Republic of Nigeria. Lagos: Government Press.

Williams, G. A. 1971. *Annual Report of the Medical Officer of Health*. Lagos: Public Health Department, Lagos City Council.

World Bank. 1983. *World Development Report*. Washington, D.C.

POLAND

Marek Lubicz and
W. Cezary Wlodarczyk

Introduction and Historical Overview

In respect to geography and politics, Poland is an East-European country, sharing frontiers with USSR, East Germany, and Czechoslovakia. In respect to culture, however, the Polish people find their country to be a bridge between west and east, reflecting their relations with Roman culture, the central role of the Catholic Church, and more than one thousand years of statehood. In its history, Poland has had to struggle many times for its existence, attacked by all its neighbors; it lost its national independence for the period from 1795 to 1918.

Up to the nineteenth century, the basic form of outpatient medical service was the private practice of doctors; hospitals were operated by the church. The first attempts at organizing a public health service dated from the eighteenth century; however, the National Health Service (NHS) system was partly introduced only in 1918 after independence was regained. At that time, the Polish State adopted a number of social laws of great significance for health care, including an 8-hour workday, a 46-hour workweek, women's and juvenile labor protection, and paid maternity leaves. The health service was dispersed among a number of sectors: national, provincial, insurance, and private. In particular, the state and provincial sectors together possessed 53 percent of the beds. With regard to outpatient care, 80 percent of the services were rendered by general practitioners; there were also separate health centers for the poor and additional facilities administered by insurance companies.

After World War II and the tragic period of Nazi occupation, when the country had lost 6 million citizens (one-seventh of the total population) and a huge portion of its national wealth, important changes took place. The liberation of the country by the USSR and the subsequent triumph of the left resulted in the socialist political system of the contemporary Polish People's Republic. The changes were evident in the organization of health care as well. First, the principle of state responsibility for health care was accepted. In 1945 the Ministry of Health was established, and in 1948 the central planning system was extended to the health sector. During the years from 1950 to 1951, the private character of the medical professions was abolished. Since then, medical professionals have been employees in the national health service. In 1960 the Ministry of Health and Social Care (MHSW) was established to stress a complex set of actions in the health-care sector. In 1968 some elements of professional self-control were restored with state acceptance of a statement of ethical norms written by the Association of Polish Physicians. In 1973 the national program for the development of the health-care system through to 1990 was adopted. The program—found by the *Seym* (Parliament) in 1983 to be excessively optimistic—established ambitious goals for expending national health resources. It was designed to ensure the comprehensive and gratuitous provision of all needed health services for all Polish citizens. In order to attain these program goals, an effort was undertaken during the years of from 1973 to 1975 to integrate the NHS organizational structure and to merge all forms of health and social care into uniform institutions, the so-called Local Integrated Health Services (ZOZs). Unfortunately, this effort was an excessively formal one, although the act of 1982 modified various organizational rules to create considerably more flexibility.

The principles of state responsibility for health included not only the operation of health service institutions, but also their rules concerning patient access to services. The so-called rule of common availability, for instance, did not eliminate existing special rights within the health services but instead gradually expanded coverage to particular, previously excluded groups. In 1972 the last group, some 6.5 million agricultural workers (predominantly private farmers) received health insurance protection. Since then, 99 percent of the Polish population is entitled to ambulatory and inpatient care in hospitals without payment.

Health Status of the Population

Demographic Situation

Poland is a relatively young though aging country of over 37 million inhabitants. In 1985, the population had the following age distribution: 0 to 14 years, 25 percent; 15 to 64 years, 65 percent; and over 65 years, 10 percent of the total population. The birth rate was very high just after the war, subsequently falling in the period from 1950 to 1970, but, from the end of the 1970s, once again increasing to what may well be the highest in all of Europe (Table 1).

The mortality rate has stabilized in the last four years, after a period of growth (from 1960 to 1980). There remains greater mortality of men (11.1 for men in 1985, 9.4 for women), which appears to have increased over the last two decades. The average life expectancy for persons at ages 0, 15, 30, 45, and 60 amounted

Table 1
Key Health-Related Statistics of Poland

	1946	1950	1960	1970	1980	1985
1. Total number of inhabitants /in millions/	23.6	25.0	29.8	32.7	35.7	37.3
2. Number of live births						
in 1,000s	622.5	763.1	669.5	546.0	692.8	677.6
per 1,000 inhabitants	26.2	30.5	22.5	16.7	19.4	18.2
3. Natality rate per 1,000 inhabitants	16.0	18.9	14.9	8.5	9.6	8.0
4. Infant morality rate per 1,000 live births	119.8	108.0	56.0	33.2	21.2	18.4
5. Mortality rate per 1,000 inhabitants	10.2	11.6	7.5	8.2	9.8	10.2

in 1985, respectively, for women, 74.8, 61.3, 46.7, 32.5, 19.5; and for men, 66.5, 53.3, 39.2, 26.0, and 15.8.

Epidemiological Situation

From the epidemiological point of view, the most important diseases are as follows:

1. Cardiovascular diseases. These are the most common cause of death, as well as the cause of nearly half of all disability cases.
2. Neoplasms. These have caused increasing number of deaths in recent years (Table 2).
3. Accidents, traumas, and poisonings. The highest cause of death for children. The mortality rate for traffic accidents has, however, slightly decreased in the recent past.
4. Mental and nervous diseases. These represent a major social threat due to their frequent occurrence, upward tendency (numbers of new cases in 1981 and 1985 were, respectively, 139,000 and 146,000), and high degree of disability. Two of the most important problems in this area are alcoholism and—recently—narcomania, mainly among the young.
5. Infectious diseases. In the last fifteen years, the incidence of many diseases has considerably decreased; some have even been eliminated—poliomyelitis, measles, diphtheria, pertussis, and scarlatina. Other diseases are still significant epidemiological problems, including influenza, viral hepatitis (incidence per 100,000 population: in

Table 2
Most Common Causes of Death

Number of deaths per 100,000 Inhabitants	1975	1980	1985
1. Cardiovascular disease	378.1	439.9	492.1
2. Tumors	157.4	171.2	182.7
3. Accidents, traumas, poisonings	69.6	75.9	72.8
of which: traffic accidents	16.6	16.8	13.3
4. Respiratory diseases	57.0	54.9	56.3
5. Diabetes	10.1	12.5	15.9
6. Infectious and parasitic diseases	19.0	16.0	10.8
of which: tuberculosis	12.1	8.0	6.4

1980, 136; 1985, 115), meningitis, scabies, salmonellosis, and tuberculosis. The number of new cases of tuberculosis is 23,000 per year and is slightly decreasing.

6. Respiratory diseases, which cause most of the sick leave taken, and digestive disorders, which cause most of the incidents of hospitalization.

Health-Care System

Structure of Health Administration

Up to 1975, the structure of health administration in Poland corresponded to the four-level administrative structure of the country as a whole: The health system was divided into seventeen provinces, and those were divided into districts and communes. In 1975, the district level was eliminated, and 49 provinces were established. However, in 1973, the former districts became the basis for deriving elementary units of the modified health-care system: the ZOZs. The actual relationships among administrative (representative and executive) and NHS authorities on particular management levels may be represented as follows:

1. Central level: Parliament, government—ministry (MHSW).
2. Provinces: People's Council, *Voivode*—Provincial Health Department.

3. Former districts: no authorities—ZOZ.
4. Communes: People's Council—no NHS authorities.

The ministry is the main coordinator and executor of the health policy of the state. It is responsible for nearly all aspects of health services provided to the general population, particularly medical personnel training and financial support of the NHS. The ministry has strategic responsibilities in the field of health and social care. Moreover, it controls directly several NHS institutions: medical academies, national research institutes, the Central NHS Investment Board, and others.

The provincial authorities, responsible for organizing health care in particular provinces, manage the following NHS units: ZOZs, provincial hospitals, social welfare institutions, sanitary-epidemiological units, pharmacies, blood-collection service, and NHS transport. ZOZ authorities, in turn, are involved in various current management problems, including personnel transfers, job evaluation, and assignment of funds among the several facilities within the ZOZ.

Organization of Health Care

The main local units of the NHS system are in the general ZOZs. An average ZOZ serves about 90,000 inhabitants, but in big cities, a ZOZ may serve as many as 250,000 people. Within one institution having joint management and budget and functional departments, a typical ZOZ comprises hospital and ambulatory care units (both those offering primary and also specialist care) emergency services, social welfare units, and laboratory and diagnostic facilities. At the provincial level, there are provincial hospitals, which also offer a wide range of specialty services and some auxiliary actions (e.g., personnel training). Moreover, in certain provinces, specialized ZOZs are organized to provide ambulatory and stationary services to particular groups of people (e.g., industrial and academic ZOZs, providing primary care as well, or ZOZs for mother and child), or for particular specialities (e.g., for mental diseases). Finally, this third level of highly specialized NHS units includes clinics of medical academies and national medical research institutes. In addition, there are separate medical care systems serving military personnel, militia (police), and employees of airlines and railroads, as well as their families.

The usual point of entry to the NHS system is the primary care unit in the locality where a person lives. The patient may subsequently be referred to a polyclinic, where various specialities are engaged, to an outpatient department of a nearby general hospital, or to a higher level specialist unit, according to the case and rules of regionalization. The patients may also go on their own to a specialist unit, if they wish, without referral from a primary care unit; however, referral is the preferred arrangement. Table 3 presents statistical data on services rendered by particular types of NHS institutions.

Besides the NHS institutions, it is also possible to get medical assistance in

Table 3
Services Rendered by NHS Institutions

Services of particular health sector	1970	1980	1985
1. Ambulatory services, millions of visits per year, of:			
-generalized ZOZs	161.1	222.8	226.8
-industrial/academic ZOZs	35.7	54.5	50.9
-private/cooperative units	4.1	7.8	8.0
2. Ambulatory services per person	6.2	8.0	7.8
of which in general ZOZs:			
-primary care units in towns	4.1	4.5	4.3
-rural primary care centers	1.5	2.4	2.5
-dentists services	0.9	1.2	1.1
-specialist services	1.3	1.6	1.6
3. Hospitals:			
-numbers of patients per 1 bed	19.4	22.0	21.9
-hospital admissions per 1,000 population	99.5	122.4	124.3
-average length of stay per patient in days	16.0	14.0	13.1
4. Emergency medical services: millions of calls to:			
-accidents	0.3	0.4	0.4
-sickness emergencies	2.8	4.1	4.5
-transfers of patients	1.3	2.6	3.5
5. Social care: thousands of people receiving social benefits:			
-financial/tribute assistance	949.0	625.0	1,111.0
-stay in social care houses	47.4	59.8	62.0
6. Pharmacies: thousands of people per one open pharmacy	12.7	11.0	10.8

medical cooperatives (i.e., private group practice clinics) and also in private consulting rooms (see Table 3). Hospitalization, however, is available only in NHS facilities. Activities for the benefit of the health and, above all, social care, mainly in the care of the chronically ill, prevention of alcoholism, and social welfare are also performed by the Roman Catholic Church, other religious organizations, and numerous social organizations (e.g., the Polish Red Cross).

Primary Health Care. Primary Health Care in Poland is considered to include adult internal medicine, pediatrics, obstetrics-gynecology, and dentistry. Two main types of ambulatory care facilities offer primary care within each generalized ZOZ: rural health centers (RHCs) and urban primary care centers (UPCCs). A typical RHC is staffed by one general practitioner, who gives primary care to men, women, and children, as well as by one dentist. Both of them are aided by two or three nurses. Occasionally, a gynecologist-obstetrician (described simply as gynecologist) visits for a session. In towns, the UPCCs usually serve a larger population of from 6,000 to 24,000 persons and they are more fully staffed. Theoretically, two general practitioners (GPs), one pediatrician, two dentists, and a part-time gynecologist are supposed to serve a population of 10,000. A UPCC is typically divided into four units, corresponding to the four primary care disciplines.

Every doctor in an RHC or a UPCC gives therapeutic and also preventive service. Activities of the first kind include first-contact health service and home visits (by GPs and pediatricians). Preventive care includes periodic check-ups on those with chronic conditions or high-risk adults and children. This policy, known in Poland as "dispensarization," focuses in particular on serious cardiovascular diseases, tuberculosis, and for children, serious visual defects, developmental problems, and mental retardation. The pediatricians also offer systematic well-baby examinations and health surveillance for school children. The gynecologists provide preventive care directed at early detection of organ cancer and perform periodic prenatal and postpartum examinations. The postpartum patients are also visited at home by a midwife a few times up to six weeks after childbirth.

Specialist Health Care. Specialized secondary-level services are provided by the following institutions:

1. Polyclinics or specialist care units, tied to larger primary care centers of general ZOZs, which offer services in major specialities (surgery, laryngology, etc).
2. Outpatient departments of ZOZ hospitals, provincial hospitals, and medical academy clinics, which provide a wide range of highly specialized services (e.g., cardiology, psychiatry, or orthopedics).
3. Dispensaries of specialized ZOZs, which—as described before—offer specialities for particular subpopulations.

Inpatient Health Care. The main NHS institutions offering inptient health care are general hospitals. There are four principal levels of such hospitals: (1) highly specialized clinics of medical academies, (2) provincial integrated hspitals, (3) local hospitals for each ZOZ area, and (4) a wide variety of smaller hospitals, both in towns and rural areas, limited to basic specialities. In addition, there is a great diversity of specialized hospitals for particular diseases or specialities. There are, for instance, psychiatric hospitals and other institutions of mental health care (sanatoriums for psychoneurotic patients, separate for children and adults, and convalescent institutions for alcoholic and drug addiction patients); antituberculosis sanatoriums; special units for rehabilitation of the orthopedically disabled; and so on. All hospitals of specialized ZOZs must be included here as well. Moreover, there is a variety of "health resorts sanatoriums," intended first of all as places for convalescence of patients discharged from a hospital.

In 1985 general hospitals had 210,000 beds at their disposal; psychiatric hospitals, 38,400; health resorts sanatoriums, 44,600; and the remaining somatic care facilities, 16,000. This amounted to 55.5 beds per 10,000 population for general and, in addition, 10.1 beds per 10,000 in psychiatric hospitals (the corresponding figures in 1970 were 51.3 and 11.6). (See also Table 3.)

Emergency Medical Services. Emergency medical services (EMS) are typically included in the scope of the generalized ZOZs and are offered by all 404 EMS departments, which both provide medical assistance in the outpatient rooms of EMS facilities and respond to telephone calls for ambulance service. The great part of all cases are not true emergencies (about 90 percent); some ambulance trips are transfers of patients to or from hospitals (about 40 percent) and some are calls of nonurgent nature (another kind of "home visits"). In principle, there is always a physician in each EMS team. Thus that form of medical assistance is very attractive for the patient—each call must be answered—but it is very expensive for the NHS system.

Social Welfare. The last type of major service in local ZOZs is provided by more than 440 social welfare units. They deliver social care for the aged, the disabled, retarded children, and other handicapped persons. The social care service provides benefits to those living at home (financial as well as food, fuel, and so on) as well as institutional benefits to social welfare institutions for the aged or special care houses for the chronically ill (nursing homes). (See Table 3.) There are also social welfare agencies directed at social and professional rehabilitation for the disabled and the blind (for instance, numerous cooperatives with more than 200,000 workers in all these agencies in 1983).

Occupational Health Services. The occupational health services provide primary, specialist, and sometimes also somatic health care for nearly 5.5 million employees (75 percent) working in different types of industry and enterprises. The majority of them are served by industrial health centers (IHC), subordinated to specialized "industrial" ZOZs. Those working in small plants or firms are usually served by multiplant IHCs which often belong to general ZOZs. The industrial physicians give treatment service and perform preemployment and periodic health examinations (dispensarization as well) and supervision of the working environment.

Other Services. The activities of basic health and social services institutions are supported by a number of functional services, including:

1. Blood-collection service, which comprises the provincial blood stations. In 1985, nearly 550,000 liters of blood were collected from 1 million honorary and family donors, and from 33,000 paid donors.

2. State sanitary supervision (sanitary-epidemiological service) which performs environmental sanitation, particularly communal, occupational, water, and school hygiene; food and nutrition control; and prevention of communicable diseases.
3. Drug production and distribution institutions, which include pharmaceutical companies, mainly within the Polfa complex, as well as hospitals and open pharmacies (see Table 3).

Medical Personnel

The actual supply of Polish medical personnel must be evaluated in relation to the critical lack of health manpower in the postwar period. The ratio of physicians, for instance, declined to 3.2 per 10,000 population in 1946 as nearly half of all doctors died during the war. As a result, taking into account the goals of the new health-care programs, great efforts were applied to the intensive training of medical personnel, especially physicians. The state established rapid but full pledged (and free of charge) professional education for physicians, dentists, and pharmacists at the university level, as well as intensive training of nurses at the vocational level. The effect of these actions is evident in Table 4.

The legal rules that guide the Polish health-care system emphasize a dominant role of the physicians, who are the only medical workers allowed to make independent therapeutic decisions. Physicians have lawful monopoly on the rendering of health services just as only dentists are permitted to do restorative work in a patient's mouth. It should be noted that there are also providers from outside the medical profession (for instance, bioenergotherapists) who render services and have considerable support from some customers. However, there is an MHSW instruction that forbids NHS employees to cooperate with such unlicensed providers.

Upon graduation, a physician has the right to practice after completing a one-year internship and registering with provincial-level health authorities. Then he is engaged typically in medical work in the public system and also (quite often) in a second type of medical work, either in the NHS agencies or in private practice. The only condition for private practice, carried on also by dentists, is simultaneous full-time employment by an NHS institution. The private practice concerns ambulatory services only; surgical interventions, except simple interventions, critical emergencies, and abortions must be performed in hospitals (there are no private hospitals in Poland). A strong tendency to acquire speciality qualifications is evident among Polish physicians: nearly 70 percent of all doctors are either first or second degree specialists (the first degree may be equated with an American speciality candidate), mainly in internal diseases, 20 percent; pediatrics, 15 percent; and surgery, 13 percent. A similar tendency exists among dentists.

The proportion of physicians and other academic graduates in the health force is as follows: pharmacists and dentists make up 15 percent of all health workers; nurses, midwives, and other middle-level health personnel constitute nearly one-

Table 4
Medical Personnel

	1946	1955	1965	1975	1980	1985
1. Total number of NHS employees thousands	x	x	355	522	599	716
2. Fractions of qualified personnel per 10,000 inhabitants						
-physicians	3.2	6.7	12.6	15.9	17.8	19.6
-dentists	0.7	2.5	3.6	4.4	4.7	4.7
-pharmacists	1.0	2.3	3.2	4.1	4.3	4.3
-nurses	2.5	17.9	24.4	35.9	43.9	48.1
-midwives	2.6	2.8	3.4	3.9	4.5	5.4
-feldshers	0.3	2.0	1.8	1.2	1.0	0.9
3. Percentage of total NHS personnel in the total number of employees in socialized sector				4.5%	5%	5.9%
4. Salaries of NHS personnel, in thousands zlotych,						
-average for the sector				3.1	4.8	15.5
-average for physicians				6.4	8.8	26.3
-average for whole country/ socialized sector/				3.9	6.0	20.0
5. Distribution of qualified NHS personnel - standard deviation from mean fraction per 10,000 people in particular provinces				1975	1980	1983
- physicians				7.3	7.3	6.4
- dentists				1.7	1.3	1.3
- nurses				10.0	8.4	8.2

half of all health manpower; the balance are housekeeping, clerical, or maintenance workers. The majority of all nurses are fully qualified (R.N.) nurses; the supply of assistant nurses has been declining since 1970 as a result of particular social and economic conditions. As noted, nurses perform most activities on the doctor's recommendation or under his surveillance. This principle concerns also midwives who, however, handle most normal maternity cases; only complicated deliveries are undertaken by physicians. The numbers of the allied health workers (laboratory technicians, dieticians, health educators, and others) are rising, but their combined number constitutes only half of the nursing personnel.

The Polish medical personnel are salaried public employees. They are paid permanent salaries which, however, increase with speciality qualifications, with seniority, with medical positions, and with undertaking work in rural areas or in primary care units. Moreover, physicians and also some other health workers may get additional pay for emergency duties (during night or weekend hours) in hospitals or EMS stations, as well as fees from private patients.

Financing and Planning Functions

Given the principle of state responsibility for health and social care, planning for the NHS is an integral part of the nationwide central planning system. Also financing of the NHS goes, in most part, through the state budget. Plans in the domain of health and social care (HSC) are contained within the National Social-Economic Plan, defining general directives for NHS; the Central Annual Plan, determining particular major projects or intentions in the area of HSC; and also of local/provincial or communal plans. Planning is based upon centrally fixed normative, financial, and numerical indices. The hierarchical competence system decides then which problems are incorporated in particular plans in the budget structure. The central budget finances only those health institutions that are subordinated to the ministry. Other institutions are financed by provincial budgets that comprise 84 percent of all health-related budget funds. Apart from funds originating from the budget, the government has some additional funds at its disposal (Table 5). These include voluntary contributions of citizens to the National Health Fund and other public funds as well as contributions from companies (for setting up health facilities in the workplace). Moreover, there are other budgetary funds not included in Table 5 (for instance, for the production of drugs); those funds are at the disposal of other ministries.

Despite declaring the fundamental principle of the free public medical services, there are some costs (approximately one percent of personal income) to be paid from the patient's pocket. These include partial payments for drugs prescribed by public ambulatory care agencies (30 percent in most cases) or for health resorts treatment and, of course, full payment for all services outside the NHS. Moreover, aged pensioners, persons with serious chronic diseases, railroad employees, and NHS personnel (approximately 15 percent of the total population) do not pay for medicine.

Major Problems Confronting the Health Sector

The main problems confronting the Polish health and social care system may be classified into the following categories: problems related to the health status of the population, to the organization and performance of the NHS, to the actual financing system, and to the availability of manpower and material resources.

Among the problems related to health status are the gradual aging of the population and certain unfavorable death-rate tendencies, particularly with regard to average life expectancy and the significant high mortality among men. Increases in morbidity and mortality from the "diseases of civilization" (especially

Table 5
Financing of Health and Socal Care

	1975	1980	1985
1. Structure of NHS budget funds coming from particular sources /in milliards zlotych, actual prices/			
-Central budget	60.0	105.2	479.7
-Contributions from enterprises	0.8	1.7	6.0
-National Health Fund and other public funds	0.8	1.4	5.2
-expenses form the patient's pocket /costs of private consultations not included/	9.1	15.9	38.4
Total /in actual prices/	70.7	124.2	529.3
Total /constant prices 1982/	271.9	343.5	328.0
2. Fraction of personal expenses in total NHS expenditures	12.9%	12.8%	7.3%
3. Fraction of total NHS expenditures in Distributed National Income /not equal to GNP/	5.2%	6.1%	6.2%

cardiovascular diseases and tumors) and a significant alcoholism problem must be noted as well. Despite the reduction in morbidity from a number of preventable infectious diseases of early life, tuberculosis and some diseases related to unsatisfactory sanitary conditions still generate epidemiological problems. It should also be noted that changing demographics result in a growing demand for NHS services. This includes both increasing numbers of preschool and school children as well as of the aged, disabled, and chronically ill (the number of the aged grew twice as fast as the total population).

The second category, problems related to organization and performance of the NHS, includes the following issues: inadequate efficiency and effectiveness of primary care and, in general, lack of organizational or economic incentives for the efficient utilization of the NHS resources; high percentage of specialist consultations, which constitute nearly 35 percent of all ambulatory services; and also an overly long hospital length of stay. The latter is caused, among others, by poor work organizations by the considerable number of patients who do not need hospital treatment but stay there because of lack of places in nursing homes, and by shortages in resources.

The actual financing system influencing the NHS system is also a problem. The relatively weak position of the health sector vis-à-vis other sectors of the national economy has led to the underfinancing of the NHS. Even in the period of prosperity in the 1970s, the expenditures for health and social care (constituting an almost constant proportion of about 5 percent of distributed national income) were insufficient in relation to the goals of the health program.

The current supply of medical personnel is still inadequate to the needs for health and—especially—for social services. The shortages are particularly large in relation to middle and lower level personnel. This situation results in excessive workloads for professionals (including fully qualified nurses and doctors) and in a lower quality of services. There are also inequalities in the distribution of medical workers among the various provinces. These inequalities have been decreasing only slowly (see Table 4), and rural regions are still understaffed. Excessive speciality dispersion and weak points of health manpower education system should be mentioned as well. Finally, the actual supply of material resources, i.e., technical and medical equipment, as well as pharmaceuticals, especially in local institutions, sometimes leaves much to be desired.

Future Changes in the Health and Social Care System

A major reform of the Polish NHS system was initiated in 1981. In its first stage, coordinated by the MHSW and later by the Group for Economic Reform of the Government Planning Commission, the primary care development program was introduced in 1981, and the flexibility of organizational structures was increased, in 1982. The implementation of this reform has generated a significant growth in the number of primary care personnel, due both to financial incentives (higher salaries) and a change in the social climate concerning primary care. Moreover, application of the principle of the free choice of a primary care doctor has been initiated by selected urban health centers.

The activities of the committee for developing a Polish strategy for "Health for All by 2000" (appointed in May 1984) are a continuation of the work on reforming the NHS. At the time of writing, the committee is still working, thus it is not possible to present a final list of fixed goals or policies. The main problems considered were the following: reduction of the mortality rates of infants and mothers and of the mortality rates due to cardiovascular diseases, tumors, accidents, traumas, and poisonings, especially for youths; elimination of preventable diseases; reduction of number of young disabled persons; and further reduction in differences in health status among social groups living in particular provinces or with different living and educational standards. These health goals refer to a wide system of environmental and behavioral agents. The emphasis is thereby on the participation of other sectors in creating healthy conditions for the whole society, and thus intersectoral coordination and cooperation among numerous institutions with no formal relation to the MHSW.

The following two key questions must also be considered: the tendency toward excessive specialization, particularly at the primary care level, and the efficiency of the NHS system. In the first case, it is proposed to return (at least in part) to the family doctor pattern and to abandon (to some extent) the basic specialties at primary care level. Proposals are also being developed to connect the income of medical personnel with their job performance (elements of the capitation system provided the rule of the free choice of doctor) as well as to modify financing rules of other health institutions, in particular, hospitals.

References

Indulski, Janusz M. et al. 1984. *Health Care in Poland: Attempts of Evaluation and Trends of Rationalization*. Warszawa: Zdrowie Publiczne (Public Health).

Rocznik Statystyczny (Statistical Yearbook). 1986. Warszawa: Central Statistical Office.

Rocznik Statystyczny Ochrony Zdrowia (Health Care Statistical Yearbook). 1985. Warszawa. Central Statistical Office.

Roemer, Milton I. and Ruth Roemer. 1978. *Health Manpower in the Socialist Health Care System in Poland*. Washington, D. C.: Department of Health, Education and Welfare.

Tymowska, Katarzyna and W. Cezary Wlodarczyk. 1984. Reform of Polish Health and Social Care (in Polish). In *Social Services*. PWE.

Wlodarczyk, Cezary W. and Zdzislaw Urbaniak. 1985. Trends in Health Legislation in Poland. In *Health Legislation in Europe*. Copenhagen: WHO Regional European Office.

SAUDI ARABIA

Eva Jane McHan

Introduction

The development and character of the health-care system of Saudi Arabia has been shaped by the evolution of the country's monarchical government, the revenues derived from the oil-based economy, the ethnic flavor of the Arab population, the customs of the Bedouin tribes, and the influence of the desert climate. Virtually all aspects of development, government planning, and daily life are influenced and guided by adherence to the Islamic religion. For example, an additional influence on the health-care system is the role of the Ministry of Health in the plans for the annual pilgrimage that thousands of Muslims make to the city of Mecca in the western part of the kingdom.

The Kingdom of Saudi Arabia is the largest country in the Middle East with a total land area of 2,149,000 square kilometers (Ministry of Planning 1983). In 1980, the population estimate (Saudi and expatriate) was 9,283,000. Based on a 3.7 percent rate of national increase, the 1985 estimate is 11.15 million people (9.2 million Saudis) (Sebai 1981). In other than the major cities, the population tends to be widely dispersed, resulting in a 4.3-person density per kilometer. The Bedouin population currently comprises an estimated 10 to 15 percent of the total population. The harshness of the climate is reflected in the high mean temperatures of 97° F during the summer months and in the low average rainfall. The terrain is largely desert, but there are also extensive coastal areas in addition to mountainous regions.

History

Prior to the 1920s, the country was almost totally isolated from the western world. The area was primarily nomadic in population and culture, poverty stricken, and fraught with innumerable health problems. In 1932, King Abdul Azis Bin Saud formally proclaimed the establishment of the Kingdom of Saudi Arabia as an Islamic monarchy. Two years later, the exploration for oil was initiated with the subsequent discovery of vast oil reserves. The sudden oil wealth transformed the country into a rapidly developing society with utilization of the revenues directed toward provision of housing, electricity, sanitation, communication, and education. The health-care system, at that time, was essentially a blend of both modern and traditional forms of medicine with health-care delivery largely performed by expatriate physicians from Egypt. The governmental health system was formally organized in 1950 (Birks and Sinclair 1985). The growth rate in the health sector was initally low, but it increased to an annual rate of 5.8 percent between 1961 and 1969 (Ministry of Planning 1980a, 36). By that decade, the emphasis had been appropriately placed on provision of curative services.

Since the inception of the system in the 1950s, primary, secondary, and tertiary institutions have been established, and four medical colleges, located in Riyadh, Jeddah, Dammam, and Abha, have been founded. The emphasis in planning and delivery systems has shifted from primarily curative to a mixture of curative and preventive services.

The evolution in planning is best illustrated by the increasing emphasis on preventive health care in the last three national five-year plans. The First Five-Year-Plan (1970–1975) emphasized the development of manpower and infrastructure, but also set goals toward improving preventive health, health education, and research (Ministry of Planning 1980a, 145–157). The second Five-Year-Plan (1975–1980) targeted expansion and improvement in "preventive medicine, physical environment, health education and access to and improvment in curative treatment" (Ministry of Planning 1980b, 75–80). The Third Five-Year Plan (1980–1985) placed emphasis on health education, preventive medicine, and primary health care (Ministry of Planning 1985, 81).

With the establishment of the four medical schools (the first in 1967 in Riyadh) and the increasing numbers of Saudis who have been and are being educated abroad, the percentage of indigenous Saudi medical personnel is increasing steadily. Saudis who receive their medical education abroad typically prefer to return to Saudi Arabia to practice.

Health Indications

The growth and development of the Kingdom of Saudi Arabia's economic resources are reflected by the population's improved health status and the increase in health resources. A good country-wide database system does not now exist. As a result, health statistics still must be estimated from selected samples that may not adequately reflect the actual situation in the population. While the health indices for the urban areas are probably better than those shown in Table 1, those for isolated rural areas may be far worse. Beginning in March 1984, the

Table 1
Health Related Statistics for Saudi Arabia, 1960 and 1980

	1960	1980
Crude birth rate per 1000	49	45
Crude death rate per 1000	23	13
Infant mortality rate per 1000 live births	185	111
Child deaths (age 1-4) per 100	48	17
Daily per capita calories		2,895
Literacy rate of adult population	3%	25%
Per Capita GNP		$12,600

Source: World Bank, *World Development Report*, New York: Oxford University Press, 1983, pp. 149, 187, 193, 197.

Ministry of Health established the computerization mechanisms required to improve reporting for health-related indicators. The most recent data released by the ministry dramatically illustrate the rapid development of health-related resources. For example, officials reported in February 1985 that preliminary calculations of 1982 data show a decrease in infant mortality of 84 per 1,000 live births and a decrease in the crude death rate to 10 per 1,000 population. Selected statistics are shown in Table 2.

Despite improvement in many economic and health-related sectors, other health indices have not improved at the same rate as those shown in Table 2. The crude birth rate is still one of the highest reported in developing countries, and the population pyramid resembles that of the developing world in that approximately 45 percent of the total indigenous population is under the age of 15 years (Ministry of Planning 1983).

There is moderate agreement among major authoritative sources concerning hypothesized causes of mortality and morbidity in the kingdom. By far, the greatest burden falls on infants (birth to 1 year) and children (from 1 to 5 years); gastroenteritis is the major cause of death for both groups. During infancy, prematurity, infectious diseases, and congenital malformations (possibly related to the high rate of consanguinity) are leading causes of morbidity. In addition to the prevalance of gastroenteritis, respiratory illnesses are a major factor for

Table 2
Provider Statistics, 1970 and 1980

	1970	1984
Number of Hospitals	74	145
Number of Hospital Beds	9000	26,000
Number of Physicians	1 per 4,950	1 per 840
Number of Health Care Centers	519	1,430

Source: Ministry of Health, Riyadh; Arab News, "Greater Attention Given to Health Care—Hujeilan," November 19, 1984, p. 2.

the children from 1 to 5 years of age. Most of these illnesses decrease in frequency as age increases until adolescence and young adult years, when traffic accidents become the leading cause of mortality and morbidity of males. Females in the reproductive age groups are prone to problems associated with pregnancy, particularly eclampsia and preeclampsia, hemorrhage, and shock. The maternal mortality rate has decreased in urban areas such as Riyadh and is reported to be less than 0.5 per 1,000 due to improvement in maternal child health care and the establishment and availability of blood banks. Some of the more common health problems in adults are communicable diseases including pulmonary tuberculosis and hepatitis B, heart disease, and kidney problems (Al-Bakr 1983; Arabian American Oil Co. 1980). There is an extremely high prevalence of blindness, which is generally attributed to the effects of trachoma, a disease that has decreased in incidence in recent years.

Health Services Structure

The governmental health services of the kingdom are provided by thirteen departments or agencies; the Ministry of Health (MOH) has the greatest responsibility for both provision of care and setting of overall policies for the entire health-care system. Every Saudi citizen is entitled to comprehensive and free health care at MOH facilities. Guest workers, i.e., expatriates, are entitled to the same care at MOH facilities if they are employed by companies or institutions with fewer than 50 employees. Companies with more than 50 employees are required to make their own provisions for their employees' health care, usually in the form of an agreement with a hospital or institution, or by hiring their own physician and providing an infirmary on their premises.

The MOH is divided into four major levels: the national level located in Riyadh;

the regional level with eleven regions, each of which is responsible for public health and statistical functions as well as the management of teritary care hospitals and primary health care centers; a district level with management functions; and a municipal (local) level that consists of health-care centers and secondary institutions. Speciality hospitals have been set up for treatment of infectious diseases such as tuberculosis, and for areas such as psychiatry, pediatrics, ophthalmology, and leprosy. Referrals are supposed to be made only by physicians in the MOH and governmental health facilities.

The national level is headed by the minister, who is appointed by the king. There are two deputy ministers; one is in charge of planning and development, and the other is responsible for the implementation of both curative and preventive health policies. The director generals who head the regional health departments report directly to the deputy minister for implementation. The current emphasis at the ministerial level is on preventive medicine and expansion of the primary health-care system. The 1985 organization chart for the ministry is shown in Figure 1.

The control of drugs and the establishment and maintenance of a pharmaceutical policy are responsibilities at the national level. There is a ministry laboratory for the testing of drugs prior to registration, and there are regulations regarding both the production and importation of drugs. Plans have been made for local production of certain categories of drugs.

In addition to the MOH facilities, health care is also provided by a number of other governmental institutions. The intersectoral relationships between these various providers of health care are briefly listed in Table 3 along with the major responsibilities assumed by each.

There is also governmental involvement in environmental health by Meteorology and Environment Protection Agency and the Ministry of Municipalities and Rural Affairs. The Ministry of Industry and Electricity and the Ministry of Labor and Social Affairs set and enforce occupational health standards. The Ministry of Labor and Social Affairs is also responsible for rehabilitation services. The General Organization for Social Insurance administers a compulsory insurance system for employees in the private sector and the state-owned corporations that provide retirement pensions and also financial aid for workers temporarily disabled due to occupational causes.

The financing mechanisms for all governmental agencies originate in the Ministry of Finance. Recommendations are included in the five-year plans, and requests are made by each of the various sectors. However, the final decisions regarding allocations are made by the Finance Ministry. The growth of the Ministry of Health budget as a percentage of the total budget of the kingdom is shown for selected years in Table 4.

In addition to the governmental health-care system, a sizable and significant number of providers operate in the private sector both as dispensaries and hospitals. In 1984 approximately 32 percent of the total hospital beds in the kingdom were allocated to the combined category of "private plus other governmental

Figure 1
Ministry of Health Administrative Structure

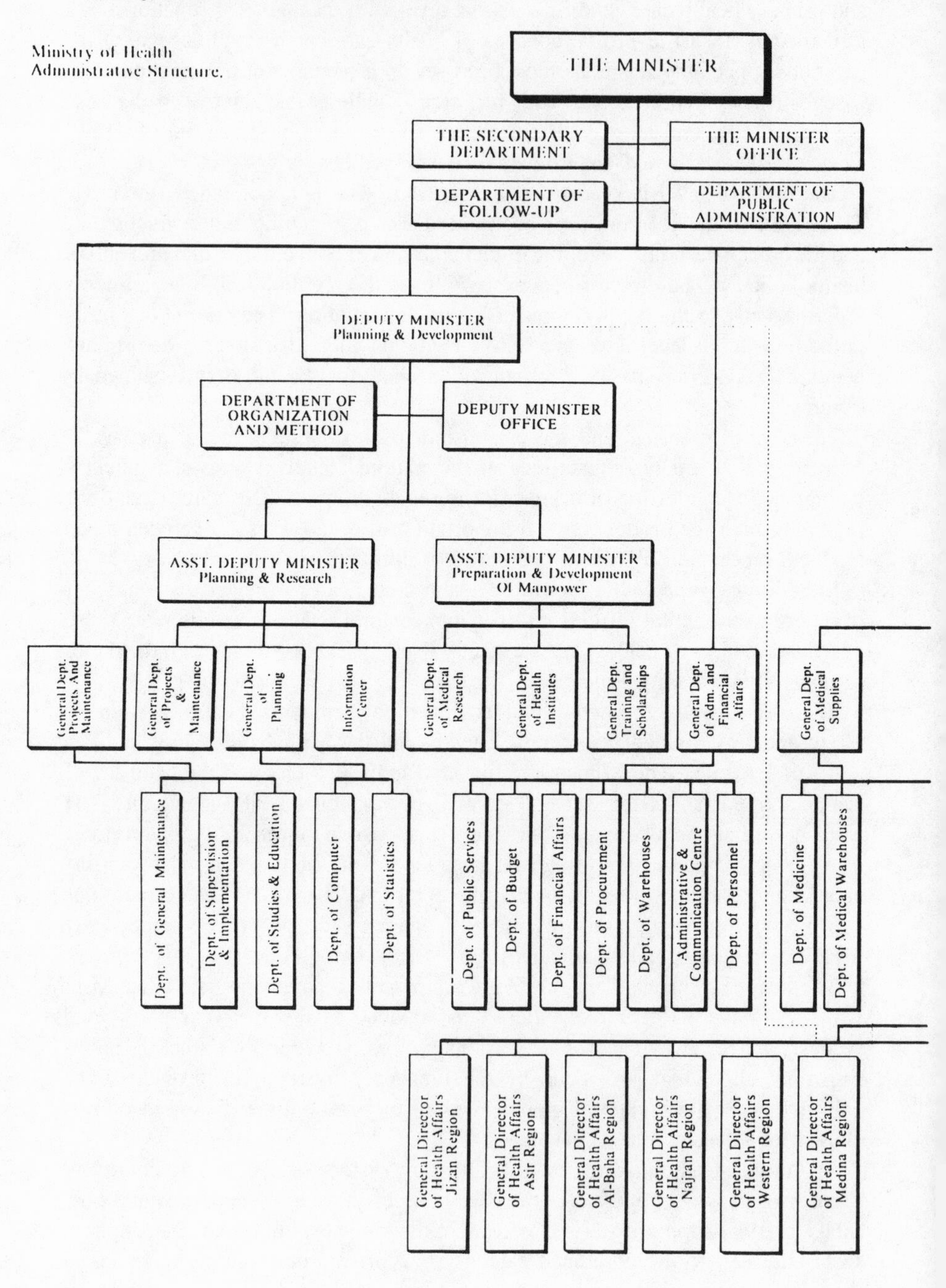

Figure 1 (continued)

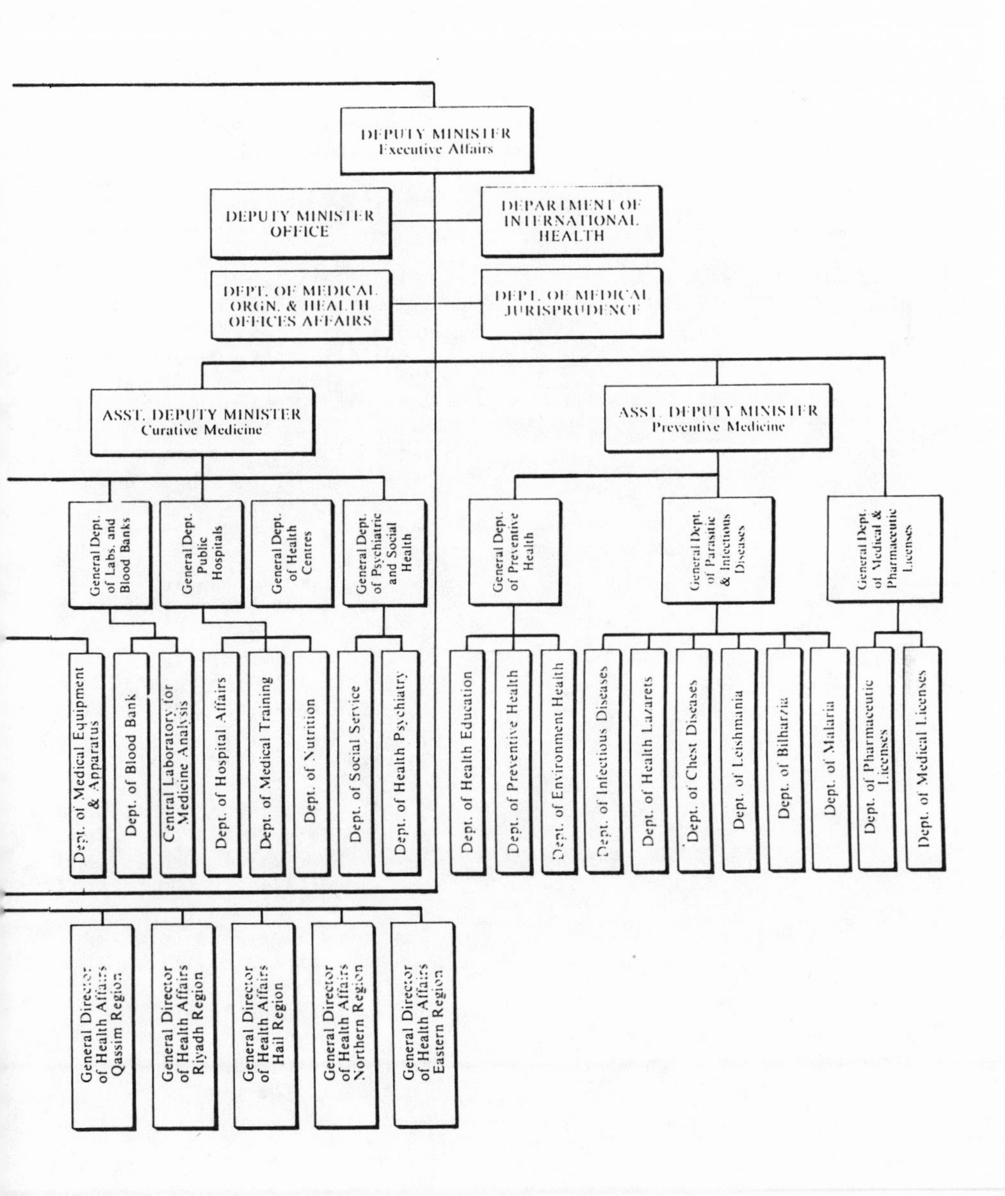

Table 3
Governmental Health-Care Providers

Agency	Responsibility
1. Ministry of Health	Provision of health care through primary care centers and hospitals; preventive health services; Hajj health services; curative and preventive health policies and goals; medical licensure; and pharmaceutical standards.
2. Ministry of Education	Provision of school health for male students.
3. Presidency of Girl's Education	Provision of school health units for female students.
4. Ministry of Higher Education	Responisbility for all phases of the four medical schools in addition to the University Hospitals. The four schools are located in Riyadh, Jeddah, Abha, and Dammam.
5. Ministry of Defense and Aviation (MODA)	Responsibility for the medical care of their personnel and administration of their hospital.
6. Ministry of Interior	Medical care for their personnel and administration of their hospital.
7. National Guard (NG)	Responsibility for medical care for their personnel and administration of their hospital facilities.
8. Specialist Hospitals	Highly specialized treatment at hospitals such as the King Faisal Specialist Hospital and the King Khalid Eye Hospital.
9. Red Crescent Society	Emergency ambulance services; special responsibilities during Hajj; operation of emergency road centers.
10. Royal Commission of Jubail and Yanbu	Medical care and hospitals located in the two industrial cities.

Source: *The Third Developmental Plan*, Ministry of Planning, 1700-140 AH, 1980–1985, Riyadh.

Table 4
Ministry of Health Budget (in Billion Saudi Riyals)

	Health Budget	Total Budget	Health Budget as percentage of of total Budget
1970/1971	177	6,380	2.8
1975/1976	3,197	110,935	2.9
1979/1980	4,177	185,800	2.2
1984/1985	10,743	260,000	4.1

Sources: Central Department of Statistics, *Statistical Year Book*, 1977, p. 415; Ministry of Health, *Statistical Review*, 1982, p. 25; Ministry of Health, interview data, for 1984–1985.

agencies.'' The private facilities charge fees according to a schedule formulated by the Ministry of Health and they must also be approved by the medical licensure department in the ministry. These physicians do not have hospital admission privileges for either MOH or other governmental hospitals. Private companies such as Aramco also operate large-scale health systems solely for their own employees. There is a modified Health Maintenance Organization (HMO) health-care system being developed, which is located in the industrial city of Jubail. Private insurance may be available in the near future, but it is currently only in the planning stage. Current data regarding the private sector are shown in Table 5.

The staffing of the hospitals and primary health-care centers is still largely expatriate for both the public and private sectors, although each year the total number of Saudi physicians increases. Cultural bias against female employment in the nursing field persists, and, although there are Saudi female administrators and physicians, there are very few Saudi nurses, which requires the continued recruitment of nursing personnel from such countries as India and the Phillipines.

The kingdom has in the past relied upon international consulting groups and hospital corporations to recruit staff for the specialist hospitals and some of the government hospitals, such as the military hospitals and the university hospitals.

Table 5
Health Services Structure

	Private Sector	MOH	Other govt. Agencies	TOTAL
A. Physicians (1983-84)	3,234	7,529	3,504	14,267
B. Nursing Staff	4,548	14,982	4,255	23,785
C. Hospital Beds	3,440	18,913	4,057	26,410
D. Outpatient Visits (1982-83)	N.A.	43.6 million	N.A.	N.A.

Source: Ministry of Planning, Riyadh, January 1985.

Another form of recruitment has been through agreements with foreign medical schools to assist in supplying staff for the university hospitals. With the growing number of Saudi administrators and Saudi physicians, however, the trend is increasingly toward less dependence upon such external agencies.

Salaries for health-care workers depend upon the sector in which they are employed. MOH has a salary schedule that is employed throughout the kingdom and is based upon experience and education. Faculty at the medical colleges are considered governmental employees and they are paid on the same schedule as other professors. They can, however, earn additional allowances for clinical work. It has been fairly standard to also provide free furnished housing and annual round-trip airline tickets for expatriate workers and their families.

Continuing education is provided for all levels in the health field in the form of seminars and conferences offered by both major hospitals and universities. There is also an annual Saudi medical meeting covering the major areas of medicine.

There are no health workers' unions, nor are there any country-wide associations analogous to such organizations as the American Medical Association. There are, however, speciality clubs that meet regularly in the major cities.

Future Issues

Overall, viewed in terms of education, personnel, and facilities, the kingdom has made significant gains in the provision of curative medical care in a relatively short time span. There are major problems the health-care system must still confront in logistical areas, manpower levels, basic infrastructure, and in the future direction of policy emphasis.

The geographic diversity, population density, and distance between many settlements are factors that continue to complicate the health delivery system. The morbidity data differ greatly according to geographic location. Continued improvement in both communication and transportation is essential to increase the accessibility and quality of health care in remote aras of the kingdom.

The current policy is toward the increase of the number of Saudi personnel. This trend is increasing steadily and should be reached by the year 2000 for the occupational categories of physicians, administrative personnel, and advanced technical levels. Expatriates will probably continue to constitute a large proportion of the manpower requirements in nursing and at all levels of the geographically isolated settlements.

A second area of concern that has been identified for emphasis is that of public attitudes and perceptions toward illness and health care. There are currently studies of the traditional practice of treatment in the country in regard to efficacy and also reasons for preference by certain groups within the population who opt to attend traditional healers either in conjunction with modern medical treatment or instead of seeking professionally trained health workers. Herbal preparations and cautery are reported to be among the more popular forms of traditional treatment (Molony 1982, 87–98). In addition to ascertaining both the beneficial and possibly deleterious aspects of treatment, the findings of these studies will be important in the design of health educational programs, and also in the promotion of primary care facilities and preventive medicine.

Third, psychological and psychiatric services are yet another area that has been identified for expansion and improvement. The cultural biases toward physicians majoring in psychiatry have begun to disappear even though the majority of specialists in the mental health areas are still expatriates, and the negative perceptions regarding mental illness and treatment are also slowly changing. Social work services, generally based in hospitals and dispensaries, are available in major cities. Counseling personnel, though, have yet to be placed within the primary and secondary school systems.

A fourth and crucial policy area is coordination between the various sectors that provide health care. Both the Third and Fourth-Five-Year Plans included recommendations for a coordinating and integrating body. There is general agreement that improvement in management is essential to avoid overlap and to increase efficiency at all levels.

The Saudi government is committed to the improvement of the health sector as demonstrated by the rapid growth of curative medical facilities, equipment, and personnel. Plans are being formulated to increase the system's emphasis on preventive and promotional health services. Consistent with WHO's Health for All by 2000 goals, the Ministry of Health has announced specific plans to expand primary health care and the number of family health centers. Indeed, this attention has also been demonstrated by the establishment of the first Saudi master's degree programs in postgraduate medicine in the primary care and family medicine areas. Socioeconomic problems have also been singled out for improvement, particularly in the areas of safe water, drug management, food availability and production, communication, and education, to name just a few of the major expansion projects.

In conclusion, the kingdom is a rapidly developing society where the health-care system can be characterized as having established curative services and having moved toward a transitional phase of expansion and improvement in these facilities along with the initiation of preventive agencies. The current plans are oriented toward an integrated health system that will include preventive and promotional services. The realization of quality health care is at this stage dependent on successful implementation strategies and also on effective administrative decision making and management skills.

References

Al-Bakr, Mohammad Salim. 1983. ''An Exploratory Study of the Efficacy of Health Care in Saudi Arabia: Objective and Subjective Assessment.'' Ph.D. diss., University of Southern California.

Arabian American Oil Co. *Morbidity and Mortality*. 1980. Dhahran: Arabian American Oil Co.

Birks and Sinclair. 1985. ''Population Projections for Saudi Arabia, 1975–1985.'' Riyadh: Allied Medical Group Ltd.

Geographical Factors and Disease Patterns. 1980. *Saudi Medical Journal* 1:184–186.

Ministry of Planning. 1980a. ''Development Plan, 1390.'' Central Planning Organization.

———. 1980b. ''Second Development Plan, 1395–1400 AH, 1975–1980.'' Riyadh, KSA.

———. 1985. ''Third Development Plan, 1400–1405 AH, 1980–1985.'' Riyadh, KSA.

———. 1983. ''CK Health Planners Report.'' Riyadh, KSA.

Moloney, George E. Local Healers in Qasim. In *Community Health in Saudi Arabia*, ed. Zohair Sebai, 87–98. Riyadh, KSA.

Sebai, Zohair A. 1981. *The Health of the Family in a Changing Arabia*. Jeddah: Tihama Publications.

———. 1985. *Health in Saudi Arabia*. Jeddha: Tihama Publications.

SPAIN

Pedro J. Saturno

Introduction

Spain is situated on the southwestern tip of the European continent. In 1981, it had a population of 37.6 million inhabitants, a figure which has been slowly but steadily increasing during the last decade. The density of population in Spain, however, is lower than the European average; only Greece has a lower density among similar southern European nations (WHO 1983). In contrast to the density data, the proportion of urban population is higher in Spain than the European average (75.8 percent vs. 71.6 percent) and among the highest in the southern European group (WHO 1983). This combination of a relatively low average density with a high proportion of urban population suggests a concentrated spatial distribution of the population.

Spain ranked eleventh in the world according to 1981 gross national product (GNP), but only thirty-ninth in terms of GNP per capita, at $5,640 (World Bank 1983). Spain's wealth is not well distributed among its different regions—the per capita income of the wealthier regions (Madrid, Catalonia, and the Basque provinces) are almost double that for the poorest areas (Andalusia, the Mancha, Estremadura). Similarly, the national unemployment rate, which is currently close to 20 percent, is a greater problem in some areas (where it reaches 25 percent) than in others (where it is 10 percent). The unemployment rate has a major impact on the health-care system, whose main component, the National Health Insurance, has historically been tied to Spain's system of social benefits for employees.

Health Statistics

The general mortality rate in Spain was 7.8 in 1983, a figure that is among the lowest in Europe. Infant mortality was 9.6 percent of live births in 1982.

Table 1
Demographic Indicators, 1983

Death Rate	7.8
Infant Mortality*	9.6
Birth Rate	12.5
Natural Increase	4.7
Life Expectancy**	Male: 72.4
	Female: 78.6

*1982.
**1980.
Source: WHO, *World Health Statistics Annual 1986*, Geneva, 1986.

Life expectancy at birth was 72.4 for males and 78.6 for females in 1980 (Table 1).

Age-specific death rates for 1979 show a peak for infant mortality, followed by a decreasing pattern until the age of fifteen. From that age, rates are steadily increasing, reaching values similar to the infant mortality figure beyond age 64. Death rates are consistently higher for males than for females in all age groups. In the last 30 years, Spain has considerably reduced the mortality rates for the age groups below 44 years, with particular success among the youngest groups: Mortality reductions for the period 1950–1980 ranged from 87.3 percent (age group 1–4 years) to 57.7 percent (age group 40–44 years). Reduction in the mortality rate of those older than 70 years was a smaller 15.9 percent.

According to 1980 data, the most important group of causes of death in Spain is diseases of the circulatory system. They account for more than 45 percent of all deaths; the leading cause is cerebrovascular disease (35.8 percent of the group). The second major group is neoplasms, most commonly in the respiratory tract, which caused 20 percent of deaths. Three other important causes of death were diseases of the respiratory system; accidents, poisonings, and violence; and diseases of the digestive system; however, these three groups altogether account for fewer deaths than neoplasms alone. Diabetes mellitus accounted for fewer than 2.5 percent as the primary cause of death. All other groups of causes represented 2 percent or fewer of the total deaths (Table 2).

The only available information on morbidity at the national level is for certain infectious diseases, specifically those subject to compulsory reporting (Table 3) and to causes of hospital admission. It must be borne in mind that reported figures are only the tip of the iceberg. Spain's hospital morbidity pattern resem-

Table 2
Percentage Distribution of Causes of Death,* 1980

	Total d.	Total group
1. DISEASES OF THE CIRCULATORY SYSTEM	45.8	
Leading cause: Cerebrovascular disease		35.8
2. NEOPLASMS	20.1	
Leading cause: Neoplasms of trachea, lung, and bronchius		15.1
3. DISEASES OF THE RESPIRATORY SYSTEM	9.3	
Leading cause: Pneumonia		34.8
4. DISEASES OF THE DIGESTIVE SYSTEM	6.0	
Leading cause: Cirrhosis of liver		48.3
5. ACCIDENTS, POISONING, AND VIOLENCE	4.6	
Leading cause: Motor vehicle accident		45.8
6. SYMPTOMS AND ILL-DEFINED CONDITIONS	3.5	
7. ENDOCRINE, NUTRITIONAL, AND METABOLIC DIS.	2.7	
Leading cause: Diabetes mellitus		88.5
8. DISEASES OF GENITO-URINARY SYSTEM	1.9	
Leading cause: Nephritis and nephrosis		73.4
9. INFECTIVE AND PARASITIC DISEASES	1.4	
Leading cause: Tuberculosis of Resp. Sys.		33.3
10. CERTAIN CAUSES OF PERINATAL MORTALITY	1.1	
11. DIS. OF NERVOUS SYSTEM AND SENSE ORGANS	1.2	
Leading cause: Meningitis		6.8
12. ALL OTHER CAUSES	2.4	

*ICD-9 groups of causes.
Source: WHO, *World Health Statistical Annual 1986*, Geneva, 1986.

bles that of other developed countries, and it is likely to become closer still. The trend is toward relative decreases for currently more frequent causes (normal delivery, appendicitis, hernia, tonsilectomy), and yearly increases in hospital use due to cardiovascular diseases, neoplasms, and osteoarticular diseases (Saturno 1987).

Spain has recently performed a national health survey for the first time, but the findings have not been published as of this writing. Therefore, there is no reliable data upon which to estimate disability days, nor any other direct measure of health status.

Table 3
Selected Infectious Diseases Subjected to Compulsory Reporting, 1986 (Annual Figures, New Cases and Crude Rate per 100,000 Population)

MEASLES	
cases	220,109
rate	553.8
BRUCELLOSIS	
cases	6,255
rate	15.7
PULMONARY TUBERCULOSIS	
cases	13,755
rate	34.6
SHIGELLOSIS	
cases	50,484
rate	127.0
TYPHOID AND PARATHYROID FEVERS	
cases	5,437
rate	13.7
STREP. SORE THROAT/SCARLATINA	
cases	13,135
rate	33.1
TRICHINOSIS	
cases	124
rate	0.3
DIPTHERIA	
cases	2
rate	0.01
ACUTE POLIOMYELITIS	
cases	2
rate	0.01

Source: Ministerio de Sanidad y Consumo, *Boletimes Epidemiologicos Semanales, 1986*. Madrid, 1986.

Historical Development

National Health Insurance (NHI) in Spain originated in 1947 as a paternalistic provision of the Franco regime to those "weak" industrial workers who lacked private insurance. It was presented as a charitable program to protect them from the depredations of diseases. In fact, though benefits were initially very limited, NHI did increase accessibility to health services for the newly insured. However, funds for the program came from compulsory premiums paid by employers (75

Table 4
Percentage of Population Covered by Social Security Health Insurance, 1975–1984

1975	1980	1984
85.2	82.4	93.0

Sources: 1975–1981: Memoria Estadistica INP/INSALUD 1975–1981; 1982–1984: *Boletin de Indicadores Sanitarios*, No. 11, November 1984; data for 1983 and 1984 are provisional estimations.

percent) and workers. Consequently, critics argued that the NHI system was directly (premiums) or indirectly (less salary, higher prices of goods) financed exclusively by the working class, since general tax revenues had no role in the new program. Further, NHI surpluses were used mainly to subsidize other government institutions like the revenue-losing National Industry Institute (INI). Accordingly, a frequent criticism of Spain's NHI was that it worked like a compulsory savings program in which only the government was entitled to use the funds. The fascists called the program *Seguro Obligatorio de Enfermedad* (Compulsory Sickness Insurance), or SOE; prevention and health promotion were explicitly not included. It was part of the *Instituto Nacional de Prevision* (INP), an institution within the Ministry of Labor, tied not to other health-care institutions but to Social Security programs for pensions, family subsidies, and unemployment benefits. As the SOE grew, its provision solely of curative care, its structural isolation from other health institutions, and its funding scheme all became seen as important flaws in its organization.

The SOE scheme was expanded to cover increasing numbers of workers, particularly following the 1972 reform (Table 4). The name of the program was changed also: the traditional *Seguro Obligatorio de Enfermedad* was to be known simply as Social Security (SS), and in 1978 an autonomous institution (Instituto Nacional de la Salud, INSALUD) was created for the management of the SS medical care services. During this period, partly in response to real need and professional pressure, partly due to the preference of the fascists for big public construction projects, and partly to absorb surplus NHI funds, thousands of hospital beds were built by and for the Social Security health-care system. From the mid–1960s to the mid–1970s, with an increase of over 32,000 new beds, the SS share of the total hospital beds in the country jumped from 9.1 percent in 1963 to 23.2 percent, in 1977 (De Miguel 1983). Most of the new beds were in large, sophisticated, and fully equipped modern hospitals. This growth in the hospital sector reinforced the curative bias of the system, particularly since the the growth in beds was not complemented by similar improvements in ambulatory care. At the same time, hospital size and location were decided with an evident lack of rational planning considerations: Even a very superficial analysis suggests that these new institutions were too big and that their location was often questionable (for instance, the two biggest NHI hospitals in Madrid are located across the street from each other).

Certain characteristics of the SOE, however, act as cost-containment mechanisms that are compatible with high levels of equity and effectiveness. These include the tradition of salaried health personnel at all levels and the global budget approach to hospital financing. Most importantly, the SOE/SS experience has forged an apparently irreversible social agreement that access to health care is a right for the whole population, and one strongly felt by the population.

The health system created by the Franco regime was described in the *Ley de Bases de Sanidad Nacional* (National Health Basis Law) in 1944 and complemented mainly by the *Ley de Bases del Regimen Local* (Local Administration Basis Law) in 1945. These legal texts established the paternalistic responsibility of the government in health care, limited almost exclusively to public health activities mainly through provincial *Jefaturas de Sanidad* structurally dependent on a central *Direccion General de Sanidad* within the *Ministerio de la Gobernacion* (a form of Ministry of the Interior). At the same time, the *Ley del Regimen Local* established provincial and municipal health care to the official poor (a special card of indigency was devised). Provincial councils were obliged to operate a general hospital, a maternal institute, a psychiatric hospital, and social shelters for children, the elderly, and indigents. After the SOE institutionalization and development, provincial councils remained responsible for mental inpatient care, for an important part of the social services, and for hospitalization of the uninsured population.

In addition, the Ministry of Education built its own teaching hospital attached to schools of medicine; the Ministry of Justice has its own health-care network, including some hospitals, for inmates; the military forces have a separate health-care system; and the private sector, as a complement to public institutions, includes for-profit hospitals, religious, and (in theory) charitable medical care institutions, and Red Cross hospitals (theoretically semipublic, but in practice most of them working as private). In sum, Spain was, and remains, a structural health delivery nightmare, which has fortunately been overwhelmed by the enormous growth of the Social Security NHI system.

After almost 40 years of dictatorship, 1977 was the first year of full democracy in Spain. One of the newly elected government's first initiatives was to create a Ministry of Health, a change for which there was broad consensus. Previously, five different ministries had direct administrative responsibilities in the health-care area. Public health had been in the *Ministerio de la Gobernacion*, and most health-care resources and health services delivery were managed by the Spanish Social Security, a powerful autonomous public entity formerly in the Ministry of Labor. The process of organizing the Ministry of Health, defining administrative boundaries, and delimiting responsibilities remains unfinished as of this writing.

Spain is currently undergoing a process of decentralization in all types of public activities. The timing, content, and mechanisms of the decentralization process have been uneven across the country, reflecting the fact that Spain has a number of different culturally and historically defined regions. These different regional cultures were repressed by the fascist regime, particularly in the Basque country. After Franco died, the process of decentralizing authority to local governments began—rather rapidly for the so-called "historic communities" (Catalonia, Galicia, the Basque country, Andalusia), but subsequently in the rest of Spain as well. There are now seventeen *Comunidades Autónomas* that reflect past regional boundaries and are entitled to varying levels of actual autonomy. The long-run tendency seems to be to equalize the decentralization for legislative and executive activities across all seventeen autonomous regions. An important element of this decentralization process will involve the organization of the health-care system.

Under the new 1978 Constitution, the Spanish people's right to health care is explicitly recognized. This right also is the legal basis for a proposed National Health Service (NHS), which would cover the whole population without distinction and would include the whole range of health services. This Spanish NHS is intended to replace the present atomized health-care system, whose major features are discussed below.

The Current Health-Care System

At present, Spain has a mixed public-private health-care system, in which the public side predominates. The system's core is a massive NHI program which now covers over 90 percent of the population. Virtually all types of current and retired workers and their families are covered, and participation is compulsory for all salaried workers. NHI funds come mainly from compulsory employer and employee premiums, which provide, roughly, 70 percent and 20 percent of the funds, respectively; government subsidies amount to only about 10 percent of the system's total income). Copayments apply only to prescription drugs (30 percent on average) and some prosthesis (elderly, retired, and disabled are exempted; for them everything is free). The NHI owns hospital and ambulatory care facilities; NHI hospitals are acknowledged to be in general the best equipped and the most professionally respected by health-care personnel. However, NHI has to contract services with other public and private hospitals because—among other structural and political reasons—it does not own enough beds to satisfy the insured population's demand. On the other hand, NHI ambulatory services remain unsatisfactory: There is common agreement that they are of low quality and rather inefficient. All NHI personnel are either salaried (in hospitals) or paid through a combination of baseline salary plus capitation (ambulatory health personnel). It is important to note that the unit of payment for ambulatory care physicians is not an insured person but rather one insurance card, which may be held by a single individual or a whole family. Dental care (except extractions) and mental inpatient services are not covered.

The rest of the public sector includes: (1) a public network managed at the local level (municipality, province, autonomous community) for indigent people—its hospitals are used also by the NHI patients and its ambulatory care and public health physicians are, at the same time, NHI physicians; (2) a public network of psychiatric hospitals—mental inpatient care is a provincial responsibility and there is at least one hospital in each province; (3) public health activities (sanitation, environmental control, epidemiology, school hygiene, and vaccines), which are handled also mainly at the local level—responsibility in these activities is shared by municipal and provincial public health agencies, which are not integrated into the Social Security NHI; and (4) a network of hospitals and dispensaries for the military. Level of coordination between the NHI system and other public sector facilities and activities varies by autonomous regions, but it is not complete anywhere.

Finally, there are some private practice and some private facilities. Most of the latter survive by providing care to NHI patients under special arrangements (contracts). Hospitals are paid on a per diem rate, which varies with the hospital's level of sophistication.

Resources

Overall, Spain has a great oversupply of physicians, a limited or perhaps even an undersupply of nurses and medical technicians, a remarkable undersupply of dentists, and a fair number of hospital and ambulatory care facilities (Tables 5,6,7). The ratio of physicians to population is among the highest in Europe, while the ratio of dentists to population is the lowest among the EEC countries. This disparity reflects two concrete policies: (1) the unrestricted access to practically free medical studies versus very restricted access (partially due to the limited number of schools) to dental studies, and (2) the exclusion of dental services from SS/INSALUD coverage.

The evidence of an overwhelming physician oversupply and the difficulties in providing a reasonable education to an increasingly large number of students were officially felt by the late 1970s. Substantial unemployment among recently graduated physicians was by then already a fact. Consequently, a nationwide *numerus clausus* for new medical students was made mandatory in 1979. The number of new students was fixed at 7,320 (compared to 19,960 and 11,454 first-year medical students admitted in 1977 and 1978, respectively). In June 1983, 10,346 new physicians graduated: the highest figure in history. Given that medical studies require a six-year curriculum in Spain, the effect of the *numerus clausus* policy will be evident in the number of graduates only in 1986 and after. Even accounting for that effect, the oversupply will probably last a long while.

Regarding physician specialization, a recent official study reported that by 1978 the proportion of specialists was 57.6 percent of all physicians. However,

Table 5
Health Personnel, 1979–1982

	1979	1982	1986
PHYSICIANS			
number	81,658	104,759	130,574
per 10,000 pop.	22.1	27.8	33.5
DENTISTS			
number	3,532	4,065	5,722
per 10,000 pop.	1.0	1.1	1.5
PHARMACISTS			
number	21,986	26,117	31,118
per 10,000 pop.	5.9	7.0	8.1
VETERINARIES			
number	7,922	8,037	9,237
per 10,000 pop.	2.1	2.1	2.4
NURSES AND MEDICAL TECHNICIANS			
number	111,107	136,892	143,762
per 10,000 pop.	29.9	36.3	37.4
PHYSIOTHERAPISTS			
numer	2,072	2,648	2,876*
per 10,000 pop.	0.6	0.7	0.8
MIDWIVES			
number	4,620	4,893	6,207*
per 10,000 pop.	1.2	1.3	1.6

*1985.

Sources: 1979: WHO, *World Health Statistics Annual 1983*, Geneva, 1983; 1982: INE, *Anuario Estadistico de España 1983*, Madrid, 1984; 1986: Consejos Generales de Colegios Profesionales, unpublished data.

the increase in the total number of physicians in the last five years and the restricted number admitted for residency is reducing that percentage. By 1985, only 1,336 first-year residency positions were posted in the whole nation, which is the lowest figure ever offered. Furthermore, the explicitly stated policy of the Ministry of Health is (1) to increase the number of specialists in family and community medicine; (2) to increase the number of specialists in public health (for a target ratio of 1: 25,000, the total number of has to increase by approximately 1,500); and (3) to increase the number dentists (an estimated 15,000 new dentists are needed) (Ministerio de Sanidad y Consumo 1984).

Table 6
Hospital Resources, 1976–1983

	1976	1979	1983
TOTAL			
number	1,226	1,135	976
beds	194,097	203,819	181,794
average size	158	180	186
beds/1,000 pop.	5.4	5.5	4.7
GENERAL HOSPITALS			
number	842	781	422
beds	126,735	137,399	113,141
average size	150	176	268
beds/1,000 pop.	3.5	3.7	3.0
SPECIALIZED HOSPITALS			
number	270	243	443
beds	23,684	24,951	33,380
average size	88	103	75
beds/1,000 pop.	0.7	0.7	0.9
PSYCHIATRIC HOSPITALS			
number	114	111	111
beds	43,678	41,469	35,273
average size	383	374	318
beds/1,000 pop.	1.2	1.1	0.9
PUBLIC HOSPITALS			
number	476	436	391
beds	132,907	139,050	121,748
average size	279	319	311
beds/1,000 pop.	3.7	3.7	3.2
% total beds	68.5	68.2	67.0
PRIVATE HOSPITALS			
number	750	699	585
beds	61,190	64,769	60,046
average size	82	99	102
beds/1,000 pop.	1.7	1.7	1.6
% total beds	31.5	31.8	33.0

Sources: 1976–79: WHO, *World Health Statistics Annual 1983*, 1983; 1983: INE, *Anuario Estadistico de España 1986*, Madrid, 1987.

Table 7
Hospital Utilization, 1976–1979

	1976	1979
TOTAL		
admissions/1000 pop.	85.3	91.8
hospital days/person	1.4	1.4
GENERAL HOSPITAL		
admissions/1000 pop.	77.9	84.0
hospital days/person	0.9	0.9
SPECIALIZED HOSPITALS		
admissions/1000 pop.	6.7	6.2
hospital days/person		
PUBLIC HOSPITALS		
admissions/1000 pop.	54.1	58.8
% total admission	63.4	64.1
% total hospital days	68.5	67.9
PRIVATE HOSPITALS		
admissions/1000 pop.	31.2	33.0
% total admissions	36.6	35.9
% total hospital days	31.5	32.1

Source: *World Health Statistics Annual 1983*. WHO, Geneva, 1983.

The number of hospital beds per 1,000 population has not increased since 1979. However, bed distribution is uneven, with higher ratios in urban areas than in rural areas, and in rich industrialized provinces than in poor agricultural provinces. This reflects the preference of SS/INSALUD authorities to build large centers in areas where the proportion of active industrial workers was high. Additionally, the public/private mix is uneven.

INSALUD owns 179 hospitals totaling 56,266 beds, but it represents only 26 percent of the total beds in the country and 38.2 percent of the public beds. In

1982, INSALUD itself was the employer of 55,207 physicians, 53 percent of all Spanish physicians, making INSALUD by far the major health personnel employer in the whole country. Sixty-six percent of INSALUD physicians work in primary health settings (31 percent as general practitioners, 7 percent as pediatricians, 4 percent in emergency services, and 25 percent as some other type of specialist); 34 percent of the INSALUD physicians work in INSALUD hospitals (of whom 28 percent are staff and 6 percent are interns and residents) (Ministerio de Sanidad y Consumo 1984). Although these figures suggest that primary health care is the major focus within INSALUD, overall INSALUD expenditures indicate that hospital care consumes the largest portion of available resources.

Organization and Management

The baseline for the 1986 health reform is a complex system composed of (1) three separated subsystems for medical care (SS/INSALUD, the provincial councils' general and psychiatric hospitals, and the municipal medical care network for the poor); (2) two subsystems for public health activities; and (3) private hospitals, clinics, and ambulatory care facilities. There are some connections among them: for instance, municipal physicians—who are supposed to be family physicians for the poor and public health practitioners of the whole population of their municipal district—are, at the same time, SS/INSALUD family physicians, and are the main human resource for the central and provincial public health programs. Yet, each system has its own independent administration, which usually is highly centralized, with the exception of the provincial councils' system and—particularly—the municipal network. In the SS/INSALUD network, all the relevant decisions had to be approved in Madrid; local INSALUD institutions had only administrative power. Since the decentralization process started, INSALUD decision making has been transferred only to four of Spain's seventeen autonomous communities, two of them starting January 1, 1987.

Organizationally, the simplest structure of these concurrent health systems is that of the provincial councils. Its only geographical unit is the province, and its single institutions (one general hospital, one psychiatric hospital, one nursing home, and one orphanage house) are expected to cover the entire provincial population. For the municipal health-care network, township territory is divided into districts. A physician and a physician assistant (PA) are assigned to each distict; a midwife and basic dentistry services are also provided but at a more aggregate level. In relatively big townships (usually over 10,000 to 20,000 inhabitants), there is also a *Casa de Socorro*, an emergency center for ambulatory care. Some big townships have also a municipal hospital, which usually is old and poorly equipped. Overall, vaccinations and school health are probably the two most important tasks of a municipal physician.

The smaller structural unit of the huge SS/INSALUD network is the so-called *zona* (zone). In the early years of the system, SS/INSALUD zones and municipal districts had the same boundaries, and the physician serving both networks was the same. As the NHI population grew, the initial zones/districts were further divided into smaller areas, and new health personnel were appointed. Currently, most municipal districts contain more than one INSALUD zone, and there is more than one physician in each of them. The basic health team in the INSALUD network is a general practitioner, a PA, and a pediatrician. They work either in small INSALUD-owned or rented rural offices, *consultorios* (ambulatory general practice facilities), or *ambulatorios* (where there are usually both general and specialized ambulatory care physicians). The next structural unit is the subsector, which has more specialized ambulatory care, and the sector, which has the whole range of ambulatory care and a general hospital. A sector may have some subsectors attached or only zones.

Each specialist is assigned a certain number of general practitioners (GPs) for his or her specialized ambulatory care referrals. The whole structure is strictly pyramidal, with the family insurance card as the basic planning unit. Cards may include the whole family, but they can be also individual: Each worker or retired worker has his or her own card; thus in families where more than one member is working, there is more than one insurance card (although dependents are included on only one of them). This system reflects the fact that health benefits were traditionally included, with retirement pensions and other social benefits for workers, in a single Social Security package. Physicians are assigned (and paid for) a number of insurance cards rather than individual persons. Depending on family size and frequency of single-person insurance cards, a physician's actual workload for the same number of insurance cards may vary considerably. In general, a GP has from 700 to 1,200 insurance cards.

Access to ambulatory care specialists is strictly restricted to referrals from GPs or pediatricians. About 20 GPs (actual 1983 data: from 20.5 to 22.4) refer to one specialist in general surgery, ophthalmology, ENT, traumatology, digestive system, respiratory and cardiovascular systems, and odontology. About 40 GPs are assigned to one specialist in gynecology, urology, dermatology, and neuropsychiatry. From 65 to 70 GPs are assigned to one endocrinologist. Ambulatory radiology and laboratory services may receive referrals from both GPs and specialists; there are one radiologist and one clinical analyst for approximately 25 GPs. In areas with over 5,000 insurance cards, the INSALUD ambulatory care network has an additional network for ambulatory emergency care.

Access to hospital care for INSALUD patients is usually restricted to referred patients. In case of emergency, people can go directly to the hospital; however, many people go directly to hospitals in nonemergency cases as well. Hospital discharges, either from inpatient services or emergency room, may be referred to their ambulatory care specialists or GPs for follow-up treatment; in some cases, they are required to attend the hospital outpatient clinics. Typically, hospital and ambulatory care physicians work separately; they usually feel they inhabit different worlds, and professional relationships among them are usually nonexistent.

In general, INSALUD ambulatory care is viewed by both physicians and population as poor, whereas its hospital care is highly esteemed. It seems that the system itself makes efficient ambulatory patient care almost impossible to provide. One of the more frequent complaints among INSALUD ambulatory care physicians is the amount of purely bureaucratic work they have to do, particularly single-item prescriptions and the need to certify a sick worker weekly.

The 1986 health reform is expected to introduce three main innovations in the health system structure: First, all the existing public subsystems are to be integrated into a single, publicly managed health-care system. Second, the highly centralized INSALUD is to be further decentralized, and full managerial power is to be given to local governments. This process started in July 1981, when Catalonia received INSALUD competence from the central government. In February 1984 the same procedure was applied to Andalusia, and in January 1987 to Valencia and the Basque country. Legal instruments will be devised shortly for the rest. Third, primary health care (PHC) is to be the basis of the new health care system. Accordingly, old INSALUD ambulatory care facilities are to be converted into new PHC centers, better staffed and better equipped, and with a different health-care mission. Anticipating this future structure, INSALUD has created 200 new PHC centers (*Centros de Salud*) nationwide. However, the attempt to impose the new structure within an otherwise unchanged INSALUD system has been difficult.

Health System Financing

The cost of health care is hard to measure in Spain, given the complex relationship among different subsystems and a lack of readily available data. Attempts have been made, but the results are always expressed with caution. Official data give the figure of 6.3 percent as the proportion of health-care consumption in total national expenditures for 1982 (OCDE 1985).

Municipal and provincial councils' health expenses are difficult to assess at the national level. Some estimates have been made, though, in particular regions (Rodríguez 1986, Saturno, Gol 1983). For Catalonia, for example, they were estimated to account for 5.5 percent of total health-care expenditure in 1981 (2 percent, provincial councils; 3.5 percent, municipal). Municipal health expenses in the Madrid province averaged 1 percent (ranging from 0.1 percent to 4.5 percent) of total municipal expenditure in 1981, and psychiatric inpatient care accounted for 11 percent of total provincial council health expenses (86.5 percent of nonpsychiatric health expenditure). INSALUD expenses totaled 60 percent of total health expenditure in Catalonia, and around 70 percent in the Madrid province. These figures, while region specific, indicate tht INSALUD has the dominant role in health system finances.

The INSALUD budget is part of the Social Security budget, which is a well-differentiated and autonomous part of the national general budget (NGB). The

SS budget amounted to 25.1 percent of the NGB in 1984, but SS benefits include cash benefits (pensions, unemployment and sickness salaries, family incentives and subsidies, etc.) and social services (services for the aged and handicapped, occupational health, special educational programs, etc.) as well as medical care benefits managed by INSALUD. The 1984 INSALUD budget was 28 percent of the total SS budget (7 percent of the NGB). Comparatively, the 1984 Ministry of Health budget (37,934 million pts.) was 0.3 percent of the NGB, equivalent to 1.2 percent of the total SS budget, or 4.4 percent of the INSALUD budget. It is to be noted that INSALUD, though theoretically included within the Ministry of Health, has in practice a great deal of management autonomy and total financial dependence on the SS budget.

SS income comes mainly from direct employers and employees quotas. However, the government's subsidy is increasing: Although it was only 3.8 percent of the total SS income in 1975, it increased to 8.8 percent in 1978, and it reached an estimated 20.2 percent in 1984. For this same year, direct levies were expected to be 78.2 percent of the total SS income, of which 73.7 percent was from employers and 25.5 percent was from workers (Saturno, Gol 1983).

The whole SS system showed a small 0.6 percent deficit in 1975, but that has increased to a 14.6 percent deficit in 1984. However, the health-care component is not the central cause; in fact, SS health insurance was in surplus until 1978. The increasing government subsidy is almost entirely to fund SS cash benefits. Medical care, although 28 percent of the 1984 SS budget, was close to 50 percent of the SS expenditure in 1975 (Saturno, Gol 1983).

When one disaggregates SS medical care expenditure (Table 8), the following become visible: (1) Contracted services still account for 15–20 percent of the total expenses, despite the stated policy of trying to reduce utilization of privately owned services. (2) The goal of progressively decreasing pharmacy expenses is being achieved. Pharmacy is an area with well-defined policies at the national level, which appear to have been successfully implemented. (3) Primary health care is not receiving an increased share of INSALUD resources. Indeed, the proportion of resources devoted to PHC has actually been steady or decreasing in the last few years, despite policy preferences to the contrary. (4) Operating expenses are consistently over 90 percent of the total expenses, with salaries and wages around 45 percent. Such a low proportion of capital expenditure is a fair indicator of a relatively stable institutional structure. Similarly, the rather low proportion of personnel expenses suggests that a policy of low-paid personnel and/or low staffing patterns is being used as an effective cost-containment mechanism. (5) Actual (inflation adjusted) expenses decreased by almost 15 percent in 1980, in relation to the previous year's figure, and, still, the 1984 INSALUD is less than the total 1977 expenses. Given (and in spite of) the intended expansion of population coverage, inflation adjusted expenses per covered person are budgeted to be, in 1984, 8.2 percent less than in 1977. Private medicine does not seem to be expanding concurrently. Though the precise extent to which private

Table 8
Social Security Health Services (INSALUD) Expenditures, 1977–1984

	1977	1980	1983*	1984**
TOTAL (millions)	346,336	519,791	844,526	875,215
Inflation adjustment	346,336	324,667	359,838	345,370
% total SS exp.	43.3	--	30.8	28.2
% GNP	--	--	3.7	3.5
% SS owned facilities	54.4	53.8	55.9	57.9
% contracted services	19.8	21.7	22.0	20.5
% pharmacy	24.3	22.7	20.1	19.0
% other	1.4	1.7	2.0	2.6
% PHC (exc. pharmacy)	--	22.4	18.4	21.7
% hospital care	--	53.0	58.5	56.3
% operating expenditure			96.7	96.0
(wages and salaries)	--	--	44.8	47.7
% capital expenditure			3.3	4.0
(investments)	--	--	3.0	3.9
Pts/insured p.	10,483	16,710	25,349	24,383
Inflation adjustment	10,483	10,437	10,800	9,619

*provisional.
**budgeted.

Sources: *Memoria Estadistica* INP/INSALUD 1977, 1978, 1979, and 1980. INSALUD, Madrid; *Boletin de Indicadores Sanitarios No. 6* (May 1984), pp. 3–8 and *No. 7* (June 1984), pp. 3–7, INSALUD, Ministerio de Sanidad y Consumo, Madrid, 1984; *Anuario El Pais 1984: Economia Española*, pp. 332–36, Madrid, 1984.

medicine is being used by the population at large is still to be assessed, people were not spending a greater share of their family budget on medical services in 1981 than they were in 1974, according to national surveys (INE 1980, 1983).

The Future: Toward a PHC-Based National Health Service

The 1986 health law established a public, decentalized, PHC-centered National Health Service to provide integrated health services for the whole population. Given the current system's features and history, change undoubtedly will not be easy. The main innovations and likely conflicts include universal coverage, a decentralized system, and a PHC-based system.

Universal Coverage

Universal coverage implies dramatic changes in both financing mechanisms and the integration of public and private facilities. A higher (perhaps majority) proportion of general tax revenue would appear to be unavoidable. At the same time, financial responsibility for the present INSALUD network will have to be transferred to central and local health authorities. Comprehensiveness implies the creation of a new integrated structure, where non-INSALUD-covered services (namely, psychiatry, dentistry, and health promotion and education) will have to compete with traditional curative activities. Problems here undoubtedly could be organizational, educational (health personnel are almost exclusively curative oriented), and budgetary (comprehensive coverage, which includes curative services plus social and preventive services, is unlikely to cost less than present services).

A Decentralized System

According to the 1986 health law, the central government in Madrid will establish mostly general policies, while most planning and management activities will take place at the local level. Town councils keep most of their environmental health activities, but they do not provide medical care; former provincial councils' medical care responsibilities and facilities are to be integrated into the regional autonomous community health-care system. All autonomous communities (the higher level of local government) are to be divided into geographical units called health areas having at least one general hospital and including from 10 to 25 primary health centers (HCs). HCs are staffed with physicians, PAs, social workers, and administrative and clinical auxiliary personnel, and they give comprehensive primary health care to from 5,000 to 20,000 inhabitants. HCs will have directors/coordinators designed by area and regional (autonomous community level) health authorities, from the list of physicians working at each HC. HCs are expected to be relatively autonomous in designing their activities. Politically, this tridimensional process of decentralization/integration of health-care activities network construction and management will probably be difficult to establish because it endangers traditional attitudes and power relationships. Additionally, it is becoming apparent that the decentralization process, as it is evolving so far, may impede eventually the equity of the system at national level. The country may result in having as many different health systems as autonomous communities.

A PHC-Based System

Preventive versus curative and PHC versus hospital care issues have been discussed for many years, yet they remain unresolved in practice. The newly designed health-care system will have to deal with both in the near future. Health personnel education, the current system's tradition and history, and prevalent power structures in the health sector all work against innovation on either front. It will be probably very difficult to achieve substantial success in the short run. However, it seems that despite the many obstacles the Spanish health system is determined to move in the above described direction.

References

De Miguel, J. 1983. *La Estructura del Sistema Sanitario*. Madrid: Tecnos.

I.N.E. 1980. *El Consumo de las Familias Españolas*. Madrid: INE.

I.N.E. 1983. *Encuesta de Presupuestos Familiares 1980–1981*. Madrid: INE.

Ministerio de Sanidad y Consumo. 1984. *Oferta y Demanda de Médicos en España (una primera aproximación)*. Madrid: S.G.T., Ministerio de Sanidad.

OCDE. 1985. *Measuring Health Care 1960–1983*. París: OCDE.

Rodríguez, M. 1986. *El Gasto Sanitario en Cataluña, 1981. Estimación y Análisis Descriptivo*. 1987. Barcelona: Generalitat de Catalunya, Dep. Sanitat y SS.

Saturno, P. J. 1987. *La Función Hospitalaria*. Murcia: Sec. Pub. Universidad Murcia.

Saturno, P. J. and Gol, J. 1983. *El Gasto Sanitario en la Provincia de Madrid como base y complemento de la evaluación Estructural del Sistema*. Madrid: Diputación—Provincial de Madrid.

World Bank. 1983. *World Bank Atlas 1983*. Washington D.C.

WHO. 1983 *World Health Statistics Annual 1983*. Geneva: WHO.

SWEDEN

Richard B. Saltman

Introduction

The Swedish health-care system is a regionally based, publicly operated national health service. Although broad policy decisions are taken at the national level, the implementation of policy and the administration of most health-related services—and nearly all curative medical services—are the responsibility of the county council (*landsting*). This relationship between state and country has been described as one of rider and horse: The rider—or state—may seek to guide the horse, but ultimately it is the horse—the county—that must decide where to go and how to get there. Additionally, it should be noted that health-related decision making, like political decision making generally in Sweden, is typically characterized by a consensus-based process that ensures overall agreement prior to policy implementation (Twaddle and Hessler 1986). The combination of Sweden's formal state-county relationship with its highly rationalized policy formulation process creates what can be viewed as a very deliberate approach to health system development. Indeed, this basic model has continued to operate even within the relatively highly charged policy environment in Sweden of the 1980s.

Health Statistics

Sweden's aggregate mortality and morbidity indices reflect the high standard of living in Sweden as a whole. At birth, a male baby had an average life expectancy of 73.8 years in 1984 (compared to 72.1 between 1971 and 1975). The infant mortality rate in 1984 was 6.4 per 1,000 live births (10.0 between 1971 and 1975), and the rate of legal abortions per 1,000 live births was 327.6, down from a 1979 high of 360.9 per 1,000 live births (NOMESKO 1986).

The most common causes of death in Sweden, reflecting its advanced industrial status, were quite clearly the "diseases of affluence." In 1984, in order of importance, they were (1) ischemic heart disease, 34 percent; (2) diseases of the central nervous system, 10 percent; and (3) other diseases of the circulatory system, 5.7 percent (NOMESKO 1986).

Historical Overview

The Swedish health-care system has been predominantly public in nature from its inception. Although a system of state-paid district physicians was established in the 1700s, the basic present-day structure was first set out in a 1864 decision that gave county government the responsibility for operating the hospital sector. The Swedish health system's development since 1864 can be viewed as a more-or-less continual expansion of county responsibilities in nearly all health-related sectors.

A crucial step in providing universal coverage for physician consultations, prescription drugs, and sickness compensation occurred in 1946, when a national health insurance act was voted by Parliament, and in 1955, when this act was implemented. Subsequently, in 1959, private beds and fee-for-service payments for hospital physicians were abolished. The so-called Seven Crown Reform of 1970 prohibited hospital physicians from taking private payment for ambulatory care—with the result of making Swedish hospital specialists fully salaried civil servants. In 1971, the retail drug distribution industry was nationalized, and it was reorganized into a separate, state-owned company called *Apotekbolaget* (Heidenheimer and Elvander 1980).

In a similar pattern, a number of national health-related obligations have been transferred to the counties. In 1960, the counties became responsible for all hospital-based outpatient care. The district medical officers were transferred to the counties in 1963. In 1965, ambulance services became a county responsibility. In 1967, mental hospitals were transferred to county control (Ministry of Health and Social Affairs 1985). Most recently, the 1983 Health and Medical Services Act gave the counties "full responsibility" for health-delivery-related matters, and, in 1985, the Dagmar Reform consolidated previously retrospective fee-for-service payments from the national insurance system for ambulatory physician visits into a prospective, capitation-based system channeled exclusively through the county councils.

Perhaps the most important policy development within the Swedish health-care system has been the development, acceptance, and subsequent implementation of a primary-care-based strategy. Although such an approach was first sketched out in the Höjar Report in 1948, the concept did not come to legislative fruition until the Primary Care Act of 1974, which stipulated that increased emphasis was to be placed on the development of primary and preventive modes of health care. Since 1974, there has been a major effort to develop the necessary administrative and service delivery tools to operationalize this primary health care (PHC) based policy. These efforts have included a variety of attempts at the county level to reconfigure the hospital-based administrative structure to facilitate the movement of increased resources into the primary care sector. One technique implemented by Skaraborgs Country Council in 1975, and since adopted in modified form by a number of Swedish counties, was to create separate subcounty political districts for primary care.

A second major policy thrust over this same period has been an effort to identify and remove barriers that obstruct equal access to health services. While this effort initially concentrated on the distribution of service sites (including the development, from 1958 onward, of a regional system of six subspeciality referral hospitals), in recent years emphasis has been placed on intersectoral and social barriers to adequate medical and/or health services. It is as much a measure of the difficulty of achieving these policy goals in an advanced industrial county as it is of Swedish persistence and determination that both issues remain, a decade later, on the current policy agenda (Brogren and Saltman 1985).

Health System Structure and Personnel

The Swedish health system has components that pursue activities on four different governmental levels: national, regional, county, and municipal. Although broad issues of overall health policy, service standards, and operating procedures reflect a complex intermingling of interests at the national level among professional organizations (in particular, the Swedish Medical Association), employee unions, the Federation of County Councils (*Lanstingsförbundet*), and quasi-independent national bodies like the National Board of Health and Welfare (*Socialstyrelsen*) and the Swedish Planning and Rationalization Institute (SPRI), service delivery is now almost exclusively a county-level responsibility. Each of Sweden's 23 counties and three separate municipalities (Göteburg, Malmö, and the island of Gotland) defines and administers its own selected service mix. These include tertiary and secondary hospital inpatient services; outpatient clinics; primary care centers; maternal and child health centers; nursing, rehabilitation, and chronic care homes; inpatient and outpatient mental health services; and visiting nurse services. Regional university hospitals, with subspecialist and other intensive clinical facilities, are also administered by the county in which they are located. Moreover, Swedish counties raise over 60 percent of all health system revenue through an income tax levied on county residents.

Primary Care

The primary care services deliver both first-level curative as well as preventive services through an increasingly comprehensive network of public primary care centers. These health centers provide services to from 20,000 to 50,000 inhabitants of a demographically defined district, and they are staffed by at least three physicians and an equivalent number of nurses. Often, these health centers perform rudimentary laboratory and X-ray services. Many centers have or share services from consulting specialist physicians, typically pediatricians, but occasionally gynecologists and psychiatrists as well.

The primary care sector in Sweden also has management responsibilities for a variety of ambulatory and/or non-hospital-based services. These include a well-developed network of nursing homes; a decentralized community-based program of mental health services; facilities and programs for the mentally retarded, physically disabled, and chronically ill; and such disparate services as alcohol treatment centers and visiting nurse services.

Up until the early 1980s, most primary care services were administered by the counties as part of so-called hospital districts, often by the same administrative staff that managed the county's tertiary hospital. This agreement led, for numerous structural and political reasons, to the continued preeminence of hospital-based care in the distribution of health-related resources and personnel. As part of a series of experiments dating back to 1975 (in Skaraborgs County), Swedish counties now are developing politically and financially independent mechanisms through which to administer their primary care sectors. The goal is perceived as one of creating an independent organizational base for primary care activities that will be more attuned to its needs and, equally important, can compete more effectively for new resources against the established hospital sector of the system.

Hospital Sector

Each county typically provides two levels of inpatient hospital care. The district hospital, which provides secondary care, usually has available specialists in four areas (internal medicine, surgery, pathology, and radiology), as well as some specialized services like emergency and maternity care. The central hospital, of which there may be two in the larger counties, provides tertiary level services in from fifteen to twenty clinical specialities in a relatively large, 600- to 1,000-bed facility.

For highly specialized and/or intensive forms of care, Sweden has six large, university-affiliated regional hospitals. These institutions—which also serve as major teaching facilities—provide the full range of medical specialities, and are available for referral patients with particularly complex conditions requiring both collaboration among subspecialists and sophisticated diagnostic and/or treatment facilities. Although the national government defrays those regional hospital costs associated with teaching and research, the hospitals are administered by the county within which they are located, with adjacent county councils reimbursing the administering county (usually on a per diem basis) for care provided to their respective inhabitants. It should be mentioned that the national Federation of County Councils administers a financial clearing house among the counties to facilitate various reimbursements between and among the counties for out-of-county emergency care, shared services, and other prorated financial undertakings.

Sweden is considered to have a relatively high ratio of beds to population (7.2 per 1,000 population in 1984), despite the fact that this figure has fallen dramatically from the figure of 10.7 per 1,000 population in 1975. Although the recent emphasis on primary care has begun to increase the number of ambulatory visits provided at health centers, it should be noted that, in 1982, a full 50 percent of all physician consultations were provided in hospital outpatient clinics (NOMESKO 1986). In this regard, Swedish citizens retain the right to self-refer to hospital outpatient specialists, although hospital-based physicians can no longer have private patients (1970), and private beds were abolished, as noted above, in 1959.

Municipal Health-Related Services

The 284 municipalities in Sweden engage in a variety of preventive activities in environmental areas (prevention of communicable diseases and supervision of food and water supplies) along with school health programs. In addition, the municipalities are responsible for social welfare services in Sweden, including income maintenance and—most importantly for the primary care sector—home care services and support staff. As this administrative split between primary health (county) and home care (municipal) services suggests, the issue of coordinating patient care across separately organized and budgeted bodies is a crucial issue in Sweden.

One interesting innovation in this area, termed Medical Care Program (*Vårdprogramme*), seeks to coordinate hospital, primary, and social service sectors for a specific common disease or condition. As of 1985, Medical Care Programs have been written for a variety of conditions, including such major health-care management problems as essential hypertension, breast cancer, diabetes, and alcohol disorders. These Medical Care Programs have not always been adopted by county administrations since they often view these integrated programs as too expensive to implement properly.

Health Sector Personnel

Until recently, Sweden has devoted an increasing percentage of its manpower to the health sector. The total number of health sector employees grew from 115,000 in 1960, or 3 percent of the labor force, to 405,941 in 1983, or approximately 9 percent of the work force. This total fell to about 380,000 in 1985, or about 8.5 percent of the total employed—a reduction that reflects successful efforts in the last few years to reduce the rate of health sector growth to below that of the Swedish economy as a whole. While a portion of this long-term growth can be attributed to a shortening of working hours and a growing proportion of part-time employees, there has nonetheless been a considerable increase in the number of full-time employees over the past twenty-year period (Brogren and Saltman 1985).

A large segment of these new workers continue to be absorbed by the hospital sector. Over the period from 1970 to 1977, for example, 75 percent of the new workers were absorbed by hospitals. While the increasing emphasis on primary care during the first half of the 1980s could be expected to reduce this percentage, the reduction is likely to have been only marginal.

Sweden had 17,726 physicians in 1982. Similarly, the 1984 figures indicate that there were 71,300 fully trained nurses and midwives and 8,803 dentists (NOMESKO 1986).

Virtually the entire Swedish health-care sector is unionized. Depending upon their educational level and training, health sector workers belong to SACO/SR (physicians and administrators), TCO (nurses and physiotherapists), or SKAF (support personnel). It is worth mentioning that SKAF is one of the largest unions in Sweden, with considerable influence in national health-policy formulation.

Wage agreements are negotiated at the national level in Sweden, between the national offices of the several unions and the Federation of County Councils in Stockholm. With the passage in 1977 of a national codetermination act (Medbestämmandelagen or MBL), the Swedish health-care system has initiated a program of codetermination between the unions and management. Under this MBL system, county administration is obligated to notify the affected union of decisions that materially affect hospital employees, and to consult with those workers as to the suitability of the proposed changes. After a specified waiting period, however, the administration is entitled to implement decisions over employee objection. While neither management nor union is fully satisfied with the codetermination system's present structure (administration says privately that MBL delays hospital retrenchment, while unions say they cannot prevent undesirable changes), the system represents a unique effort to introduce shared decision making within Swedish hospitals.

Health System Finance

Health-care expenditures in Sweden are financed through four interrelated sources: 1) direct county taxes on personal income, 2) the national health insurance system (for ambulatory physician visits), 3) national grants (to support teaching and research at university hospitals and to equalize income among well-off and less-well-off counties), and 4) small user fees for outpatient physician consultations, inpatient care, and some drug prescriptions.

The major source of health system funding is, as noted, the county councils' direct tax on the personal income of its inhabitants. This tax, which provided 61.8 percent of total county income in 1985, has risen from an average of 4.5 percent of personal income in 1960 to 13.50 percent in 1985, a level which will severely restrict any increases in this source of revenue in the future. Equivalent revenue figures for 1985 show that state tax equalization grants provided 6.2 percent of total county income and that state university-hospital-related grants provided another 12.1 percent. Additionally, in 1985 the counties received 6.5 percent from charges to patients and certain national social compensation combined; 3.4 percent from compensation from other authorities; and 9.3 percent in miscellaneous income (largely rents and financial revenues) (Landstingsförbundet 1987).

Out-of-pocket medical costs, including user fees, are tightly restricted in Sweden. The patient fee for an outpatient phyisician visit is 40 Swedish crowns (approximately US $7); the per diem fee for inpatient hospital care is 50 Swedish crowns. Prescription drug costs are shared between patients and the national health insurance, with all charges above 40 Swedish crowns for drugs prescribed by a doctor on any one occasion paid by the insurance fund. It is worth noting that such fees do not restrict access to care, since a comprehensive network of child allowance, social security, and pension systems ensures sufficient income to all citizens. Additionally, drugs for chronic and acute conditions are covered entirely by the national insurance, and, in all cases, further patient charges are waived for both physician visits and prescription drugs after a patient has made fifteen visits within a calendar year.

There has been a major emphasis on increasing hospital cost-effectiveness and overall health system productivity during the last several years. This effort was further spurred by the release in 1985 of a controversial Ministry of Finance report indicating that overall productivity in the Swedish health-care system had declined by 3 percent per year since 1960 (Finansdepartmentet 1985). Although the methodology and the conclusions of this report remain the subject of considerable debate, the report heightened pressures for increased efficiency just as initial cost-containment efforts were beginning to take effect—demonstrated by a reduction in total percentage of gross domestic products (GDP) consumed by the health sector from 9.7 percent in 1982 to 9.4 percent in 1984 (OECD 1987), with an equivalent drop in the total number of health sector employees.

One interesting experiment undertaken by several counties was to decentralize responsibility for the annual operating budget to the clinical department level. In Älvsborg County, for instance, day-to-day budget responsibility in one of its tertiary care hospitals was parceled out to eight blocks, each composed of services that had similar clinical characteristics (the surgical block, for example, included general surgery, orthopedics, eye surgery, and the operating theater). The designated block chief received a monthly statistical breakdown from hospital administration showing the portion of the annual block budget expended that month, the proportion of the total annual budget remaining unspent, and a comparison of these figures with equivalent percentages from the prior year. The block chief, usually a senior physician, could, if the figures so indicated, discuss expenditure ratios with the block's several department chiefs. Moreover, with agreement of these other department chiefs, the block chief could reallocate funds between clinics and also between activities: Savings on the use of overtime nursing personnel, for instance, could be transferred to the small capital equipment or continuing education accounts. This form of decentralization has now been discontinued, however, in the belief that it reinforced inertial tendencies toward the development of isolated minihospitals.

Future Issues

There has been a growing debate in Sweden about the future development of the health-care system (Rydén and Bergström 1982). While there is widespread consensus about the appropriateness of a primary-care-based delivery system, there is little certainty as to how best to achieve it. There is, further, concern that the present organizational structure is unable to satisfy the present conflicting pressures for simultaneously higher standards of internal productivity, worker participation, and patient satisfaction. This last is particularly complicated, reflecting a growing unwillingness among Swedes to accept long queues for certain elective surgical procedures (typically for elderly patients) or time-consuming appointment scheduling mechanisms.

Proposals for change currently include a wide variety of decentralized and/or privatized delivery formats. Within the public sector, there have been attempts to restructure administrative responsibilities inside the county councils—as with the Skaraborgs County experiment described above. There also are efforts to decentralize responsibilities from county to municipal levels in an effort to conjoin primary care with municipally run social services within a single administrative unit—the so-called Free Commune experiment.

There are, rather differently, a growing number of experiments with private sector providers. In the area of ambulatory care, for example, the success of a privately operated walk-in clinic in downtown Stockholm, called City Akuten, which first opened in 1983, has triggered a number of experiments in outpatient care. In 1986, conservative-run county councils in Stockholm and Malmö have begun to contract out the management of several local health centers to privately run physician group practices on a trial basis. It should be noted that, thus far, these experiments have involved a uniquely Swedish arrangement in which public resources—buildings, patient insurance funds, and the off-duty time of fully-salaried public sector physicians—have been reorganized under private management. While Sweden has also seen the first incursions of privately financed health care—in the form of a business class service offered as a corporate benefit by a private Swedish hospital working with a large insurance company—there has been little interest thus far in this type of wholly private delivery system among the public at large.

Behind these structural issues, there also are continuing efforts to rationalize and integrate the overall delivery of health services in Sweden. For example, there are continuing efforts to "break down the walls" that divide the different clinical departments from each other, and to encourage more efficient use of scarce resources such as beds and nursing personnel. There also are national consensus conferences on specific clinical problems in an attempt to encourage specialists to revise their medical practice patterns in a more clinically effective and financially efficient direction. Finally, there is a growing recognition of the necessity of intersectoral cooperation in improving the health status of the population, and hence reducing the long-term resource requirements of the clinical sector of the health system.

Overall, the evidence would appear to suggest that Sweden will continue to experiment with new modes of health-care organization and delivery, and will continue to approach asymptotically the ambitious health sector goals it has set for itself. Whether Sweden or indeed any advanced industrial country is now capable of achieving these goals, despite heroic efforts to do so, remains an open question.

References

Anderson, O. 1972. *Health Care. Can There Be Equity? Sweden, Britain, and the United States*. New York: Wiley and Sons.

Brogren, P. O. and R. B. Saltman. 1985. Building Primary Health Care Systems: A Case Study from Sweden. *Health Policy* 5, 4: 313–29.

Finansdepartmentet. 1985. *Produktions-, kostnads- och produktivitets- utveckling inom offentligt bedriven hälso- och sjukvård 1960–1980,* DsFi 3 (*Production, Cost, and Productivity Development in Public Health Care*). Stockholm: Liber Allmänna Förlaget.

Heidenheimer, A. J. and N. J. Elvander, eds. 1980. *The Making of the Swedish Health Care System*. New York: St. Martin's.

Landstingsförbundet. 1982. *Swedish County Councils 1987*. Stockholm.

Ministry of Health and Social Affairs. 1982. *Health in Sweden*. Stockholm.

National Board of Health and Welfare. 1985. *The Swedish Health Services in the 1990s*. Stockholm: Liber Tryck.

Nordic Medical Statistical Committee (NOMESKO). 1986. *Health Statistics in the Nordic Countries*. Copenhagen.

OECD. 1987. *Financing and Delivering Health Care*. Paris: OECD.

Rydén, B. and V. Bergström, eds. 1982. *Sweden: Choices for Economic and Social Policy in the 1980s*. London: George Allen and Unwin.

Saltman, R. B. and C. von Otter. 1987. Re-vitalizing Public Health Care Systems: A Proposal for Public Competition in Sweden. *Health Policy* 7:21–40.

Strömberg, L. and J. Westerståhl. 1984. *The New Swedish Communes: A Summary of Local Government Research*. Stockholm: Liber Publishers.

Twaddle, A. C. and R. M. Hessler. 1986. Power and Change: The Case of the Swedish Commission of Inquiry on Health and Sickness Care. *Journal of Health Policy and Law* 11, 1 (Spring): 19–40.

TURKEY

M. Rahmi Dirican

Background Information

Turkey is a rectangular country stretching 1,600 kilometers from east to west and 725 kilometers from north to south. It lies 97 percent in Asia and 3 percent in Europe, sharing common borders with Greece and Bulgaria in the northwest, the USSR and Iran on the east, and Iraq and Syria on the south.

Administratively, Turkey is divided into 67 provinces. Each province has a specific number of districts to which villages are attached. At present, there are 572 district centers and 35,995 villages in Turkey. According to 1980 census (State Institute of Statistics 1984a), the total population of Turkey is 44,737,000, of which 56 percent lives in the rural areas. Percent distribution of the population in three broad age groups is given in Table 1.

Almost all developing countries suffer from insufficient health statistics. In Turkey, reporting of births, deaths, and causes of deaths are incomplete and inaccurate. Relevant, reliable, complete, comparable, and up-to-date morbidity data are scanty and approximate, not least because physicians and other health personnel attach little importance to reporting vital events. Under these conditions, special surveys are required for accurate definition of the health situation. Only a few such studies have been done in Turkey. Some health-related statistics obtained from these surveys (Hacettepe Institute of Population Studies 1978) are given in Table 2.

Historical Overview

Health services in Turkey passed through several stages of evolution. Prior to the nineteenth century, the health care of the population was in the hands of

Table 1
Percent Distribution of Population by Age Groups, 1980

Age Groups (in years)	Percent of Population		
	Male	Female	TOTAL
0 - 14	20.1	18.9	39.0
15 - 64	28.3	27.6	55.9
65+	2.3	2.8	5.1
TOTAL	50.7	49.3	100.0

Table 2
Some Health-Related Information

-Birth rate (per 1,000 population)	31
-Death rate (per 1,000 population)	10
-Annual natural increase (percent)	2.1
-Infant mortality rate (per 1,000 live births 1972-77)	134
-Life expectancy (at birth)	62 years
-The most common causes of death for children (aged 0-4 years) in cities and towns (1982).	Birth injuries and pneumonia
-The most common causes of death for adults (aged 15+ years) in cities and towns (1982)	Heart Diseases

private physicians who had completed their apprenticeships by working with experienced physicians. Immediately after the foundation of the first western-type medical school in 1827, the directors of this medical school, with the help of a special medical council, became responsible for the organization and administration of health services until a General Directorate of Health attached to the Ministry of Interior was established in 1912 (Dilevurgan 1946). Since World War I, the Turkish government has taken an active part in rendering health-care services to its citizens (Fisek 1971).

When the Republic of Turkey was created in 1923, the state was given the responsibility of improving the health conditions of the country, of combatting all diseases and other harmful factors detrimental to the health of the population, of ensuring healthful living for future generations, and of providing medical and social assistance for the people. These responsibilities have been rendered through the Ministry of Health and Social Welfare (MHSW).

The MHSW is the highest organ and supervisory authority for all health services in Turkey with the exception of those operated by the Ministry of Defense. The MHSW is responsible for improving the health conditions of the country; implementation is delegated to municipal and local health authorities (Government of Turkey 1930). The MHSW is the main provider of medical and health-care services in Turkey. Medical care is also provided by other ministries, state economic enterprises, the State Insurance Institution, medical schools, and the private sector, but their activities have not been extensive compared to the work of the MHSW.

The administrative organization of the MHSW is divided into two parts: central and provincial. At the central level, the minister, who is chosen by the prime minister from among the members of the Parliament, is ultimately responsible for all health services. The undersecretary is the chief executive officer and handles routine administration. Assistants to the undersecretary are in charge of various general directorates such as basic health services, personnel, curative services, and Maternal and Child Health (MCH), and family planning. At the provincial level, there is a director of health appointed by the MHSW. He is the highest official in the province; however, he is officially under the administrative control of the governor (*vali*). Each province is divided into districts (*kazas*) with a governor (*kaymakam*) as the highest administrative officer. In every *kaza*, there is a medical officer of health who acts as health advisor to the *kaymakam*. In cities, medical officers work directly under the provincial director of health, but, in the *kazas*, they are under the administrative control of the *kaymakam*. The MHSW appoints municipality doctors, but they are paid by the municipal authorities. Drawbacks of this central-authoritarian administrative structure of the MHSW has been repeatedly discussed, but, so far, only limited attempts have been made to change it.

From 1923 until 1950, state-provided health services and preventive medicine had priority. Since priorities and policies were set carefully, Turkey was able to overcome many of the prevalent communicable diseases, although there were great constraints in financial and manpower resources. However, due to a lack of cooperation and coordination among the various health agencies and organizations, the health services as a whole were not as efficient as they should have been.

From 1950 onward, along with increased rates of urbanization and industrialization, the emphasis shifted to medical rather than health care. Many hospitals were built, and private practice began to flourish. The rural population and the urban poor living in shanty towns were neglected. Health indices began to deteriorate. Demand for medical care increased, and environmental conditions worsened. The organizational arrangement set up in the early years of the republic was not able to cope with the increasing needs.

In 1960 a new constitution was accepted by the Turkish people. According to this constitution, it is the responsibility of the government to secure the highest possible level of health for the citizens. The parliament formulated the objective of the health program as follows:

> The main objective of the health program is to improve the health of the people. Priority is therefore given to the expansion of public health (preventive) services in the plan. These services include the improvement of environmental sanitation, health education, control of contagious diseases, improvement of nutrition and family planning. Curative health services are considered as complementary to preventive services. Priority is given to the establishment of health services which will extend to the smallest communities and will lay stress on home and out-patient treatment rather than on the more expensive system of hospitalization from which fewer people benefit (Fisek 1971).

Other major principles laid down by the Turkish parliament are as follows:

1. The health services will be financed mainly from the national budget, but the compulsory insurance system organized by the Government will also be developed. Compulsory health insurance for workers, excluding agricultural ones, is the first step taken in this direction.
2. A national health service will be developed stepwise, starting from the less developed provinces.
3. Health personnel, medical doctors included, will work full-time in the national health service, will not practice privately and will receive a fixed salary from the Government.
4. Medical care, including life saving drugs but excluding other drugs and supplies will be free in the national health services (Fisek 1971).

The Current Health-Care System

Health-Care Structure

In 1961 a new system of Turkish national health services was formulated and accepted by parliament (Government of Turkey 1961). This marked a milestone in the history of health services in Turkey. The design of the national health services is based on teamwork and cooperation. The characteristics of the planned national health services are summarized in the following paragraphs.

The organization at the ministerial and provincial levels has not been changed. The main organizational unit of the national health services at the provincial level is the health unit. A rural health unit is staffed by one physician, two nurses, one medical secretary, and three or four rural midwives who reside at health stations. Three or four health stations established at the grass root level are attached to one health unit. A health unit services an average of from 7,000 to 10,000 persons. In cities and towns, two to four health units are combined in one unit, and the staff is increased accordingly. From five to seven health units are under the administration of the head of the health district who is also the head of the district hospital. In a province, there may be many health districts depending upon the population of the province. Heads of the health districts are responsible to the director of health of the province (Figure 1).

The health unit physician is the leader of the team, who with his paramedical workers practices comprehensive medicine. He is responsible for ambulatory and home care, for all preventive work, for in-service training of the staff, and for the health education of the public. As a responsible member of the community, he is expected to motivate the people for community development. The health unit physician not only works in his office, but also visits health stations and other villages regularly.

One of the two public health nurses is responsible for supervising the work of the rural midwives and training them in service. The other public health nurse, a man, is responsible for environmental sanitation, school health, and health education of males. In outbreaks of communicable diseases, he takes part in the effort to control them.

Rural midwives are the most important members of the team in preventive work. They spend most of their time visiting villages and houses regularly. They are responsible for maternal and child health care and family planning education. They also report births and deaths to the health unit.

With regard to medical care, patients are examined first by the health unit physician, and those who need further examination or hospitalization are referred to the district or provincial hospital. Chronic cases are followed up by both specialists in the hospital and a health unit physician.

The activities of the health units are supported and complemented by district hospitals. The specialists in district hospitals are expected to visit health units regularly for consultation and in-service training. The hospital laboratory provides help for health unit physicians in the diagnosis of the patients attending the health units.

The director of health is the top health official in the province. He, with the assistance of his staff, carries out all the planning and directs the work of the heads of health districts, hospitals, and health units (Figure 2).

According to the Law on National Health Services (Government of Turkey 1961), when the national health services are applied to a province all the other health services extant in that province and supported either by the state or by the Social Insurance Institution will be united. Turkey will be divided into sixteen health regions administratively and each region will cover four or five provinces. The regional health director will be responsible for planning, administering, supervising, and evaluating all health activities in his region supported by the state or by the Social Insurance Institute.

Although the national health services have expanded over the years and now cover the whole country, the system does not work as it was planned. At present,

Figure 1
National Health Services at District Level (Approximately 1 Health District for 50,000 Persons; 1 Health Unit for 7,000–10,000 Persons, and 1 Health Station for 2,500 Persons)

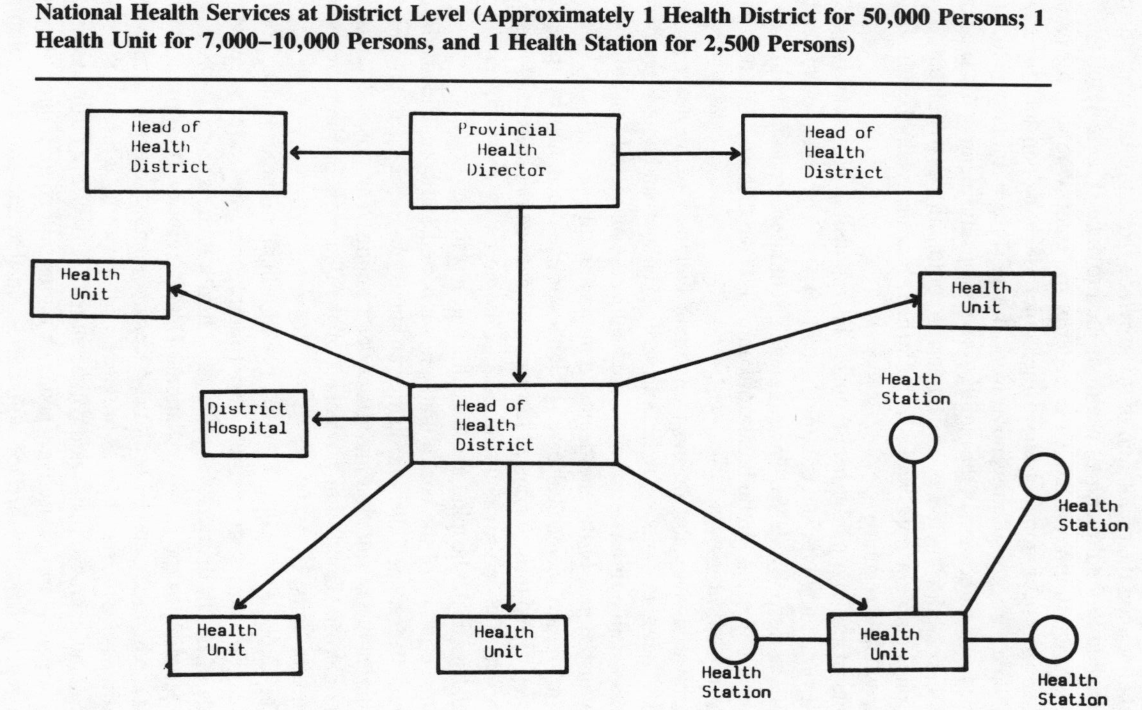

Figure 2
Provincial Organization of the National Health Services

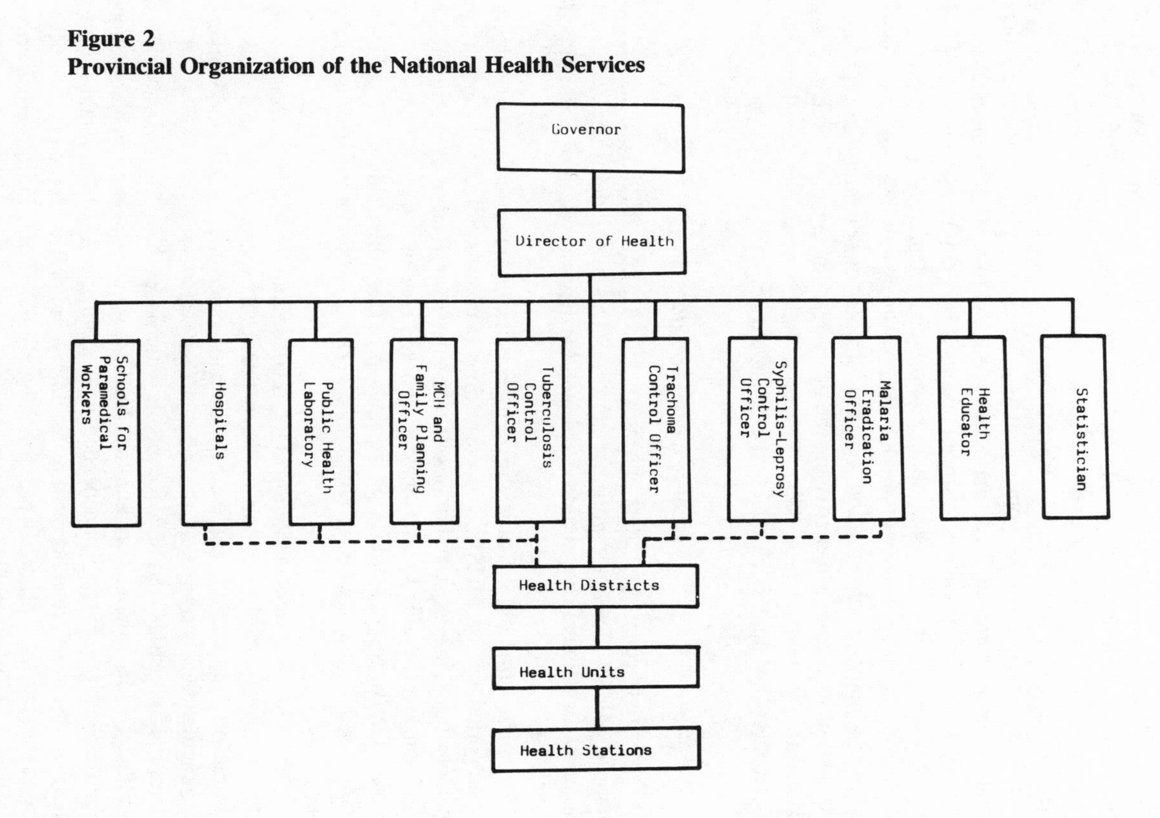

health policies are mainly geared toward enlarging the private sector. The budget of the MHSW has been reduced to a low minimum level. Community care and state medicine have lost their priority. The general health status of the public has become worse not only because of a decline in the health system as a whole, but also because of a decrease in real income and purchasing power and the deterioration of housing conditions and the nutritional status of the people. In order to increase the effectiveness of health services, however, some steps have been taken. Salaries of health personnel have been increased a little, and integration of some vertical programs such as tuberculosis control and family planning have been completed. A compulsory service of two years for medical school graduates and for specialists has been accepted by the government.

The Turkish Medical Association was established in 1953 (Government of Turkey 1953) and, although all physicians and dentists must register as members, it is not a powerful organization. It is responsible for defending the rights and interests of its members and advising the official health agencies about problems related to the medical profession. The other health personnel also have their associations but none is as effective as it should be.

Health-Care Providers

There are five main providers of health care in Turkey. All the providers other than the MHSW deal only with medical care. Therefore, their relative responsibilities for medical care could be assessed by their provision of hospital beds (Table 3).

Using this criterion, the largest part of the medical care services (60.1 percent) is supported by the MHSW with very limited contributions (1.0 percent) by municipalities and local authorities. The limited contribution at the municipal and local levels is due to poor organization and lack of funds.

The relative responsibilities of the main providers of health care could also be assessed on the number of physicians working in their organizations (Table 4).

The Social Insurance Institution is the second main provider of medical care. This scheme, started in 1946, has been financed by employers and workers. Insurance for all workers and their dependents, other than agricultural workers, is compulsory.

Several ministries and state economic enterprises have their own medical facilities for the persons they employ. Medical schools have particular responsibilities and considerable independence. Certain medical care establishments are nonprofit institutions operated by voluntary and philanthropic organizations. Private hospitals are primarily profit-making establishments built in urban areas.

There is another sector of health-care providers—quacks, traditional birth attendants, medicine men, religious healers, bonesetters, and so on. A study done in 1963 (Taylor et al. 1968) showed that there were about 85,000 of these traditional practitioners compared to 21,000 paramedical health personnel in the

Table 3
Bed Capacity of Health Institutions by Main Health-Care Providers, 1983

Health-Care Providers	Bed Capacity	
	No. of beds	%
-MHSW, Municipalities and Local Authorit. .	60,759[x]	61.1
-Social Insurance Institution	17,352	17.5
-Other Ministries, State Economic Enterprises, and Medical Schools	16,786[xx]	16.9
-Private Sector, Philantropic and Voluntary Organizations	4,499[xxx]	4.5
TOTAL	99,396	100.0

Note: Health institutions belonging to the Ministry of Defence are not shown.

[x]976 beds belong to municipalities and local authorities.
[xx]13,803 beds belong to medical schools.
[xxx]2,564 beds belong to private sector.
Source: MHSW, General Directorate of Curative Services; *Bulletin of Health Institutions with Beds* (Turkish), 1983.

country. Their numbers are probably much lower now. The type of medical care provided by these traditional health workers is often preferred by people who are poor and live in relatively neglected areas. Although these health-care providers are officially illegal, they are more accessible and acceptable than state health service for some rural settlers.

Cooperation between the various health-care providers is rather poor. They have different health service systems and belong to different ministries. The private sector is powerful and almost completely independent. Traditional medicine is both illegal and ignored. Medical schools cooperate to some degree with the MHSW. Except for the Red Crescent, the voluntary organizations are rather poor and do not contribute much to the provision of health care.

Coordination of health-related activities with other sectors is not much better. Some parts of the preventive services, especially those that have to do with environmental sanitation, are the responsibilities of municipalities and local authorities. Municipal leaders, being elected, give priority to those fields of activity that get more votes than do health-related activities.

Services related to occupational health, water supply, sewage systems, and housing are carried out by other ministries. MHSW has only supervisory responsibilities in these fields. School health and occupational health services are insufficient. On the other hand, in terms of health education, not enough use is

Table 4
Distribution of Physicians by Main Health-Care Providers, 1983

Health-Care Providers	No. of Physicians		TOTAL	
	Practitioners[x]	Specialist	Number	%
-MHSW, Municipalities and Local Authorit.	4,242	3,692	7,934[xx]	24.6
-Social Insurance Inst.	1,536	2,370	3,906	12.1
-Other Ministries, State Economic Enterprises and Medical Schools	3,852	3,975	7,827[xxx]	24.3
-Private Sector, phil. and Voluntary Org.	3,493	9,105	12,598[xxxx]	39.0
TOTAL Number	13,123	19,142	32,265	
TOTAL %	40.7	59.3		100.0

[x]Residents are included.
[xx]719 physicians employed by municipalities and local authorities.
[xxx]2,653 practitioners and 2,498 specialists (total 5,151 physicians) employed by medical schools.
[xxxx]Almost all are full-time private physicians.
Source: MHSW, General Directorate of Curative Services, *Bulletin of Health Institutions with Beds* (Turkish), 1983.

being made of the many primary and secondary schools spread all over the country. Nevertheless, some voluntary organizations partly financed by the government are doing useful work.

National development plans have a section on the health sector. The plans are prepared by the State Planning Organization with contributions from universities and the MHSW administrators. The Department of Planning and Coordination of the MHSW makes the annual plan of the MHSW according to the national development plan. For almost 25 years, the national health services have been considered the only long-term health plan for Turkey. Unfortunately, national development plans are not mandatory; they are mainly in the form of recommendations. This usually results in their being disregarded. Moreover, political parties may have different priorities and policies than those set in the development plans. Thus, plans may be altered by each new government. Therefore, while the plans for the national health services have always lagged behind, targets for hospital beds have been surpassed.

Financing Mechanisms of Health Care

Budgeting is performed by the MHSW at the end of each year, and the budget is presented to the parliament for approval. After discussions on different items of the budget, it is finalized and allocated to the MHSW. Both budgeting and distribution of funds are accomplished centrally without involving the provinces in the planning process. In the last few years, the percentage of funds allotted to the MHSW from the government budget has been decreasing. It was 4.2 percent in 1980; 3.6 percent in 1981, and 2.9 percent in 1983. The budget of the MHSW shows a 20-percent decrease from the 1981 year's budget. If the 35 percent annual inflation rate and about 25 percent salary increase to the MHSW employees are also considered, the real decrease in the budget of the MHSW reaches a much higher percentage. About 65 percent of this budget is spent annually for salaries and wages.

To get a more comprehensive view of health expenditure, the money spent for medical care by the Social Insurance Institution, the state economic enterprises, and the medical schools as well as the costs related to private and traditional sectors should be added to the budget of the MHSW. However, these are very difficult, even impossible, to quantify and therefore cannot be included in this chapter.

According to a field survey carried out in Ankara in 1974, a middle-class family spent one-fifth of its monthly income for ambulatory medical care (Eren 1974). When expenditure for inpatient care is added, the figure reaches a surprising amount. Preventive services like immunization are excluded since they are free of charge. This study also showed that in Ankara, the capital of Turkey, one patient out of every three seeks medical care from the private sector. Although they have to pay for the services, many people still prefer a private physician to a government physician.

Ambulatory care, apart from drugs, is free in national health services, but payment is made for outpatient and inpatient care and surgical interventions both in state hospitals and in medical school hospitals for those who are not insured and are able to pay. The government employees, insured workers, and dependents of both groups obtain free medical care. It is estimated that about 45 percent of the population is not covered by any official health insurance scheme and has to pay for any curative care. Recently, a health insurance program to cover all the population and financed by a special tax has been under discussion by top-level decision makers, but no attempt to implement it has yet been made.

Supply of Health Manpower

Undergraduate training of health personnel is undertaken by universities and by the MHSW. Schools for paramedical personnel (nurses, midwives, laboratory technicians, and environmental technicians) are called health colleges and most of them are operated by the MHSW. In addition, medical schools and some

Table 5
Number of Students Attending Different Schools for Health Personnel, 1983–1984, and Number of Graduates, 1983

Kinds of School	Total No. Of Schools	Total No. Of Students Attending (1983 - 1984)	Total No. Of Graduates (1983)
a-University Level			
Medical	23	21,628	2,779
Dental	8	3,745	694
Pharmacy	7	3,553	837
Higher Nursing	4	883	162
Health Administr	1	125	35
Health Education	1	319	95
Physiotherapist	1	293	54
b-Lycee Level			
Health Colleges[x]	93	17,278	3,203

[x]70 are operated by the MHSW, and the others, which train nurses, by medical schools and voluntary organizations. Of those attached to the MHSW, 27 are nursing and 34 are midwifery schools; 3 for male public health nurses, 2 for laboratory technicians, 2 for environmental sanitarians, 1 for X-ray technicians, and 1 for orthopedic technicians are also operated by the MHSW.

Source: MHSW, General Directorate of Professional Training.

voluntary organizations have their own medical colleges for nurses. All the other health personnel (physicians, dentists, pharmacists, senior nurses, physiotherapists, health administrators, and so on) receive their training at universities. Table 5 shows the total number of schools and the students attending different schools for health personnel during the 1983–1984 academic year together with total number of graduates for the year of 1983.

Systematic manpower planning is not practiced in Turkey, and, therefore, at present there is a shortage of physicians and midwives but a surplus of pharmacists and dentists. Recently, steps were taken to overcome these shortages by establishing new schools and by increasing the annual number of students admitted to these schools. However, such steps might carry the obvious detrimental effects on the quality of education due to the enormous pressure on the facilities. There also has been no planning for the specialization of physicians, which has resulted in great shortages in certain specialties and an abundance of physicians in the more lucrative specialties. Although, for a number of years, it has been stressed that general practitioners should be responsible for primary care and should play a key role in the delivery of health services, there has been no corresponding change in medical education suitable to the fundamental needs of the country.

Almost three-quarters of physicians are specialists and they usually work in cities and big towns. Compulsory service of two years for medical graduates and specialists was initiated in 1981. It is hoped that this measure will alleviate temporarily the shortage of physicians in remote areas. The shortage of public health physicians is a chronic problem. It is due mainly to relatively low salaries and the discredit attached to administrative tasks and preventive medicine. These results have such factors as the intrinsic complexity of the health sector, the strong professional tradition that emphasizes individual and institutional autonomy for medical rather than health care, and a failure to grasp the manpower aspects of health-care problems.

Nursing in Turkey has moved to approach professional standing in only the last six decades. Nurses are now obtaining university diplomas and holding responsible positions in hospitals and as directors in health colleges, as well as serving in official capacities in the government and on committees which advise the government on policies concerning nursing. However, only a relatively small group of nurses have been granted this new professional stature.

Almost 80 percent of the dentists and pharmacists work privately. There are no trained technicians who work as either assistant dentists or assistant pharmacists in Turkey.

Major Problems

The most important health-related problems in Turkey can be summarized as follows:

1. *Health-status related*. Infectious diseases are still prevalent in the country. The number of cases of tuberculosis and malaria is on the increase. Gastrointestinal infections are endemo-epidemic. Pneumonia is one of the major causes of death of children under five years of age. An effective, well-planned, country-wide immunization program is still a dream of a rationalist public health worker. Environmental sanitation is far from being perfect.
2. *Institutional organization*. Lack of coordination and cooperation not only among the different health-care providers but also among the various general directorates of the NHSW hamper health services. From 1961 to now, no government has sought to unite and to decentralize (regionalize) the administration of the health services belonging to the state and to the Social Insurance Institution. School health and occupational health services have not been organized effectively.
3. *Financing*. At present, less than 3 percent of the government budget is devoted to the MHSW. Unless larger parts of the government budget (about 10 percent) are allotted for the NHSW, financing will be considered as one of the important obstacles hampering the national health services.
4. *Personnel and other issues*. The present teaching and training of physicians and other personnel is not relevant to the needs of the country. Health facilities and personnel

are distributed unevenly. In addition to the above-mentioned problems, a very strong private sector, the commercial attitudes of many physicians and dentists, the advantageous health benefits enjoyed by certain groups of the population, and short-sighted politicians and lack of health education of the public have all played a role in hindering the establishment of an effective health-care service.

Neither top-level health administrators nor physicians in health institutions receive any management training during their undergraduate or postgraduate education. This deficiency of managerial skills at all levels of the health service creates problems in planning, implementation, and evaluation. Modern management techniques and the systems approach are hardly ever practiced.

To reach the goal of "Health for All by the Year 2000," the basic principles of a primary health-care approach should be practiced in Turkey. The already existing organization of the national health services could create a good network of primary health-care services provided that the above-mentioned problems are tackled seriously. Furthermore, an effective chain for support and referral should be arranged clearly among the primary, secondary, and tertiary levels of health-care institutes; active community participation must be developed; the value of the primary health-care work must be enhanced; and, last but not least, top-level decision makers must wholeheartedly believe that primary health care will contribute to the country's general development along with education, agriculture, industry, and transport, which also use local resources and which, acting in combination, play a part in promoting health and in enhancing the quality of life.

References

Dilevurgun, H. 1946. *Saglik Memurlari Icin Halk Sagligi Bilgisi*, S.SY. Bakanligi Yayin No: 122. Istanbul Güven Basimevi. In English, *Information on Public Health for Sanitary Technicians*, MHSW Publication, No. 122. Istanbul: Güven Basimevi.

Eren, N. 1974. "Developing a Data Collection Method in the Center of Ankara Province for the Planning of Health Services." [In Turkish.] Ankara: Hacettepe Medical School, Institute of Community Medicine. (mimeographed)

Fisek, N. H. 1971. *An Example of an Integrated Approach to Health Care: The Turkish National Health Services*. In *Ciba Foundation Symposium on Teamwork for World Health*, eds. J. London and A. Churchill, 55–76.

Government of Turkey. 1930. *General Public Health Law*, no. 1593 [In Turkish].

———. 1936. *Law on the Organization and Personnel of the Ministry of Health and Social Welfare*, no. 3017 [In Turkish].

———. 1953. *Law on Turkish Medical Association*, no. 6023 [In Turkish].

———. 1961. *Law on the Nationalization of Health Services*, no. 224. [In Turkish].

Hacettepe Institute of Population Studies. 1978. *Turkish Fertility Survey 1978*. vol. I. Ankara: Hacettepe University Institute of Population Studies.

Prime Ministry State Institute of Statistics. 1984a. *Census of Population 12.10.1980, Social and Economic Characteristics*. Publication no. 1072. Ankara: Prime Ministry State Institute of Statistics.

———. 1984b. *Death Statistics in Province and District Centers 1982*. publication no. 1073. Ankara: Prime Ministry State Institute of Statistics.

Taylor, C. E., R. Dirican, K. W. Deuschle. 1968. *Health Manpower Planning in Turkey*. Baltimore, Md.: The Johns Hopkins Press.

UNION OF SOVIET SOCIALIST REPUBLICS

Mark G. Field

Background

The Soviet health-care system was born in the turmoil of the 1917 Bolshevik revolution. As such, it then reflected not only the ideological precepts of those who made the revolution, but also the realities of the times. Ideologically, the view was that illness and premature mortality were but expressions of a ''sick'' sociopolitical configuration, i.e., capitalism. With the advent of socialism (the first phase on the march to communism), the roots of most illnesses would be extirpated. This would come as a result both of changes in society (for example, the elimination of the exploitation of man by man) and of measures of a preventive nature. These measures would, in the long run, lead to the diminution in the significance of clinical, or remedial, medical services. In addition, the basic egalitarian nature of that future socialist-communist society would also lead not only to the elimination of unequal and antagonistic classes, but also to the disappearance of differences between specialists, particularly professionals, and the rest of the population. Health services would be made available to all on an equal basis, and at no cost at the time of the service. Private practice, whether in medicine or in any other profession, would disappear, to be replaced by public practice. In the early phase, immediately after the revolution, health care would be made available to the new ''ruling classes'' (the workers, peasants, and soldiers) ahead of the former owners and exploiters, as the simple retributive justice that must accompany any revolution: Those who had nothing before, including decent medical care, now would get it before their former masters.

The realities of the situation immediately after the revolution were stark. At the time Lenin seized power, the country was on the verge of collapse. A ruinous and inconclusive war against Germany and Austro-Hungary had produced a deteriorating health situation aggravated by the lack of food and disinfectants, including soap, which would lead shortly to epidemics with a high mortality rate. The situation would be made worse by the presence on Soviet soil of Allied troops dispatched to bolster a sagging front against the Central Powers, a bitterly fought and destructive civil war, and widespread famine. In 1919 Lenin stated at the Seventh Congress of the Soviets that either socialism would defeat the louse (carrier of typhus) or the louse would defeat socialism (Field 1967, 52). Thus, the early years of the regime were dominated by the problem of epidemic diseases.

A nucleus of the organization of a medical service under Bolshevik control was in place on the very first day of the revolution; two months later a Council of Medical Collegia was created to unite the health units of the commissariats (the revolutionary term for departments). Later on, on July 11, 1918, a decree over Lenin's signature established a Commissariat of Health Protection, which became the supreme organization for health care and health protection (Field 1967, 52ff.).

The term "health protection" is the literal translation of the Russian word *zdravookhranenie*. It embodies the meaning of prevention and of a lack of distinction between preventive and clinical services, between personal and public health. Although the commissariat became, in the course of time, a ministry, it is still today a Ministry of Health Protection, not a Ministry of Health or of Public Health. Its major concern, at first, was the health of the Red Army as well as the struggle against cholera, plague, typhus, and other acute epidemic illnesses that threatened the new regime.

The early years of the Soviet health system were also marked by conflicts between the organized medical profession and those few physicians who had sided with the Bolshevik regime (the first commissar had been an exile companion of Lenin) and who now were in a directing position. Before the revolution, Russian medical associations had gained wide recognition and had achieved a great deal of autonomy in professional matters. They generally belonged to the liberal intelligentsia, were eager to reform the health service along progressive lines, and after the revolution fully expected to play a leading role in the new health-care system. Bolshevik physicians, on the other hand, considered these doctors to be hopelessly bourgeois in their ideology, and they viewed their associations as a threat to the Soviet regime. The "old school" physicians, for example, resented being considered "medical workers" on a par socially and professionally with nurses, feldshers, and attendants. They also rejected the idea of giving medical care on a priority basis to members of the proletariat, insisting on the ethical universalism of medicine. The Bolsheviks rejected this as pure cant, insisting that in any (class) society physicians always treat the members of the ruling class better than others. Unable to capture the leadership of these associations or to establish control over their activities, the Bolshevik regime moved to dissolve them as counterrevolutionary. Thus, medical associations ceased to exist in the early years of the Soviet regime. Physicians became, in effect, "proletarianized" employees of the state and functionaries as they are today. As a result, there is no Soviet counterpart of the American, British, Canadian, or any other similar medical association (Field 1972).

The first ten years of the Soviet regime were years of trial in which its very existence was in question. After 1921, as the food supply improved, the epidemics gradually began to recede. By 1927–1928, the Soviet Union stood economically and demographically about where it had been immediately before World War I. It was still a relatively poor, underdeveloped nation; the majority of its population still lived from the land. In the health area, once the threat of epidemics passed, serious attempts were made to shape a health system consonant with prevailing ideological views. The emphasis in training new physicians was primarily on preventive rather than on clinical care, since most diseases were bound to disappear. The aim remained to establish an egalitarian health-care system.

By 1928 Stalin had established undisputed sway over the Soviet Union, and he launched an ambitious program to industrialize the Soviet Union and to collectivize agriculture. These gigantic plans, which produced a radical decline in living standards because of enforced savings, were also reflected in the health system. The emphasis on prevention and egalitarianism that had dominated the first ten years was abandoned as the regime concentrated on the provision of clinical services to those deemed central to the regime's production goals. In essence, the health system became an adjunct in the drive for production by maintaining the health of the labor force and by imposing labor discipline through strict control over the issuance of medical certificates to curb absenteeism and malingering (Field 1953). A system of differentiated health care for different members of the population began to emerge (Field 1984; Golyakhovsky 1984; Knaus 1981). In the last fifty years, the health-care system has not experienced any major restructuring. The Soviet Union has been a pioneer in devising what was meant to be a comprehensive system of socialized medical care, financed by the state, and available to the entire population. Both the original blueprint and the resulting Soviet delivery system deserve closer scrutiny than they have received so far.

Basic Philosophy and Principles of Soviet Health Care

Formally, the Soviet health-care system may be called "socialized medicine." The basic assumption on which it rests is that society, through the polity, has an obligation to provide preventive and clinical services to the population. Health care is thus a "public service," and the population's health is a "public utility." In fact, Lenin called public health a public asset, or "public property" (Petrovsky 1973). The Soviet health system operates according to a definite philosophy and a set of basic principles that provide an important sense of the overall system's orientation. The fundamental law of the present system of socialized medicine is found in Article 42 of the 1977 Constitution:

> Citizens of the USSR have the right to health protection. This right is ensured by free, qualified medical care provided by state health institutions; by extension of the network of therapeutic and health-building institutions; by the development and improvement of safety and hygiene in industry; by carrying out broad prophylactic measures; by measures to improve the environment; by special care for the health of youth, including prohibition of child labor, excluding the work done by children as part of the school curriculum; and by developing research to prevent and reduce the incidence of disease and ensure citizens a long and active life (Sharlet 1978).

The above objectives are to be achieved through health legislation, the fundamental principles of which were first enunciated in 1969 (until then, surprisingly enough, such principles had not been formally spelled out) (Ryan 1978). The first section of these principles enumerates the major objectives of health legislation: It is to ensure the harmonious physical and mental development of the population; health, a high level of working capacity and a long active life; the prevention and reduction of morbidity, a further reduction in the incidence of disabilities, and a reduction of mortality; and the reduction of factors and conditions having an adverse influence on the citizens' health (*Vedemosti* 1969).

Note should be made of the "working capacity and long active life" provision. Almost from the beginning, and particularly with the inception of the five-year plans, the Soviet regime's first priority has been that of productivity and industrial production. The contradiction that observers sometimes perceive between a society insensitive to human rights and the existence of comprehensive medical care vanishes when the utilitarian needs of production are considered. Morbidity and premature mortality have a profound impact on the individual's ability to work and to fight. Titmuss, in fact, characterizes the Soviet health system as an "industrial-performance-achievement" type, adding that the USSR has fashioned a system of social welfare based on the principle of work performance, achievement, and meritocratic selection (Ryan 1978, 110). Socialized medicine, Soviet style, is said to be a socialist system of governmental or collective measures having, as their general purpose, the protection of the health of the citizenry.

The above provisions, general and declamatory, are translated into reality through a series of well-articulated operating principles:

1. *Public responsibility for the health system.* Public health and personal medicine are a state concern and the responsibility of the government.
2. *Planning of the health system.* The unfolding of the health system of the nation reflects a deliberate planning process. Planning has been a feature of Soviet society since the end of the 1920s. Not only is the health system centrally planned, but its development must be integrated with the general planning for the entire nation. It thus must fit into the overall commitments, goals, programs, and other priorities of the regime. The enforcement of decisions regarding the health system is possible because it is a responsibility of the government, financed almost entirely through the state budget.
3. *Bureaucratic centralization.* The health system (both public health and medical care, as well as education, training, and research) is the overall responsibility of a central

national organization called the Ministry of Health Protection USSR, which operates either directly in matters of national importance or hierarchically through counterpart health ministries of the republics, and through health departments located at the different levels of the governmental structure (see Figure 1).

This permits a high level of centralization, standardization, coordination, and uniformity. There are also other health administrations that formally operate outside the health ministry's jurisdiction, but all health agencies are expected to operate on the basis of the same principles.

4. *Gratuity of services*. Medical and allied services are made available to the population at no direct cost at the time of the service. The health system is financed through general revenues and transfer payments from productive enterprises. There are some exceptions: A few polyclinics exist where, for a set fee, a patient may see a better qualified physician than is usually available and with less wait. Pharmaceuticals prescribed for outpatients (with the exception of those specified for use on a chronic basis, like insulin) are purchased by the individual at a state-controlled price. The private practice of medicine is legal, but it is heavily taxed and is subject to certain restrictions. Given the housing shortage, only a few physicians (usually professors) have the space and thus the possibility to see patients at home. There are not private medical or hospital facilities, although there is an equivalent, which is discussed later.
5. *Prevention as the official cornerstone*. Theoretically, prevention is the cornerstone of the Soviet health system.
6. *Unity of theory and practice*. The official emphasis in Soviet medical care and research is on the close connection between theory (in this case, Marxism-Leninism) and practice. This orientation holds that research cannot and should not be carried out without a specific and practical application; it must be oriented to the solution of actual problems caused by morbidity and premature mortality, particularly as it affects workers in production.
7. *Role of the people*. In official theory, the health system "belongs to the people" and could not operate without the constant support of the people, for example, through the efforts of voluntary and community or collective efforts. In this, it rejoins the populist or socialist ideology that undergirds the Soviet system.
8. *Priority*. As long as medical resources remain scarce, access to medical care is governed by a priority order that is determined by the regime's evaluation of the importance of the individual (or, more likely, a group of individuals) to the fulfillment of state goals and programs. Thus members of the different elites (political, scientific, artistic) have access to medical facilities reserved for them and their families of the highest quality available (Field 1984, 135). Below them, in descending order, are other members of Soviet society down to collective farmers and other rural inhabitants where care tends to be spartan if not primitive, and is often given by feldshers, or physician assistants, rather than by physicians.

The Current Structure of the Soviet Health-Care System

Soviet socialized medicine is a state run, state financed, and state managed prepaid scheme for the provision of both preventive and clinical health services to a population of about 280 million (1986). The apex of that system is the

Figure 1
Structure of the Health Ministry and Supervising Organs (All Levels)

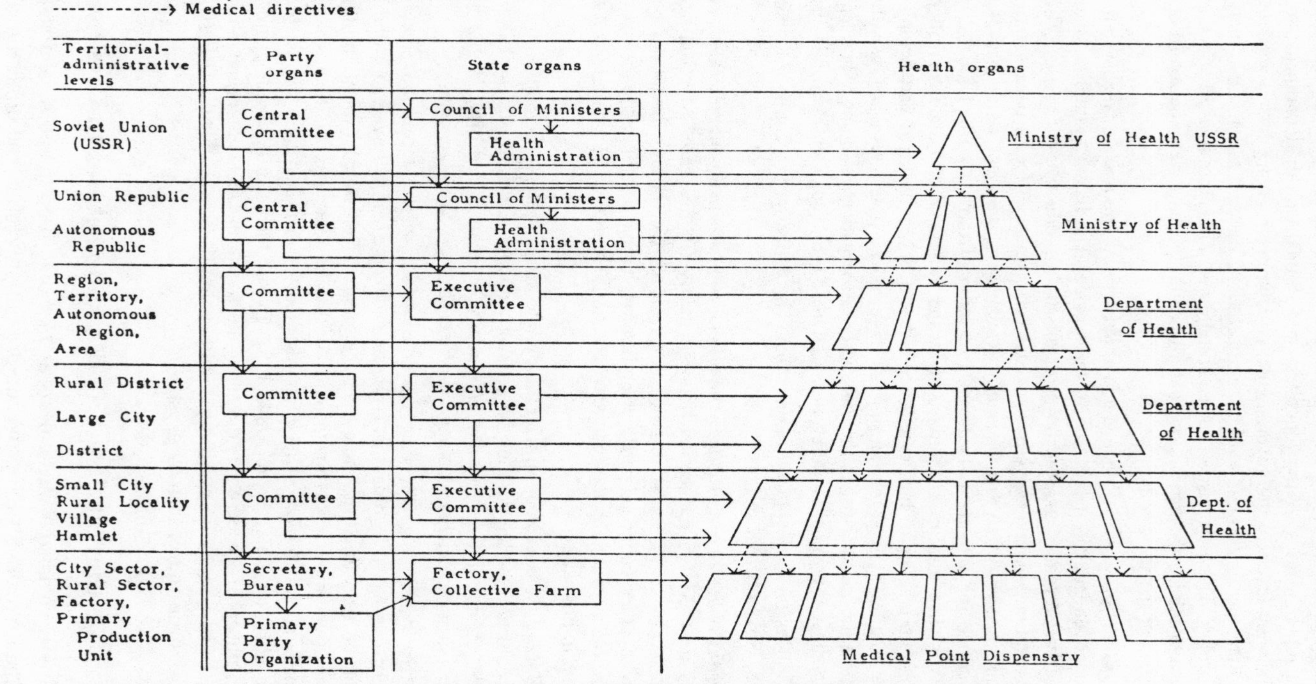

Source: Mark G. Field, *Doctor and Patient in Soviet Russia*. Cambridge, Mass. Harvard University Press, 1957, 36.

Table 1
Distribution of Population Between the Six Subsystems of Medical Care, 1975

Type of Subsystem	Number of population (thousands)	Percent Distribution
1. Elite	200	0.1
2. Departmental	12,700	5.0
3. Capital City	49,900	19.7
4. Industrial	20,200	8.0
5. Medium City	40,900	16.1
6. Rural District	129,400	51.1
Total	253,300	100.0

Source: Christopher Davis, "The Economics of the Soviet Health System: An Analytical and Historical Study, 1921–1978." Ph.D. dissertation for Degree in Economics, Cambridge University, 1979.

Ministry of Health Protection USSR, which is located in Moscow, and the key figure is that of the Health Protection Minister USSR. Formally, the minister is a member of the Council of Ministers USSR, and thus has cabinet rank. His responsibilities as the chief health officer of the country are formidable. In fact, however, not all health personnel and facilities are directly subordinate to the ministry. The ministry, however, has under its control the largest number of personnel and facilities and sets the tone for most Soviet health services. The ministry has under its jurisdiction five subsystems of health care. The sixth one (the Departmental Health System) is not formally its responsibility. These five subsystems are facilities: for the elites, also known as the Ministry's Fourth Directorate; for the capital cities; for the provincial cities; for the rural districts; and for industries (see Table 1).

The Departmental Health System consists of health facilities reserved for the employees and workers of specific ministries, presumably with special medical and health needs. Among these, we can note the Ministries of Foreign Affairs, Trade, Finances, Higher and Intermediate Education, and Aviation and the Academy of Sciences and the KGB (internal police). Furthermore, the Ministry of the Railroads has its own network of clinics and hospitals, as do the Ministries of the Merchant Marine, Island Waterways, Transport, and Civil Aviation. Last, but not least, the Ministry of Defense maintains its own medical facilities. The armed forces have their own medical schools, which train career military medical officers. Since these would be insufficient to supply medical cadres in a conflict, civilian physicians must take courses in military medicine and are thus part of the pool of available military physicians (Golyakhovsky 1984).

Nonetheless, the Health Protection Minister and the ministry are the dominant elements in the Soviet medical establishment, along with the Academy of Medical Sciences USSR—the chief research arm of the ministry. In fact, the minister is the spokesman of the medical establishment and often represents the official medical viewpoint in the media. It is his responsibility to defend and justify the portion of the total budget earmarked for the health system. Similarly, within the republics, the health ministers fulfill the same function, and so on down the line. By tradition, the health ministers and most of their administrative staffs are physicians themselves. Administratively, the health system is subject to a dual subordination (indeed, a triple one if the Communist Party is included, as it must be).

There is first the vertical system of the Ministry of Health: a series of offices reaching from Moscow to the localities, each subordinate to the next higher echelon in that chain of command and communication. But each health administrative unit, in turn, is under the horizontal jurisdiction of the unit of governmental structure (the Soviets) to which it is attached either as a republican health ministry or as a health department. At the regional level, for instance, the regional unit of health is a department of the regional governmental unit and subordinate to it. It receives from that unit its specific mandate and assignments, as well as logistic support. At the same time, that unit reports to the republican health ministry above it and supervises the work of the health departments below it (at district or municipal levels). That dual jurisdictional arrangement, vertical and horizontal, also corresponds to a division of functions. The vertical line is more concerned with modus operandi, with issuing orders, detailed instructions, staff qualifications and assignments, and so on (Davis 1986). The horizontal line is concerned with the immediate tasks at hand: the day-to-day management, financing, and operations of the health institutions under its responsibility.

A few words need be said about the role of the Communist Party of the Soviet Union. In every sense of the word, the party is the real ruler and decision maker in the Soviet Union, and a party organization is found at every administrative level, and in virtually every organization and institution. Thus, one can look at the structure of health organizations as the implementers of party policies in health. The fact that practically all positions of importance in the health system are staffed by party members reinforces the control of the party and its ubiquitous role in the Soviet system.

As mentioned earlier, professional associations of physicians no longer exist. They have been replaced by two types of organizations, neither of which has the political power and autonomy usually associated with professional associations:

1. The Union of Medical Workers, a large organization that includes not only physicians but all those employed in the health-care system, although there are separate sections for different occupational groups. These are primarily control organizations, not aimed at representing or defending the interests of their members should these conflict with state policies. Other major functions are to provide social services or welfare services; to be concerned about the working and living conditions of their members; to resolve disputes or solve bureaucratic problems, for example, the determination of retirement provisions (Ruble 1981). But they do not shape policy; the idea of a strike is simply inconceivable in the Soviet context.
2. The other organizations are professional societies concerned with substantive matters: for example, the All-Union Society of Neurologists and Psychiatrists. Their activities are scientific or clinical (rather than political) including the selection of editors for their scientific journals.

Access to Health Care

The organizational relationships among the different components of the health sector, in spite of claims of standardization, are complex and difficult to describe in a short space. Generally speaking, two basic approaches or mechanisms are utilized to match the demand for care with its supply: One is the "territorial" principle and the territorial network of facilities; the other is the "closed" principle and the closed network in which occupation or rank, rather than geographical location, determines access. It is in that second system that the facilities for the elites are located, although the closed principle also applies, in some instances, to workers in industry.

The territorial principle operates as follows: The general population is divided into medical districts or groups of about 40,000 persons of whom perhaps one-fourth are children and adolescents, the rest adults. The district is therefore an administrative health unit and not a geographical one since its size will vary with the density of the population. A city medical district will be quite small; a rural district may cover a very large area. The core installation of the medical district is the district polyclinic, basically an outpatient institution, either freestanding or a set of rooms or offices in an apartment building. Physicians, assigned to the polyclinic, generally have office hours and see patients either at the office or on house calls. The general rule is that half a physician's day is spent at the clinic, the other in visiting patients at home.

Patients are assigned to doctors in the following manner: the district population is further divided into microdistricts (*uchastok*) of from about 2,000 to 3,000 or more persons. One or two physicians, a pediatrician, and one or two nurses may be assigned to each microdistrict, whose inhabitants become their responsibility. It is the patient's precise residential address that thus determines not only the polyclinic to which he or she will report for primary health care, but also the specific physicians and other personnel who are responsible for that care. The assignment is automatic for both personnel and patients, and, in theory, no choice is possible. When a person seeking care arrives at a polyclinic, he or she is asked the number of the microdistrict and his or her name and then is directed to the physician(s) in charge. Microdistric physicians then serve as the first contacts into the system of socialized medicine and as gatekeepers.

As might be expected in a bureaucratic system of this type, there are norms of patients to be seen per hour and minutes to be devoted to each patient. A Soviet study reported that, on the average, a physician spent 2.4 minutes interviewing the patient, 2.9 minutes examining the patient, 1.8 minutes giving advice, and 4.5 minutes on paperwork (Ryan 1978, 86). The complaint, often expressed in the Soviet medical press, is that there is not enough time to do a good job, and that paper work takes an inordinate amount of time and effort. According to Andrei Sakharov, "It takes half a day to get to see a physician at a clinic. And what can the doctor do or understand in the ten minutes he has for seeing each patient?"(Sakharov 1975, 21).

A particularly thorny point is that the physician is responsible for the delivery and the renewal of official sickness certificates, which allow the individual to stay away from work (including, in some instances, staying home to care for a sick child) and to draw part of one's salary during that absence. Usually a sickness certificate (*bolnichnii listok*) is delivered for three days, to be renewed twice more for three days on the physician's signature. Beyond that time, the patient must be seen by a group of doctors to determine whether the certificate is justified, or what additional medical measures are indicated. Sickness certificates are an important part of the health system's functions and the enforcement of labor discipline. Measures are taken to monitor the issuance of such certificates and to check the performance of physicians in that area. Physicians must be on guard for malingerers (Field 1953), and the authorities must be on guard about physicians who are too lenient or too corrupt in their issuance of certificates (Kurasov 1981).

The polyclinic also has a complement of specialists whose jurisdiction is several *uchastok*, since demand for their services will be less frequent than for general practitioners (called *terapevti*). Patients may be referred to hospitals that are affiliated with the polyclinic, and the care of the patient then passes entirely to the hospital staff. Patients who need specialized care may be furher referred up the line to more specialized hospitals and research institutes, including the better and more prestigious central institutions located in the republican capitals and in Moscow.

The distinctive aspect of the territorial principle is thus the automatic assignment of individuals to a primary care physician on the basis of the individual's address. An individual, however, may have more latitude in choosing a specialist without necessarily being referred by the general practitioner. There are, for instance, a series of more specialized outpatient facilities (sometimes called *consultations*) for pregnant women, children, psychiatric assistance, tuberculosis, cancer, dental care, and so on.

The district does not itself dispose of hospital beds except in the countryside where the distances are great, and it may be necessary to hospitalize a patient immediately. These are generally very small inpatient facilities, often referred to as "dwarf" hospitals, apparently slated for extinction because of their inefficiency. In the future, their patients will be referred to provincial hospitals. Emergency medical care, of which the Soviet Union is very proud, can be obtained by dialing 03 in most cities (Storey and Roth 1971). This system operates around the clock with a system of general and specialized ambulances, usually staffed by a physician and a feldsher in addition to a driver.

One more program deserves mention: the *dispensarizatsia*. Under this program, groups deemed to be particularly at risk (children, workers in dangerous occupations, etc.) are to be seen regularly and routinely for a health checkup, and to identify incipient conditions at their early stage. The plan is that, eventually, the entire population will be placed under that system. The extraordinarily high number of physicians is often justified in terms of the needs of such a program, which is essentially preventive. Evidence, however, suggests that such examinations are often more myth than reality, and that the reporting of such examinations is done through filling statistical forms rather than examining people (Knaus 1981, 224). It may be noted that such mass surveys have been found to be of dubious value in the west. A Soviet physician doing routine electrocardiograms told a western visitor in 1982 that they were not worth the time, money, and effort invested, but such doubts so far have not been publicly expressed (Raffel 1984).

Let us now turn to the closed network of which there are several kinds. Probably the largest one caters to industrial workers. Industrial plants with more than a certain number of workers (usually 4,000) are required to establish, at their own expense, medical facilities for their workers. The larger the number of workers, the more elaborate these facilities, which may include not only outpatient clinics but also hospitals. Workers are assigned to a shop physician who is responsible for their primary care. The shop physician is thus the analog of the microdistrict doctor, except that the individual is assigned to a doctor on the basis of his place of work. The shop physician is also expected to concern himself with occupational safety. Thus, the worker may have the option of either going to the plant polyclinic and doctor, or to the physician who serves his residential area, a duplication that is sometimes deplored by Soviet commentators. At the same time, apparently, workers prefer to consult the "residential" to the "occupational" physician, perhaps because the plant physician is associated with management and labor discipline. The establishment of plant medical facilities originally was part of the special priority that workers enjoyed during the early years of industrialization, when the medical care available to the general population was poorer. According to Christopher Davis, about 8 percent of the total population had access to the closed industrial network in 1975 (Davis 1979).

In addition to the medical facilities reserved for industrial workers, there are other medical systems that cater to the members of the elites, whether political, artistic, or intellectual. For example, members of the prestigious Academy of Sciences USSR, top-rated writers, artists, and ballerinas, all have access to special medical facilities reserved for them and their families. The same is true of the political elites who have their own facilities, including the complex of medical installations generally referred to as the Kremlin hospital, or *Kremlinovka*.

In most cities, there are restricted medical institutions reserved for the local elites either freestanding (if it is a larger city), or part of regular hospitals or clinics not accessible to the general public. These facilities fall under the purview of the Ministry's Fourth Directorate. They, and all the amenities they offer, are to some degree the equivalent of private hospitals or wings in hospitals, or pay beds (for example, in Great Britain) but with one important distinction: In the west, private care, special facilities, or more luxurious accommodations are usually available for payment. In the Soviet Union, these services and facilities are part of the prerequisites of rank, for which no payment need (or may) be made. The funding thus comes from the state treasury, and the taxes are paid by the population. Promotion and demotion entail a corresponding change in one's medical category, also the medical category of the members of one's immediate family. Thus, the stratification of medical care parallels the unequal distribution of most other components of the standard of living (housing, including secondary residences, transportation, access to exclusive stores, rest homes, vacations, and so on). According to an American physician writing about the Kremlins' health-care system, certain blood tests that cannot be performed in the Soviet Union are routinely air-shipped to a laboratory in Helsinki, and the results are flown back to Moscow the next day. Furthermore,

> Deputy ministers and persons of lower rank are seen in regular private cubicles, but ministers have a special examining room. . . . There are carpets on the floor, book cases, a leather couch, and heavy red drapes over the windows. It is like a living room, not a clinic (Knaus 1981, 300).

The facilities reserved for the different elites are far superior in medical equipment, pharmaceuticals, accommodations, food, and other amenities. There is more ambivalence, however, on the quality of physicians who work there: Some feel that security considerations are so strict that those who can pass such screening are not necessarily the best qualified physicians. Lenin, a man who harbored few illusions, had written in a letter to Gorki (1913),

> God save us from doctor-comrades in general, and doctor-Bolsheviks in particular! But really, in 99 cases out of 100, doctor-comrades are asses. . . . I assure you that except in trivial cases, one should be treated by men of first class reputation. (Wolfe 1964, 613).

This was, of course, long before the birth of the Soviet health-care system. When their welfare is at stake, Soviet elites, like elites elsewhere, presumably follow

Lenin's advice and seek out the best. If the best specialists are not on the staff of the *Kremlinovka*, they will be called in as consultants (Golyakhovsky 1984).

It is thus this diversity and inequality in the provision of medical services that makes an overall assessment of the Soviet medical system difficult, indeed impossible, unless we differentiate it by the population served. Excellent care for a few may coexist with terrible care for the many. Davis attempted to divide the Soviet population in 1975 by their access to the different subsystems of health care as shown in Table 1 above.

We can thus assume that one-tenth of 1 percent of the population receives superlative attention, probably equal (or almost equal) to the best in the west. Twenty-five percent have access to care of a relatively high quality in departmental and capital city facilities. Another 24 percent obtain, again according to Davis, decent service in medium city or industrial subsystems. And about half of the population receives low-quality care in the rural subsystem. It is thus clear that the unity, integration, and rational organization of Soviet medicine is more myth than reality (Ryan 1978, 8). It is rather a collection of loosely related medical fiefdoms.

On the other hand, we should not lose sight of the fact that the health system is a creature of the Soviet state. Since practically every aspect of the system is state financed, it is relatively easy (compared to many countries in the west and to the United States in particular) to monitor the proportion of resources allocated to the health system. It is thus possible, for instance, with a high degree of precision, to determine from year to year what will be the income levels of medical and allied personnel since they all are on state-paid salaries. In this regard, it should be noted that health personnel are among the lowest paid occupational groups in the Soviet Union, and they continue to fall behind other occupations and the national average. In 1965 medical wages relative to the national average were 82 percent. In 1980, they were 75 percent (Davis 1986). The fact that most health personnel do receive formally illegal, under-the-table payments (Field 1984) is probably accepted by the regime as a justification for the low pay of such personnel. In effect, it nullifies the gratuity feature of socialized medicine, one of its most touted aspects of the system by Soviet propaganda. Patients, for instance, come to hospitals armed with sheafs of roubles to obtain the most elementary attention (Whitney 1978).

It is also relatively easy to increase or decrease the share of the national wealth that goes into health care. Indeed, there is evidence that in the last few years the proportion of the total state expenditures (budget) going into health protection has fallen by about 20 percent, a trend quite contrary to that experienced in the west. The percentage went from 6.5 percent of the budget in 1965, to 6.0 percent in 1970, 5.3 percent in 1975, and 5.0 percent in 1980 (Davis 1986). It is difficult to estimate the percentage of the gross national product (as against budgetary allocations) expended on health protection, and the figures vary depending on whether one uses roubles or dollars for the calculations.

Using a rouble figure, that proportion went from 2.9 percent in 1955 to 2.1

percent in 1977, or a decline of about 28 percent. Using a dollar estimate (which unrealistically inflates the cost of personnel), the percentage went from 9.7 percent in 1955 to 7.5 percent in 1977 or a decline of about 23 percent (Field 1984, 133). Thus, compared to most developed countries around the world, not only does the Soviet Union spend, comparatively speaking, little on health care, but the expenditures (measured as a percentage of national wealth) have decreased in the last years probably under the impact of higher priority areas, for example, defense. This decrease may well have been compensated for by allocations to health care on the part of other agencies (for example, the Ministry of Social Security, which has some chronic hospitals of its own) (Ryan 1978, 18). This may have been valid up to 1973, according to Davis, but thereafter did not apply any more (Davis 1986). One might also assume that the present Soviet budgetary crisis may well impel Soviet authorities to cut expenditures wherever feasible. Decreases in the health-care budget are less dramatic and certainly less visible than, for example, raises in taxes, the price of consumer goods, or the price of food (Eberstadt 1981).

Budgetary figures, expressed in roubles, may not by themselves be very meaningful to western analysts. More interesting, perhaps, in a comparative dimension, are the percentages allocated to the various parts of the health system. Some idea may be gathered from the figures listed on Table 2, which gives a breakdown of republican health budgets (thus excluding expenditures of the central Health Protection Ministry USSR, which account for less than 10 percent of the total expenditures for health). More than half of the monies went for salaries, followed by food (10.6 percent), drugs and dressings (8.4 percent), and administration and maintenance (7.9 percent). Other rubrics accounted, on the average, for less than 4 percent.

Major Problems Confronting the Soviet Health System

It is difficult to separate the major problems faced by the Soviet health system from those of Soviet society in general. In one sense, what goes on in that system reflects the major dilemmas faced by that country—a country that is sometimes characterized as the least developed among the developed nations. As Shipler observed:

> The system of medical care expresses the full range of strengths and weaknesses of Soviet society: it is a model of the country's hierarchy, reflecting the instinct of authoritarianism, conservatism and elitism that pervades all areas of life (Shipler 1983, 216).

This is perhaps best illustrated by the question of infant mortality (Davis and Feshbach 1981; Field 1986). Infant mortality is an important proxy measure because it tells us something about both the medical system and the general standard of living of the population. In 1971, the Soviet Union officially gave its infant mortality as 22.9 per 1,000 live births, the lowest level ever reported.

As such, it stood at less than one-tenth of what it had been before the revolution, when more than one-fourth of all children born alive died before their first birthday. Soviet writers commenting on the drastic drop in infant mortality usually added that this was, in itself, a demonstration of the superiority of the Soviet political system and of Soviet socialized medicine. Unaccountably, after 1971, infant mortality began to climb. By 1974, it was 20 percent higher than it had been in 1971 (Field 1986). Thereafter, official publication of figures was discontinued, to be resumed, and only partly, in October 1986, when the rates for 1980, 1983, 1984, and 1985 were reported, presumably as the result of the "openness" policy of Gorbachev (*Ekonomicheskaia Gazeta* 1986). They showed an infant mortality still considerably higher than what it had been in 1971.

Infant mortality was not the only suppressed statistic: Life expectancy data since 1971–1972, age and sex specific death rates for any year since 1973–1974, age-specific death rates (for both sexes combined) for any year since 1976, the cause of death data for age groups since 1971–1972, the number of doctors by specialty for any year since 1975 (including rural-urban distribution), as well as most results from the 1979 census, have been embargoed. When a major nation with an elaborate arrangement to provide health care to the entire population decides to withhold vital statistics, there is reason to believe that something is terribly wrong. The Soviets have provided no rationale nor defense for withholding data except to state, as did the first deputy minister of health when queried on the subject in May 1982: "a government has the right not to publish whatever it chooses" (Raffel 1984, 512).

A variety of hypotheses can be ventured to explain the rise of infant mortality in the absence of traumatic events such as war, famine, or epidemics. These range from the possibility that the increase is to some degree a statistical artifact (due to improved reporting); to a shifting in the proportion of births toward the less developed regions (central Asia) where infant mortality has traditionally been high; to demographic phenomena such as the shortage of manpower requiring most women to work and thereby creating difficulties in the care of infants; to an increase in family instability, for example, a rise in illegitimacy, teen-age pregnancies, and divorce; to a possible degradation in health services, particularly pediatric care due to poor training of personnel and their lack of concern at work; to a shortage and poor quality of medical equipment and pharmaceuticals, reflecting the fact that money placed at the disposal of health authorities and hospital directors is often of no use since it is impossible to find labor and to purchase materials or equipment; to problems in the food supply (including milk); to insufficiency of housing; to environmental (including radiation) pollution; and to a stagnant economy. Soviet sources, in addition, report an increase in alcoholism among women (now termed the third most important disease after heart disease and cancer), a rise in female smoking (although warning labels now appear on cigarette packages), the continued use of abortion as the main means of birth control (an estimated six per woman in non-Moslem areas), changes in infant feeding (shift to bottle feeding rather than breast), and

Table 2
Expenditures on Health Protection by Major Categories in Republican Budgets, USSR, 1970

	Millions of roubles	%
TOTAL*	8,675.3	100
Out of which		
Salaries	4,675.6	53.9
Additions to Salaries **	243.2	2.8
Administration and maintenance	685.7	7.9
Official assignments and duty travel	20.9	0.2
Food	919.5	10.6
Drugs & dressings	773.4	8.4
Equipment and appliances	192.9	2.2
Centralized capital allocations	383.8	4.4
Non-Centralized capital allocations	68.6	0.8
Soft furnishings, uniform and clothing	232.2	2.7
Repairs to buildings and plants	258.2	3.0

*Expenditures under the jurisdiction of the All-Union budget would add another 532.2 million roubles to that figure. It is not available broken down by categories of expenditures.
**This presumably covers social security payments to staff.

crowded and understaffed infant day-care institutions with high infection rates. All these elements have a bearing on infant mortality, and they have been reported at some length in the Soviet general and medical press.

If one were to look beyond the possible reasons mentioned above, one might trace the "crisis" to the international arms race. This has led to a severe constriction of resources available to the civilian sector, and it affects all elements that have a bearing on infant mortality, as well as on general mortality and thus life expectancy. But this may not be the whole story: This constriction in resources, given the stratified nature of Soviet society and of its health-care system, does not apply equally to the whole population. Surprising as it may seem, the Soviet Union *has* a poverty problem of sizable proportion. According to Soviet studies, well summarized by McAuley (1979), somewhere between 35 and 40 percent of the population (both urban and rural) lived at or below the officially designated poverty line by the end of the 1960s. Since infant mortality is generally

Table 2 (continued)

Current Expenditures on hospitals, maternity homes, and dispensaries					
Urban & Rural areas Millions of roubles	%	Urban areas and workers' settlements Millions of roubles	%	Rural areas Millions of roubles	%
6,366.3	100	5,284.2	100	1,082.1	100
3,588.8	56.4	2,992.0	56.6	596.8	55.2
198.3	3.1	165.8	3.1	32.5	3.0
568.0	8.9	470.2	8.9	97.8	9.0
14.7	0.2	11.3	0.2	3.4	0.3
816.3	12.8	663.6	12.6	152.7	14.1
589.0	9.2	488.8	9.2	100.2	9.2
131.3	2.1	109.6	2.1	21.7	2.0
-	-	-	- -	-	-
-	-	-	- -	-	-
215.1	3.4	176.1	3.3	39.0	3.6
206.7	3.2	171.4	3.2	35.3	3.3

Source: Michael Ryan, *The Organization of Soviet Medical Care*, Oxford: Basil Blackwell, 1978, p. 27. Ryan's figures are drawn from Popov, G.A., *Ekonomika i planirovanie zdravookhranenia*, p. 293.

inversely related to income, it is quite plausible that the infant mortality rate of that population has driven the national figure to a level too embarrassing to publish. (Similarly, in the United States, it is the nonwhite infant mortality—twice that of the white one—that strongly affects the country's standing in international comparisons.)

Major Trends and Issues

In the light of the above factors, it is possible to examine some of the specific problems the Soviet health system faces.

The health-care system is undercapitalized; it is labor intensive, but it lacks modern technology and supplies (including disposables) that have become standard in most developed nations. As noted by Davis: ''In spite of funding increases in the last few years . . . the Soviet health service remains inadequately financed and operates under tight constraints which affect its performance adversely'' (Davis 1982). Thus care, both in the outpatient and particularly in the hospital sectors, suffers from endemic shortages of pharmaceuticals, equipment, and supplies (Knaus 1981, 23, 110, 140). For example, in 1977, the then Health Minister Petrovsky, writing in *Izvestiia* complained, among other things, that much X-ray equipment was obsolete, that only 75 percent of the needed X-ray film was being produced, that anesthesia equipment and respirators were being produced in only half the required amounts, and that surgical equipment was inadequate in quantity and quality (Shipler 1977, 36). As already noted, availability of funds may not be meaningful if there is nothing to buy with them. Thus, the fact that the per capita outlay for health care has more than doubled in the last few years must be qualified by other considerations. A recurrent complaint of the ministry is that the funds allocated remain in the State Bank because of the inability of health authorities to spend them (*Meditsinskaia Gazeta* 1982). The fact that the health system (for the general population) enjoys only secondary or residual priority may well exacerbate the problem. A most severe indictment is that of Andrei Sakharov when he wrote to Brezhnev that ''A free health service . . . [is] no more than an economic illusion in a society in which all surplus value is expropriated and distributed by the state.'' And Sakharov noted that the hierarchical nature of Soviet society was particularly pernicious in the health service and education (Sakharov 1974, 155). Although general assessments are difficult to make, it may be fair to say that the overall nature of Soviet medicine (with the exception of services for the elites) may be anywhere from 10 to 20 years behind the West and Japan (*Newsweek* 1977; *U.S. News and World Report* 1978).

The Soviet health-care system is heavily bureaucratized. As such, individuals who work within it tend to adopt a bureaucratic style that includes, among other things, an indifference toward clients, a ''formalistic'' attitude toward duty, an avoidance of responsibility, and a segmental sense of accountability. Again, the Soviet press reflects this situation. It often complains of the indifferent, inhuman, or formalistic attitudes displayed by doctors toward their patients, and it harks back to the golden age of prerevolutionary medical practice when physicians were seen as dedicated persons who considered themselves doctors at all times, not only when they were on ''official'' duty. Thus, the media deplore what they see as the ''nine-to-five'' mentality displayed by Soviet physicians who, when they finish their work, refuse to help even in an emergency (Field 1970). Among the remedies proposed is a better selection of those who apply to the medical schools to weed out those who are emotionally or temperamentally not suited for medicine. It is significant that, in 1971, the Soviets introduced a modified version of the Hippocratic oath, which had been abolished shortly after the revolution as symbolizing reactionary, bourgeois medicine (Ryan 1978, 160). To judge from the press, this has not yet had much of an effect. However, the complaints are not only of greedy or indifferent physicians, but also of poorly trained ones whose mistakes are glossed over and tolerated by complacent colleagues who expect the same treatment when they are at fault. Thus, erroneous diagnoses, even of standard conditions, appear to be a problem. For example, in 1970–1976, incorrect diagnoses were found in the RSFSR (the Russian Republic) in 25.8 percent of cancer cases, 18.0 percent of circulatory (heart and blood-related) diseases, and so on (Feshbach 1981).

Time and again, reports surface on the admission of students to medical school through connections or bribery rather than through examinations or test scores. In 1976, the director of a medical school in Georgia was sent to jail because 170 from a class of 200 (85 percent) had been admitted through parental payments (Whitney 1978).

The health system, because of its centralized and bureaucratic nature, is unable to react quickly, decisively, and innovatively to new or unexpected situations. Such a system is capable of orchestrating spectacular advances in public health (for example, the mass vaccination of the population, or the elimination of infectious or parasitic diseases). On the other hand, as Chesnay recently pointed out, it is much less capable of dealing with aleatory elements—an unexpected epidemic, or a new virus strain (Chesnay 1983). The preventive orientation, touted as the cornerstone of the whole system, is sadly neglected not only in the area of public health (for example, air and water pollution are increasingly recognized as definite health and genetic hazards), but is also slighted at the clinical level. Knaus, for example, has pointed out that a lack of laboratory facilities to detect streptococcal infections leads to rheumatic diseases and constitutes a definite risk for thousands of Soviet children. With regard to cervical cancer: In the United States, 70 percent of such cases are identified early in a potentially treatable stage; about 60 percent of these Soviet cancer cases are not recognized until they are terminal. It is estimated that one-third of all patients acquire postoperative infections while in the hospital; in the United States, a 3-percent rate would be considered high (Knaus 1981, 137).

The stratification of health care leads to poor care in the rural districts. This problem may well recede as an increasingly large proportion of the population becomes urbanized and as more farmers utilize urban health facilities for their care (primarily hospital care). But the bulk of primary medical care in the villages remains the responsiblity of the feldsher, or physician assistant. Slated to disappear after the revolution as a symbol of a two-class medical system, the feldsher system has remained to this day and may even be in the process of expanding (Liu 1979; Storey 1972). This reflects the unwillingness of physicians to work in the countryside and their ability through a variety of devices to escape such assignments (Field 1984b). The qualilty of diagnostic and clinical care given by the feldshers has been recognized by Soviet health authorities as considerably inferior to that of the physicians.

Although in theory the Soviet concept of socialized medicine is logical, rational, efficient, socially useful, and free at time of service and thus expresses society's concern for the sick individual, the reality is rather different. Yet, given the controlled nature of Soviet society and the vested interests of many to maintain the status quo, freewheeling public debate, of the type constantly seen in western sources, is not likely to be seen or heard in the USSR (Ryan 1978, 20). From the official Soviet view, the health system is fundamentally sound. Its problems are temporary, and most often they are due to personal failings and not to its structure.

Conclusion

The Soviets have held that their blueprint, their concepts for achieving health care for all, should serve as a model for the rest of the world. One is forced to conclude, however, that that blueprint, or at least its implementation on Soviet soil, is unlikely to become a beacon to most other nations.

It may indeed be worthwhile to speculate on the social totality of which the health system is an indissoluable part. Perhaps the Soviet health-care blueprint or design is like a generic grape, producing wines of widely different quality depending on the ground, humidity, rainfall, exposure to the sun, and nature of care. The Soviets themselves subscribe to this view. They hold, for example, that a state-provided health-care scheme such as the British National Health Service must be fundamentally flawed because it does not operate in a socialist society (Ryan 1978, 20). Thus, it may only be consistent to appraise the Soviet system of socialized medicine in broader societal terms, as Ryan has done:

> . . . the Soviet health service, inextricably interlinked as it is with the wider society, embodies and endorses a pattern of values which has been imposed by one of the most rigidly and unremittingly totalitarian of contemporary states (Ryan 1978, 126).

At the same time, we must recognize that the regime has become, in the last few years, concerned that all is not well on the health scene. The embarassing rise of infant mortality and the decrease in life expectancy, the constant complaints about poor services, the existence of substantial corruption in every aspect of the health system, the lack of pharmaceuticals (*Pravda* 1978), and so on have been noted by the party and the government in a series of resolutions and decrees (1968, 1977, 1982) aimed at improving health care and the health level of the population. At the 26th Party Congress in 1981, Brezhnev himself listed a whole series of shortcomings that require correction (Central Committee 1981, 61).

These apparently did not produce the desired effects. But there are indications that the Gorbachev regime has, at long last, recognized the results of the malign neglect of the health system. Early in 1987, it appointed a new Health Minister in the person of Dr. Evgenii I. Chazov, a prominent cardiologist and co-winner of the Nobel Peace Prize, to clean house. In a fit of *glasnost*-induced candor, Dr. Chazov has publicly criticized practically every aspect of Soviet socialized medicine, starting with the fact that it was financially undernourished to its dismal performance regarding infant mortality. In mid-August 1987, a resolution signed by the party and the government and published in three full pages of *Izvestiia* and *Pravda* outlined a series of reforms designed to bring the Soviet health system up to international standards by the end of the century or earlier (*Pravda* 1987). If the past is any indication, many of these reforms will remain mostly on paper given the nature of the Soviet bureaucracy and the limited economic resources. On the other hand, the very fact that the Gorbachev regime has officially recognized that changes were overdue in the Soviet approach to the health of the population is already some progress.

References

Central Committee, Communist Party of the Soviet Union. 1981. *Materials of the XXVI Party Congress*. (In Russian.) Moscow: Politizdat, p. 61.

Chesnay, J. C. 1983. "La durée de la vie dans les pays industrialisés." *La Recherche*. Sept., 147: 1040–1043.

Davis, Christopher, M. 1979. *The Economics of the Soviet Health System: An Analytical and Historical Study, 1921–1978*. Ph.D. Diss. in Economics from Cambridge University, U.K.

———. 1981. "The Economics of the Soviet Health System" in *Soviet Economy in the 1980s: Problems and Prospects*. Joint Economic Committee of Congress, part 2, 229–264.

———. 1982. "Economic Problems of the Soviet Health System." Washington, D.C.: Wharton Economic Forecasting Associates. September 7, 1982.

———. 1986. "The Organization and Performance of the Contemporary Soviet Health Service." In G. Lapidus and G. Swanson, *State and Welfare USA/USSR*. (In press.) Rev. paper.

Davis, Christopher and Feshbach, Murray. 1980. "Rising Infant Mortality in the U.S.S.R. in the 1970s." Washington, D.C.: U.S. Department of Commerce, Bureau of the Census, Series P–95, No. 74.

Eberstadt, Nick. 1981. "The Health Crisis in the USSR." *New York Review of Books*. February 19: 23–31.

Ekonomicheskaia Gazeta. 1986. "Naselenie SSSR." No. 43, 6–7.

Feshbach, Murray. 1981. "Issues on Soviet Health Problems and Prospects." Washington, D.C.: Joint Economic Committee of Congress. Part 2, 203–227.

Field, Mark G. 1953. "Structured Strain in the Role of the Soviet Physician." *American Journal of Sociology*, 58: 493–502.

———. 1957. *Doctor and Patient in Soviet Russia*. Cambridge, Mass.: Harvard University Press.

———. 1967. *Soviet Socialized Medicine: An Introduction*. New York: Free Press.

———. 1970. "Soviet Medical Practice: Five Case Histories." *Review of Soviet Medical Sciences* 7: No. 2:1–12.

———. 1972. "Taming a Profession: Early Phases of Soviet Socialized Medicine." *Bulletin of the New York Academy of Medicine*. 2d series, vol. 48, no. 1:83–92.

———. 1984a. "Soviet Urban Health Services: Some Problems and Their Sources." In Henry W. Morton and Robert C. Stuart, *The Contemporary Soviet City*. Armonk, N.Y.: M. E. Sharpe, 129–155.

———. 1984b. "Changements dans la profession médicale aux USA et URSS, 1970–

1980: Demande et Commande." *Cahiers de Sociologie et Démographie Médicales*, XXIV, 4: 291–319.

———. 1986. "Soviet Infant Mortality: A Mystery Story." In D. B. Jelliffe and E. F. Jelliffe, eds. *Advances in International Maternal and Child Health*. Oxford: Clarendon Press, 25–65.

Golyakhovsky, Vladimir. 1984. *Russian Doctor*. New York: St. Martin's/Marek.

Knaus, William A. 1981. *Inside Russian Medicine*. New York: Everest House.

Kurasov, V. 1981. "Face to Face with the Law: Medical Certificates for a Bribe." *Izvestiia*. December 1, 1981. English summary in *Current Digest of the Soviet Press*. XXXIII, no. 48, December 21, p. 21.

Liu, Lillian. 1979. "Rural Feldshers and the Public Health in the Soviet Union." Unpub. paper presented at the Southern Conference on Slavic Studies, October.

McAuley, Alastair. 1979. *Economic Welfare in the Soviet Union: Poverty, Living Standards and Inequality*. Madison: University of Wisconsin Press, Chap. 4, "Poverty," 70–98.

Meditsinskaia Gazeta. 1982. "Repair According to the Old Way Creates an Artificial Deficit of Hospital Beds." (In Russian.) March 10, p. 2.

Newsweek. 1977. "Medicine: A Decade Behind." October 10.

New York Times. 1981. "World Military and Social Expenditure–World Priorities." News of the Week in Review, September 20.

Petrovsky, Boris. 1973. "Health Care." *World Marxist Review*. February 1971, pp. 52–54. Cited in Samuel Hendel, *The Soviet Crucible* (4th ed.). North Scituate, Mass.: Duxbury Press, pp. 367–368.

Pravda. 1978. "A person goes to the drug-store." May 21, 1978, 3. Available in English in *Current Digest of the Soviet Press*. XXX, June 14, 1979, p. 20.

———. 1987. "Project of the Central Committee and the Council of Ministers USSR 'Fundamental directions of the development of the health protection of the population and the restructuring of health protection USSR in the 12th five year plan and for the period until the year 2000.' " August 15, pp. 1–3.

Raffel, Norma K. 1984. "Health Services in the Soviet Socialist Republics." In Marshall W. Raffel. *Comparative Health Systems: Descriptive Analyses of Fourteen National Health Systems*. University Park: Pennsylvania State University Press, 488–519.

Ruble, Blair A. 1981. *Soviet Trade Unions: Their Development in the 1970s*. Cambridge: Cambridge University Press.

Ryan, Michael. 1978. *The Organization of Soviet Medical Care*. Oxford: Basil Blackwell, 143–157.

Sakharov, Andrei. 1974. "Postscript to Memorandum Sent to Brezhnev." *Sakharov Speaks*. New York: Vintage Books, 155.

———. 1975. *My Country and the World*. New York: Vintage Books, 21–23.

Sharlet, Robert. 1978. *The New Soviet Constitution of 1977*. Brunswick, Ohio: King's Court Communications Inc.

Shipler, David. 1977. "Soviet Medicine Mixes Inconsistency with Diversity." *New York Times*, June 26, 36.

———. 1983. *Broken Idols, Solemn Dreams*. New York: Times Books, 216.

Storey, Patrick B. 1972. *The Soviet Feldsher as a Physician's Assistant*. Washington, D.C.: U.S. Department of Health, Education and Welfare, DHEW Publication No. (NIH) 72–58. February.

Storey, Patrick B., and R. B. Roth. 1971. "Emergency Medical Care in the Soviet Union: A Study of the Skoraya." *Journal of the American Medical Association*, 217, 588–592.

U.S. News and World Report. 1978. "A U.S. Doctor's Report on Soviet Medical Care: Don't Get Sick in Russia," 85:20, 65–66, November 20.

Vedemosti Verkhovnovo Soveta SSSR. 1969. No. 52 (1502), pp. 710–728. English translation in *Current Digest of the Soviet Press*. XXII, No. 1, pp. 7–13.

Whitney, Craig. 1978. In "Soviet Bribes Help to Get a Car, Get an Apartment, and Get Ahead." *New York Times*. May 7, pp. 1, 22.

Wolfe, Bertram. 1964. *Three Who Made a Revolution*. New York: Dell, 613.

Appendix: A Note on Soviet Statistics and Sources

In the Soviet context, statistics have an ideological significance. This may explain why they are provided inconsistently, and sometimes not published at all, or published with great delays. This makes it difficult to provide data comparable with those provided by other nations. For instance, infant mortality rates were not published between 1975 and 1986 when figures for the years 1980, 1983, 1984, and 1985 were released. The same befell a series of other vital data, for example, age- and sex-specific mortality rates for any year since 1973–1974, or the number of physicians by specialty for any year since 1975. We have attempted to provide here as wide a range of figures given the above limitations as well as space restrictions. All figures are derived from official Soviet handbooks and other sources, though most of the tables are based on already worked-out data in English by Mark G. Field and Murray Feshbach. More recent figures (up to 1985) have been culled from the latest Soviet statistical handbook available.

The sources in the following tables will be identified as such:

Handbook—Mark G. Field, "Health," in Ellen Mickiewicz, *Handbook of Soviet Social Science Data* (New York: Free Press, 1973), pp. 101–118.

Compendium—Murray Feshback, *A Compendium of Soviet Health Statistics*, CIR Staff Paper No. 5 (n.d.).

NK—Narodnoe khoziaistvo SSSR (Moscow: Finansi i statistika). This is the annual handbook of Soviet statistical data published by the Central Statistical Administration. Usually the information is made available in the statistical handbook for the year prior to the handbook's publication date. Data from sources other than those listed above will be identified in full.

Table A1

Population by Republics and by Urban/Rural Residence, 1940–1986 (in Thousands)

	All population					including URBAN					RURAL				
	1940	1959	1970	1979	1986	1940	1959	1970	1979	1986	1940	1959	1970	1979	1986
USSR	194077	208827	241720	262436	278784	63112	99978	135991	163586	182930	130965	108849	105729	98850	95854
RSFSR	110098	117534	130079	137551	144080	37926	61611	80981	95374	105268	72172	55923	49098	42177	38812
Ukraine	41340	41869	47126	49755	50994	14023	19147	25688	30512	33690	27317	22722	21438	19243	17304
Belorussia	9046	8056	9002	9560	10008	1925	2481	3908	5263	6319	7121	5575	5094	4297	3689
Uzbekistan	6551	8119	11799	15391	18487	1606	2729	4322	6348	7745	4945	5390	7477	9043	10742
Kazakhstan	6148	9295	13009	14684	16028	1833	4067	6538	7920	9223	4315	5228	6471	6764	6805
Georgia	3612	4044	4686	5015	5234	1106	1713	2240	2601	2833	2506	2331	2446	2414	2401
Azerbaidzhan	3274	3698	5117	6028	6708	1212	1767	2564	3200	3617	2062	1931	2553	2828	3091
Lithuania	2925	2711	3128	3398	3603	674	1046	1571	2062	2389	2251	1665	1557	1336	1214
Moldavia	2468	2885	3569	3947	4147	332	643	1130	1551	1895	2136	2242	2439	2396	2252
Latvia	1886	2093	2364	2521	2622	662	1174	1477	1726	1854	1224	919	887	795	768
Kirgizia	1528	2066	2934	3529	4051	332	696	1098	1366	1607	1196	1370	1836	2163	2444
Tadzhikistan	1525	1981	2900	3801	4648	293	646	1077	1325	1553	1232	1335	1823	2476	3095
Armenia	1320	1763	2492	3031	3362	375	882	1482	1993	2281	945	881	1010	1038	1081
Turkmenistan	1302	1516	2159	2759	3270	459	700	1034	1323	1552	843	816	1125	1436	1718
Estonia	1054	1197	1356	1466	1542	354	676	881	1022	1104	700	521	475	444	438

Source: *NK 1986*, p. 9.

Table A2
Population by Republics and by Sex 1940–1986 (in Thousands)

	Men				Women			
	1959	1970	1979	1986	1959	1970	1979	1986
USSR........	94,050	111,399	122,329	130,938	114,777	130,321	140,107	147,846
RSFSR.......	52,425	59,325	63,483	66,983	65,109	70,754	74,068	77,097
Ukraine.....	18,575	21,305	22,744	23,507	23,294	25,821	27,011	27,487
Belorussia..	3,581	4,138	4,442	4,681	4,475	4,864	5,118	5,327
Uzbekistan..	3,897	5,744	7,558	9,114	4,222	6,055	7,833	9,373
Kazakhstan..	4,415	6,263	7,084	7,760	4,880	6,746	7,600	8,268
Georgia.....	1,865	2,202	2,355	2,474	2,179	2,484	2,660	2,760
Azerbaidzhan	1,757	2,483	2,939	3,276	1,941	2,634	3,089	3,432
Lithuania...	1,245	1,468	1,603	1,699	1,466	1,660	1,795	1,904
Moldavia....	1,334	1,552	1,858	1,969	1,551	1,907	2,089	2,178
Latvia......	919	1,081	1,161	1,217	1,174	1,283	1,360	1,405
Kirgizia....	975	1,402	1,714	1,981	1,091	1,532	1,815	2,070
Tadzhikistan	965	1,426	1,878	2,300	1,016	1,474	1,923	2,348
Armenia.....	842	1,217	1,475	1,646	921	1,275	1,556	1,716
Turkmenistan	730	1,063	1,358	1,612	786	1,096	1,401	1,658
Estonia.....	525	620	677	719	672	736	789	823

Source: *NK 1986*, p. 9.

Table A3

Number of Hospital Beds, 1940–1985, and by Medical Use 1940–1979 (Excluding Beds in Military Hospitals) (in Thousands, End of Year)

Medical use	1940	1950	1960	1970	1979	1980	1982	1984	1985
Total beds	790.9	1,010.7	1,739.2	2,663.2	3,262.0	3,324.2	3,443.0	3,552.0	3,608.0
Therapeutic[1]	102.3	177.0	361.7	544.0	730.6	NA	NA	NA	NA
Surgical[2]	99.4	143.7	236.7	351.2	459.9	NA	NA	NA	NA
Oncological[3]	1.7	12.2	24.2	46.6	55.5	NA	NA	NA	NA
Gynecological	33.6	42.2	91.3	154.5	179.4	NA	NA	NA	NA
Tubercular	34.0	85.5	157.2	271.9	234.9	NA	NA	NA	NA
adult	28.7	75.3	136.3	245.2	215.4	NA	NA	NA	NA
children	5.3	10.2	20.9	26.7	19.5	NA	NA	NA	NA
Infectious	94.3	125.6	166.6	198.3	238.1	NA	NA	NA	NA
adult	62.4	81.8	91.3	105.7	120.7	NA	NA	NA	NA
children	31.9	43.8	75.3	92.6	117.4	NA	NA	NA	NA
Pediatric(excluding infectious)	52.5	79.1	163.9	324.8	401.2	NA	NA	NA	NA
Ophthalmologic	13.4	16.1	30.3	39.3	45.7	NA	NA	NA	NA
Ororhinolaryngological	6.9	8.9	20.0	39.7	48.9	NA	NA	NA	NA
Dermato-venereological	15.4	30.0	31.0	52.8	75.0	NA	NA	NA	NA
Psychiatric	82.9	71.8	162.5	267.9	365.3[4]	NA	NA	NA	NA
Neurological	10.0	15.1	30.5	71.5	114.2	NA	NA	NA	NA
Pregnant women and newborns[5]	113.5	122.2	175.3	198.0	221.8	NA	NA	NA	NA
General beds	119.7	73.2	67.9	92.8	91.3	NA	NA	NA	NA

NA. Not available.

1. Also includes beds for endocrinological and physiotherapeutic patients.
2. Beds for surgery patients includes beds for neurosurgery, orthopedic traumotology, urology, and stomatology patients.
3. Includes beds for radiology patients.
4. Including narcological.
5. Includes beds in general hospitals and in maternity homes.

Sources: *Handbook*, Table 14; *Compendium*, Table 4; *NK 1985*, p. 539.

Table A4
Hospital Beds, USSR and Republic, 1913–1985 (Excluding the Military) (per 10,000 Population)

USSR and republic	1913	1940	1950	1960	1970	1980	1982	1985
USSR	13.	40.2	55.7	80.4	109.4	124.9	127.1	129.6
RSFSR	14.8	43.3	59.2	82.1	112.5	129.6	132.1	134.6
Ukraine	13.6	37.7	52.2	79.8	107.9	125.4	128.0	131.5
Belorussia	32.6	32.6	41.2	67.9	104.1	125.2	127.0	130.4
Moldavia	12.2	24.6	45.1	72.3	99.0	120.0	121.8	124.1
Estonia	26.2	47.7	66.1	94.0	110.3	124.1	126.4	124.0
Latvia	24.9	63.0	71.7	107.2	118.9	136.8	138.0	140.0
Lithuania	7.7	30.0	42.1	77.6	102.4	119.8	121.4	125.9
Armenia	2.1	30.1	47.6	69.1	85.6	83.4	84.3	83.5
Azerbaidzhan	4.8	37.8	57.8	69.1	93.4	96.8	97.2	98.3
Georgia	8.0	36.0	54.6	72.3	91.5	107.1	107.5	106.3
Kazakhstan	3.2	39.7	52.1	80.4	118.4	130.1	131.4	133.8
Kirgizia	1.2	24.1	40.3	73.5	106.7	119.7	120.4	119.2
Tadzhikistan	.4	28.6	43.9	67.1	97.7	98.8	100.9	104.3
Turkmenistan	2.7	41.6	61.3	83.0	101.7	104.5	106.1	104.9
Uzbekistan	2.3	30.1	49.7	83.9	101.7	113.1	117.4	120.9

Sources: *Handbook*, Table 13; *Compendium*, Table 3.

Table A5

Number of Medical Physicians, Stomatologists, and Dentists, Excluding the Military, 1916–1985 (in Thousands, per 10,000 Population)

Year	Doctors and dentists of all specialties	Rate	of which, women	Share of women	of which, both sexes		
					Medical physicians	Stomatologists [2]	Dentists [3]
1913 [1]	28,100	1.5	2.3	10	23.2	NA	4.9
1940	155,300	7.0	96.3	62	134.9	6.8	13.6
1950	265,000	13.6	204.9	77	236.9	10.4	17.7
1960	431.7	20.0	327.1	76	385.4	16.2	30.1
1970	668.4	27.4	479.6	72	577.3 [4]	39.6	51.5
1975	834.1	(32.8)	583.5	70	733.7 [4]	51.6	49.9
1980	997.1	37.5	683.1	69	NA	NA	NA
1982	1,071.2	39.5	731.7	68	NA	NA	NA
1985	1,170.4	42.0	802.4	69	NA	NA	NA

NA. Not available.

1. Within contemporary borders.
2. Stomatologists are graduates of a stomatological faculty of a medical institute, i.e., dentists or mouth specialists (including dental surgeons) with a professional degree.
3. Dentists, in Russian *zubnie vrachi* (''dental doctors''), are graduates of a secondary medical or middle medical school and do not hold a professional degree.
4. Figures derived as residuals.

Sources: *Handbook*, Table 8; *Compendium*, Table 11; *NK 1985*, pp. 540–41.

Table A6

Number of Medical Physicians and Dentists by Specialty, 1940–1985 (Excluding Military, Including Stomatologists and Dentists) (in Thousands)

Specialty	1940	1950	1960	1970	1975	1980	1982	1985
Total	155.3	265.0	431.7	668.4	834.1	997.1	1,071.2	1,170.4
Therapists	42.6	56.0	96.2	132.0	175.6	NA	NA	NA
Surgeons	12.6	22.5	40.5	65.9	86.2	NA	NA	NA
Obstetricians-Gynecologists	10.6	16.6	28.7	40.5	49.6	53.0	NA	NA
Pediatricians	19.4	32.1	58.9	79.0	96.3	103.0	NA	NA
Ophthalmologists 1	3.6	5.7	10.5	15.8	18.1	18.1	NA	NA
Otorhinolaryngologists (ear, nose, and throat)	2.6	4.6	9.6	15.7	18.1	NA	NA	NA
Neuropathologists	3.2	5.1	10.5	17.9	21.4	NA	NA	NA
Psychiatrists	2.4	3.1	6.4	14.3	18.7	NA	NA	NA
Dermo-Venereologists	3.9	9.4	16.5	12.2	14.5	NA	NA	NA
Radiologists	4.8	9.2	9.3	23.8	29.0	NA	NA	NA
Phtysiatrists (tuberculosis)	2.7	6.2	15.7	23.5	23.4	NA	NA	NA
Physicians specializing in physical culture	0.3	0.8	1.6	3.2	4.1	NA	NA	NA
Physicians in the public health anti-epidemic group	12.5	21.9	31.5	40.5	49.1	NA	NA	NA
Stomatologists (dental surgeons)	6.8	10.4	16.2	39.6	51.6	NA	NA	NA
Dentists	13.6	17.7	30.1	51.5	49.9	NA	NA	NA
Residuals	13.7	43.7	49.5	93.0	128.5	NA	NA	NA

NA. Not available.

1. Prior to 1970, listed as oculists.

Sources: *Handbook*, Tables 6, 8; *Compendium*, Table 13; *NK 1985*, p. 540.

Table A7

Number of Physicians (Excluding the Military), All Specialties, USSR, and by Republic, 1913–1985 (Numbers in Thousands, Rates per 10,000 Population)

USSR and republic	1913		1940		1950		1960		1970		1980		1982		1985	
	Number	Rate	Number	Rate	Number	Rate	Number	Rate	Number	Rate	Number	Rate	Number	Rate	Number	Rate
USSR	23.2	1.5	141.7	7.2	247.3	13.6	431.7	20.0	668.4	27.4	997.1	37.5	1071.2	39.5	1,170.4	42.0
RSFSR	13.0	1.5	82.1	7.4	148.9	14.5	251.4	20.9	378.4	29.0	650.7	40.3	599.3	42.5	646.8	44.9
Ukraine	6.5	1.9	33.3	8.0	48.6	13.1	85.6	19.9	131.0	27.7	182.7	36.5	195.6	38.9	210.6	41.4
Belorussia	.9	1.3	4.2	4.7	6.2	8.0	13.5	16.4	23.4	25.8	32.7	33.9	34.6	35.3	37.8	37.8
Moldavia	.2	1.2	1.0	4.0	2.3	9.8	4.3	14.3	7.4	20.5	12.5	31.4	13.8	34.0	15.6	37.5
Estonia	.4	4.5	.8	8.3	1.4	12.7	2.9	23.9	4.6	33.1	6.2	41.6	6.6	43.6	7.1	46.3
Latvia	.5	2.1	2.0	10.9	2.8	14.6	5.7	26.5	8.5	35.9	11.1	43.9	11.7	45.7	13.2	48.3
Lithuania	.3	1.2	1.9	6.7	2.7	10.6	4.9	17.3	8.7	27.5	13.4	38.9	14.2	40.7	15.4	42.9
Armenia	*	.6	.9	6.8	2.3	17.2	4.6	24.2	7.3	28.7	10.9	34.8	11.6	35.9	12.8	37.9
Azerbaidzhan	.3	1.2	3.0	9.2	5.8	20.1	9.4	23.7	13.1	25.0	20.7	33.4	22.4	35.0	25.3	37.8
Georgia	.3	1.3	4.7	12.8	9.3	26.3	13.8	33.0	17.1	36.4	24.2	48.1	26.0	50.9	28.2	54.2
Kazakhstan	.2	.3	2.5	3.9	6.1	9.0	14.2	13.9	28.8	21.8	47.8	31.8	51.9	33.6	59.7	37.2
Kirgizia	*	.2	.5	3.4	1.6	9.5	3.4	15.4	6.2	20.8	10.6	29.1	11.7	30.9	13.5	33.4
Tadzhikistan	*	.1	.6	3.8	1.2	7.7	2.7	12.7	4.7	15.9	9.4	23.5	10.6	25.1	12.4	26.6
Turkmenistan	*	.5	.9	6.7	1.5	12.4	3.0	18.7	4.8	21.3	8.2	28.3	8.9	29.1	10.7	32.5
Uzbekistan	.1	.3	2.8	4.2	6.1	9.5	12.3	13.8	24.4	20.1	46.0	28.5	52.3	30.7	61.9	33.5

*Less than 100 physicians.

Sources: *Handbook*, Table 7; *Compendium*, Table 12; *NK 1985*, p. 540.

Table A8
Medical Education, 1960–1985 (Students and Graduates)

Medical education is organized in the following way in the USSR:

Most of medical education takes place in Medical Institutes that are not part of universities. Each institute may have from one to five faculties which are: 1) Medicine; 2) Pediatrics; 3) Public Health; 4) Stomatology; and 5) Pharmacology. Most institutes have less than five faculties. There were in 1967, 74 such institutes with the following number of faculties:

1) Medical	72
2) Pediatrics	34
3) Public Health	23
4) Stomatology	30
5) Pharmacology	13

There were also five Medical Faculties that were parts of universities, plus two free standing Stomatological Institutes and five free standing Pharmacological Institutes.

Academic year	1960/61	1970/71	1980/81	1984/85	1985/86
Medical students[1]	189,200	329,800	377,200	393,200	381,200
Graduates	30,600	43,800	59,600	63,600	64,900

1. Includes a small number of students in physical culture.

Sources: *NK 1985*, pp. 506, 515; *Handbook*, Table 17.

Table A9
Number of Mid-Level Medical and Dental Personnel (Excluding the Military), 1913–1985 (in Thousands)

Specialty	1913	1940	1950	1960	1970	1980	1982	1985
Total	ca.50	472.	719.4	1,388.3	2,123.0	2,814.3	2,963.0	3,158.9
Feldshers	37.8	82.2	160.0	334.7	475.0	NA	NA	NA
Feldsher-midwives	-	12.8	42.0	76.2	81.3	NA	NA	NA
Midwives	-	68.1	66.5	139.3	216.0	NA	NA	NA
Assistants to public health physicians and epidemiologists	-	9.7	18.5	28.2	37.6	NA	NA	NA
Nurses	10.0	222.7	325.0	623.5	1,033.8	NA	NA	NA
Laboratory technicians	-	11.7	25.3	52.5	81.8	NA	NA	NA
X-ray technicians and X-ray laboratory technicians	-	3.6	7.5	18.3	23.8	NA	NA	NA
Dental technicians	-	4.9	6.7	13.9	25.4	NA	NA	NA
Disinfection instructors and disinfectors	-	15.9	27.0	52.4	73.2	NA	NA	NA
Residual	-	35.4	43.6	49.3	75.1	NA	NA	NA

NA. Not available.

Sources: *Handbook*, Table 9; *Compendium*, Table 15; *NK 1985*, p. 541.

Table A10

Number of Mid-Level Medical and Dental Personnel (Excluding the Military), USSR, and by Republic, 1960–1985 (Numbers in Thousands, Rates per 10,000 Population)

USSR and republic	1960		1970		1980		1982		1985	
	Number	Rate	Number	Rate	Number	Rate	Number	Rate	Number	Rate
USSR	1388.3	64.2	2123.0	87.2	2814.3	105.7	2963.0	109.4	3158.9	113.5
RSFSR	817.1	67.7	1212.3	92.8	1585.0	114.0	1659.3	117.8	1730.6	120.2
Ukraine	275.6	63.9	411.5	86.9	515.6	103.1	536.7	106.7	566.6	111.4
Belorussia	44.6	54.2	73.1	80.8	94.1	97.6	100.2	102.5	-	-
Moldavia	16.4	54.0	28.0	77.2	38.1	95.2	40.8	100.6	45.7	110.1
Estonia	9.5	77.5	12.9	93.8	15.6	105.0	16.8	111.4	17.6	114.3
Latvia	15.4	71.8	22.1	93.4	29.2	115.9	30.6	119.9	32.9	126.2
Lithuania	14.9	53.1	24.7	78.1	37.2	108.3	39.8	113.9	43.8	121.7
Armenia	11.3	59.5	17.9	69.9	25.3	81.0	27.9	86.4	30.7	91.3
Azerbaidzhan	26.1	65.6	39.7	76.0	52.2	84.3	56.2	87.8	62.0	92.5
Georgia	30.7	73.3	43.2	91.7	56.5	111.9	58.7	114.8	61.3	117.6
Kazakhstan	58.4	57.1	106.0	80.2	150.2	99.8	160.8	104.1	181.1	113.0
Kirgizia	10.8	48.8	21.6	72.4	31.5	86.3	34.2	90.0	39.2	97.0
Tadzhikistan	8.4	39.7	15.4	51.4	26.1	65.0	28.4	66.9	33.3	71.7
Turkmenistan	10.6	65.5	16.1	72.2	22.8	78.4	24.9	81.7	29.1	88.7
Uzbekistan	38.5	44.1	78.5	64.7	134.9	83.5	147.7	86.7	176.4	95.4

Sources: *Compendium*, Table 14; *NK 1985*, p. 541.

Table A11
Annual Average Number of Workers and Employees in the Health Sector, 1928–1985 (in Thousands)

Year	Number
1928	399
1940	1,507
1950	2,569
1960	3,461
1970	5,080
1980	6,223
1982	6,448
1984	6,672
1985	6,784

Sources: *Handbook*, Table 11; *Compendium*, Table 10; *NK 1985*, p. 391.

Table A12
Number of Deaths, 1960–1985 (in Thousands)

Year	Number
1960	1,528.6
1961	1,563.0
1962	1,666.7
1963	1,626.9
1964	1,581.3
1965	1,689.8
1966	1,711.0
1967	1,799.0
1968	1,833.5
1969	1,957.3
1970	1,996.3
1971	2,015.4
1972	2,105.4
1973	2,164.2
1974	2,191.4
1975	2,363.4
1976	2,426.5
1977	2,494.7
1978	2,545.6
1979	2,665.9
1980	2,743.8
1981	2,742.1
1982	2,723.6
1983	2,793.4(1)
1984	2,957.0(1)
1985	2,928.7(1)

1. Estimates.
Sources: *Compendium*, Table 16; *NK 1985*, pp. 32–33.

Table A13
Crude Death Rates, USSR, and by Republic, 1960–1985 (per 1,000 Population)

USSR and republic	1960	1970	1980	1982	1983	1984	1985
USSR	7.1	8.2	10.3	10.1	10.3	10.8	10.6
RSFSR	7.4	8.7	11.0	10.7	11.1	11.6	11.3
Ukraine	6.9	8.9	11.4	11.3	11.5	12.0	12.1
Belorussia	6.6	7.6	9.9	9.6	10.0	10.5	10.6
Moldavia	6.4	7.4	10.2	10.2	10.9	11.1	11.2
Estonia	10.5	11.1	12.3	11.9	12.0	12.5	12.6
Latvia	10.0	11.2	12.7	12.2	12.5	12.9	13.1
Lithuania	7.8	8.9	10.5	10.0	10.3	10.9	10.9
Armenia	6.8	5.1	5.5	5.5	5.8	5.8	5.9
Azerbaidzhan	6.7	6.7	7.0	6.7	6.7	6.8	6.8
Georgia	6.5	7.3	8.6	8.4	8.4	8.8	8.8
Kazakhstan	6.6	6.0	8.0	7.8	8.0	8.2	8.0
Kirgizia	6.1	7.4	8.4	7.8	7.9	8.3	8.1
Tadzhikistan	5.1	6.4	8.0	7.7	7.6	7.4	7.0
Turkmenistan	6.5	6.6	8.3	8.0	8.5	8.2	8.1
Uzbekistan	6.0	5.5	7.4	7.4	7.5	7.4	7.2

Sources: *Compendium*, Table 17; *NK 1983*, pp. 33, 35.

Table A14
Age-Specific Death Rates, Both Sexes, 1896–1897, 1938–1939, 1960–1961, 1970–1971, 1975–1976 (per 1,000 Persons of Each Age Group)

Age Group	1896/ 1897	1938/ 1939	1960/ 1961	1970/ 1971	1975/ 1976
0-4	133.0	75.8	9.9	6.7	8.7
5-9	12.9	5.5	1.0	0.7	0.7
10-14	5.4	2.6	0.7	0.5	0.5
15-19	5.8	3.4	1.2	1.0	1.0
20-24	7.6	4.4	1.7	1.6	1.7
25-29	8.2	4.7	2.1	2.2	2.1
30-34	8.7	5.4	2.7	2.8	3.0
35-39	10.3	6.8	3.0	3.8	3.8
40-44	11.8	8.1	3.7	4.7	5.3
45-49	15.7	10.2	5.4	6.0	6.9
50-54	18.5	13.8	7.5	8.7	9.3
55-59	29.5	17.1	10.9	11.8	13.4
60-64	34.5	24.5	16.6	17.9	18.9
65-69	61.6	35.1	24.5	26.9	28.0
70 and over	89.0	78.9	63.1	74.9	75.0

Source: *Compendium*, Table 18.

Table A15

The Historical Course of Soviet Infant Mortality, 1913–1985 (Reported 1913–1974, 1980–1985; Estimated 1943–1981, and Adjusted 1959–1985, Deaths) (per 1,000 Live Births, Ages 0–1)

Year	Reported	Estimated	Adjusted(c)
1913	273(a)		
1913	269(b)		
1926	174		
1928	182		
1937	170		
1938	161		
1939	167		
1940	182		
1943		300(k)	
1946		140(k)	
1950	81		
1956	47		
1957	45		
1958	41		
1959	40.6		46.4
1960	35.3		40.4
1961	32.3		37.0
1962	32.2		36.8
1963	30.9		35.3
1964	28.8		32.9
1965	27.2		31.1
1966	26.1		29.9
1967	26.0		29.9

Year	Reported	Estimated	Adjusted(c)
1968	26.4		30.2
1969	25.8		29.5
1970	24.7		28.3
1971	22.9		26.2
1972	24.7		28.3
1973	26.4		30.2
1974	27.9		31.9
		28.8(g)	32.8
1975		29.4(d)	33.6
		30.8(i)	35.1
		28.8(g)	32.8
1976		31.1(d)	35.5
1977		28.8(f)	32.8
		28.0(e)	31.9
1978		28.8(g)	32.8
		28.0(e)	31.9
1979		28.8(g)	32.8
	26.0(h)	28.0(e)	29.6
1980		28.8(g)	31.9
			32.8
	27.3(l)		42.0
			31.1
1981		20.8(e)	31.9
		30.0(f)	34.2
1983	25.3(l)		28.8
1984	25.9(l)		29.5
1985	26.0(l)		29.6

Table A15 (continued)

a. Within USSR borders until 3 September 1939.

b. Within contemporary USSR borders.

c. The Soviets exclude from their statistical reporting of infant mortality live births of infants of under 28 weeks of gestation, less than 35 cm. in length and less than 1,000 g. in weight, who die within seven days of delivery. They are considered as miscarriages or abortions. Davis and Feshbach estimate that this method of computing the infant mortality leads to a 14.4 percent underenumeration. The "Adjusted" column thus reflects an upward revision of reported infant mortality by 14.4 percent. C. Davis and M. Feshbach, Rising Infant Mortality in the USSR in the 1970s. Washington, D.C.: U.S. Department of Commerce, June 1980.

d. These estimates by Davis and Feshbach based on the published figures for 1975 and 1976 of deaths in ages 0-4, and on the fact that the relationship between infant mortality and 0-4 mortality has been fairly constant in previous years.

e. Based on a statement by a Soviet official, Aleksander I. Smirnov of the State Planning Commission, to the effect that the infant mortality had been about 28 per 1,000 live births since 1978. S. P. Burenkov, Interview in Literaturnaia Gazeta, July 21, 1982, 12. In English, in Current Digest of the Soviet Press, XXXIV, 20, 10-11, 1982.

f. The London Times reported a figure of 30 per 1,000 live births based apparently on the same source (at a press conference) as in Burenkov (1982) above.

g. Estimated by the World Health Organization cited in M. L. Levy, "La Mortalité Infantile dans le Monde, Population et Sociéties," 1983, May, 169, Table 3. Figure given for 1975-80.

h. Reported in Novostii Press Agency, Soviet Economy Today, Westport, CT: Greenwood Press, 1981, 32.

i. R. Pressat, Une évolution anachronique: La hausse de la mortalité en union Soviétique. Concours Medical 105-2, 431-2434, May 21, 1983.

j. Organization Mondiale de la Santé, Statistiques sanitaires mondiales, Genève, 1982. The figure is accompanied by a subscript "corrected." This is an estimate adjusted presumably to account for the Soviet underenumeration reported above.

k. Maksudov (pseud.). Some causes of Rising Mortality in the USSR. Russia, 4.9, 1981.

l. Ekonomicheskaia Gazeta, 43, 6-7, 1986.

Table A16
Deaths from Certain Infectious Diseases, 1940–1985 (Number of Cases in Thousands)

	Incidence				
	1940	1960	1970	1980	1985
Typhoid fever and paratyphoid A,B,C [1]	121.3	47.3	22.5	16.9	17.6
Scarlet fever	251.5	671.2	469.9	230.1	277.9
Diphteria	177.0	53.2	1.10	0.35	1.51
Pertussis (whooping cough)	453.3	554.1	39.5	13.9	53.9
Tetanus		2.3	0.65	0.30	0.28
Acute poliomyelitis	1.28	7.2	0.27	0.17	0.14
Measles	1,181.9	2,083.3	471.5	355.7	272.8

	Rates per 100,000				
	1940	1960	1970	1980	1985
Typhoid Fever and paratyphoid A,B,C [1]	62	22	9	6	6
Scarlet fever	129	313	194	87	100
Diphteria	91	24.8	0.45	0.13	0.55
Pertussis (whooping cough)	232	259	16	5	19.4
Tetanus		1.1	0.27	0.11	0.10
Acute poliomyelitis	0.65	3.3	0.11	0.06	0.05
Measles	605	972	194	134	98

1. Until 1965 only cases of typhoid fever and paratyphoid A and B were registered.

Source: *NK 1985*, p. 545.

Table A17

Number of Persons and Percent of Population Hospitalized in Medical Institutions, All Ministries and Agencies, USSR and by Republic, 1960–1985[1] (Numbers in Thousands)

USSR and republic	1960		1970		1980		1982		1985	
	number	per 100	number	per 100	number	per 100	Number	per 100	number	per 100
USSR, all ministries and agencies	41,500	17.6	52,237	21.5	62,777	23.7	64,883	24.1	69,637	25.1
Urban	NA	19.1	NA	22.4	NA	23.8	NA	NA	NA	NA
Rural	NA	16.2	NA	20.4	NA	23.6	NA	NA	NA	NA
RSFSR	NA	NA	28,809	22.1	33,526	24.2	34,375	24.5	36,462	25.4
Ukraine	NA	NA	10,474	22.2	12,556	25.2	13,057	26.0	13,754	27.1
Belorussia	NA	NA	1,939	21.5	2,430	25.3	2,512	25.8	2,725	27.4
Moldavia	NA	NA	724	20.1	888	22.3	952	23.6	1,062	25.7
Estonia	NA	NA	274	20.1	299	20.3	320	21.3	330	21.5
Latvia	NA	NA	501	21.2	600	23.8	623	24.5	661	25.5
Lithuania	NA	NA	578	18.4	704	20.5	755	21.7	785	21.9
Armenia	NA	NA	397	15.7	464	14.9	481	15.0	524	15.7
Azerbaidzhan	NA	NA	821	15.9	1,015	16.5	1,040	16.4	1,125	16.9
Georgia	NA	NA	778	16.6	968	19.2	894	17.5	906	17.4
Kazakhstan	NA	NA	2,955	22.5	3,633	24.3	3,721	24.2	4,039	25.3
Kirgizia	NA	NA	642	21.7	843	23.3	881	23.5	979	24.4
Tadzhikistan	NA	NA	523	17.8	785	19.8	862	20.6	994	21.7
Turkmenistan	NA	NA	387	17.7	532	18.5	574	19.1	664	20.5
Uzbekistan	NA	NA	2,435	20.4	3,534	22.1	3,836	22.8	330	21.5

NA. Not available.

1. Data are presented for all available years.

Sources: *Compendium*, Table 6; *NK 1985*, p. 543.

Table A18

Number of Deaths Caused by Circulatory and Cardiovascular Diseases, by Age and Sex, 1966/67–1971/72 (per 100,000 Population of Corresponding Age Group and Sex)

Year	Total		Under age 20		20-29		30-39	
	Male	Female	Male	Female	Male	Female	Male	Female
1966/1967	280.5	371.2	3.9	3.9	17.7	13.8	55.3	29.2
1967/1968	291.4	384.7	4.0	3.7	17.6	13.3	57.5	28.8
1968/1969	309.4	404.5	3.9	3.6	17.7	13.0	60.7	28.4
1969/1970	325.9	425.7	3.7	3.6	17.0	12.4	62.3	28.9
1971/1972	345.3	454.4	3.7	3.5	15.9	11.2	66.6	28.7

Year	40-49		50-59		60 and older	
	Male	Female	Male	Female	Male	Female
1966/1967	148.1	71.8	459.7	225.4	2742.3	2333.6
1967/1968	158.0	73.0	482.8	233.5	2798.2	2368.4
1968/1969	170.6	75.0	521.8	246.8	2888.1	2430.3
1969/1970	180.4	77.3	549.5	252.2	3037.7	2577.0
1971/1972	196.1	81.2	574.7	265.4	3112.5	2629.5

Source: *Compendium*, Table 21.

Table A19
Number and Rate of Deaths from Diseases of the Circulatory and Cardiovascular System, by Cause, 1960–1982 (in Thousands, Rates per 100,000 Population)

	1960		1970		1980		1982	
Causes of death	Number	Rate	Number	Rate	Number	Rate	Number	Rate
Total deaths from disorders of the circulatory and cardiovascular system	529.9	247.3	933.9	384.7	1441.5	542.8	1439.4	533.0
From arteriosclerotic cardiosclerosis	167.4	78.2	388.2	159.9	599.4	225.7	590.5	218.7
From hypertension (all forms)	89.9	42.0	203.5	83.8	233.4	87.9	224.0	82.9
of which,								
with vascular disorders of the central nervous system	53.0	24.7	124.8	51.4	150.6	56.7	149.9	55.5
with an infarct of the myocardium	6.2	2.9	15.8	6.5	10.9	4.1	9.7	3.6
From vascular disorder of the brain without hypertension	96.9	45.2	176.4	72.7	294.6	110.9	311.4	115.3
From other forms of ischemic heart disease and myocardial infarction(excluding hypertension)	40.9	19.1	68.7	28.3	189.0	71.2	188.7	69.9
of which,								
from myocardial infarction	NA	NA	NA	NA	62.4	23.5	63.6	23.5
From active rheumatism and chronic rheumatic heart diseases	42.8	20.0	33.5	13.8	26.8	10.1	24.1	8.9
From all other diseases of the circulatory and cardiovascular system	92.0	42.8	63.6	26.2	98.3	37.0	100.7	37.3

Source: *Compendium*, Table 23.

Table A20
Number of Deaths Caused by Cancer, by Age and Sex, 1966/67–1971/72 (per 100,000 Population of Corresponding Age Group and Sex)

Year	Total		Under age 20		20-29		30-39	
	Male	Female	Male	Female	Male	Female	Male	Female
1966/1967	133.0	118.0	8.1	6.2	12.7	12.1	38.2	35.7
1967/1968	134.6	118.7	8.2	6.3	13.1	11.7	37.6	34.7
1968/1969	136.6	118.9	8.2	6.2	12.5	11.4	36.9	33.3
1969/1970	137.3	118.5	7.9	6.0	12.3	11.5	36.0	33.2
1971/1972	140.2	120.5	8.1	6.1	11.9	10.4	35.3	32.5

Year	40-49		50-59		60 and older	
	Male	Female	Male	Female	Male	Female
1966/1967	120.1	105.4	427.8	249.4	970.9	488.9
1967/1968	124.0	104.9	432.2	250.8	969.3	483.7
1968/1969	127.3	103.0	441.9	252.4	958.2	475.4
1969/1970	128.6	101.6	447.2	245.5	962.0	479.1
1971/1972	134.5	102.4	441.4	244.9	963.4	475.7

Source: *Compendium*, Table 22.

Table A21

Number and Rate of Deaths from Cancer, by Location, 1961, 1970, 1980, 1982 (in Thousands; Rates per 100,000 Population)

Location	1961		1970		1980		1982	
	Number	Rate	Number	Rate	Number	Rate	Number	Rate
Total deaths from malignant neoplasms	245.0	113.4	308.7	127.2	371.8	140.0	390.6	144.7
Nodules in the mouth and throat	NA	NA	4.0	1.6	7.0	2.6	7.6	2.8
Of the esophagus	11.8	5.4	15.4	6.4	15.0	5.7	14.6	5.4
Of the stomach	72.8	33.7	98.8	40.7	88.5	33.3	88.9	32.9
Of the intestines, excluding the rectum	NA	NA	10.1	4.2	16.6	6.3	18.0	6.7
Of the rectum	NA	NA	9.2	3.8	17.1	6.4	19.6	7.3
Of other digestive organs	NA	NA	25.8	10.6	29.4	11.1	34.9	12.9
Of the larynx	NA	NA	4.3	1.8	7.0	2.6	7.4	2.8
Of the bronchi, trachea, and lungs	26.2	12.1	47.2	19.5	68.8	25.9	74.4	27.6
Of other respiratory organs	NA	NA	1.0	0.4	2.0	0.8	NA	NA
Of the mammary glands	15.4	7.1	12.3	5.1	20.3	7.6	21.9	8.1
Of the cervix of the uterus	32.0	14.9	12.1	5.0	12.1	4.6	11.7	4.3
Other malignant neoplasms of the uterus	NA	NA	7.8	3.2	8.1	3.1	8.5	3.1
Of other female reproductive organs	NA	NA	9.1	3.7	12.1	4.6	12.9	4.8
Of the prostate	NA	NA	3.6	1.5	5.0	1.9	5.4	2.0
Of other male reproductive organs	NA	NA	0.8	0.3	1.0	0.4	1.1	0.4
Of the urinary glands	NA	NA	9.8	4.0	13.3	5.0	14.4	5.3
Of the skin	30.1	13.9	2.0	0.8	3.5	1.3	3.8	1.4
Of the bones and connective tissue	NA	NA	3.2	1.3	4.2	1.6	NA	NA
Of the lymphatic and hemogenic tissue	NA	NA	17.8	7.3	(20.0)	(7.4)	(21.3)	(7.9)
of which, leukemia	NA	NA	NA	NA	11.6	4.3	12.1	4.5
others	NA	NA	NA	NA	8.4	3.1	9.2	3.4
Others and undefined locations	NA	NA	14.4	6.0	20.8	7.8	24.2	9.0

NA. Not available.

Source: *Compendium*, Table 24.

UNITED STATES OF AMERICA

Milton I. Roemer

This account of the health-care system in the United States is based on a model found useful in comparative studies. Every system of health care has five main components, the relationships among which may be seen in Figure 1.

Major Features

In the perspective of the world's 160 nations, the U.S. system of health care embodies several major features. First, as an affluent, industrialized country, its health-care system has abundant resources, and it spends a great deal of money. Second, as a federated nation, the governance of its system is highly decentralized to numerous states, counties, and communities. Third, as a nation with a free market economy, it incorporates very permissive laissez-faire concepts throughout its health-care system. These concepts are apparent in the forms taken by all the five system components shown in Figure 1.

All three of these system characteristics are relative—that is, relative to the policies and practices of other countries. There are, of course, other affluent, industrialized nations, other federated republics, and other laissez-faire economies. These system attributes play a particularly important role in the United States, however. They have generated a highly complex and pluralistic system with very different meanings for various sections of its population.

The federated political structure can be traced to the American Revolution against the British monarchy and to the determination to avoid a strong central government. Even within the central government, there are checks and balances among the executive, legislative, and judicial branches, which restrain governmental actions of all types. The free market economy was emerging in Europe in the early nineteenth century, just when the new world was beginning to

Figure 1
Main Health System Components

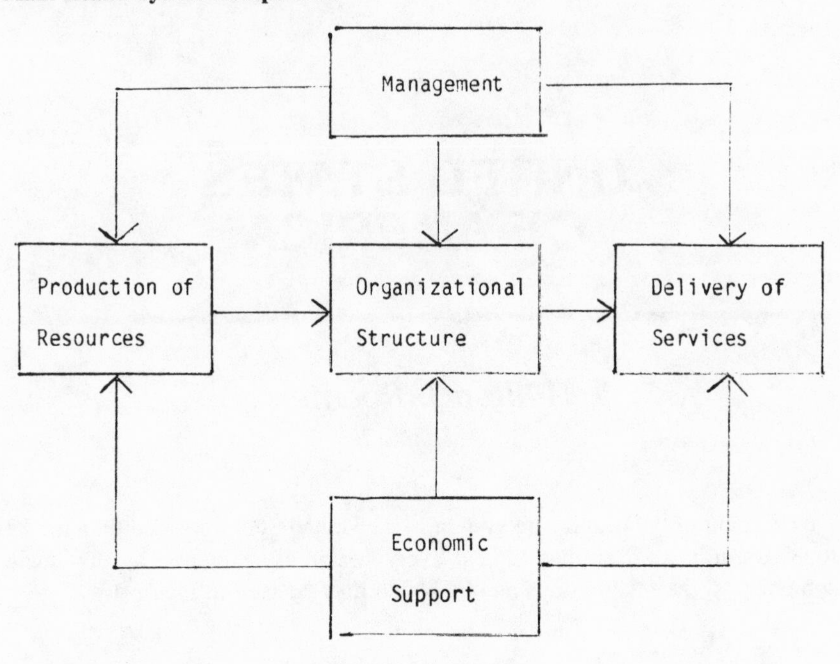

develop. Inevitably, the American health-care system was influenced by these dynamic economic processes around it.

Yet, the U.S. health-care system, like that of all countries, is not static. In spite of the dedication of national and health professional leaders to free market principles, many interventions in the operation of the market have been necessary. As the expectations of people for recovery from disease and for the maintenance of good health have risen, more initiatives have become necessary to change the contours of all five system components. Social actions have been taken to increase the quantity and quality of the resources produced, to plan and modify system management, to alter the overall system structure, to strengthen the mechanisms of economic support, and to rationalize and improve the delivery of services. The resulting profile of the U.S. health-care system today will be examined below.

Health Status

For reasons that far transcend the health-care system, the U.S. population as a whole is among the healthiest of the world's large nations. Within its 240 million population, however, there are great inequalities, and much of the excellent health service of which the nation is capable has not been made accessible to everyone.

Examining first the overall picture, life expectancy for U.S. residents was 74.5 years at birth, as of 1982. The difference is substantial for the sexes—70.8 years for men and 78.2 years for women. More indicative of the differences in the standard of living, as well as in health services, is the contrast of life expectancies for the white and black races. On the whole, blacks suffer disadvantages in virtually every condition affecting health; their life expectancy at birth is 69.5 years (as of 1982), compared with 75.1 years for whites.

The U.S. infant mortality rate in 1982 was 11.2 per 1,000 live births. While this, of course, is low, it is higher than that of fifteen other countries including those in Western Europe, Canada, Japan, and the German Democratic Republic. It is perhaps significant that these countries have less wealth than the United States (as measured by gross national product per capita), but they all have systems of national health care which make services freely accessible (or nearly free) to virtually everyone.

Tuberculosis and other serious infectious diseases have been greatly reduced in the United States. The leading causes of death are the noninfectious disorders that are prevalent in the later years of life, followed by deaths due to violence. Adjusting disease-specific death rates for the nation's age composition in 1940, the leading causes of death in 1982 were as follows:

Causes	**Deaths per 100,000**
Diseases of the heart	190.8
Malignant neoplasms	133.3
Accidents and adverse effects	37.1
Cerebrovascular diseases	36.1
Suicide	11.5
Pneumonia and influenza	11.3
Chronic liver disease and cirrhosis	10.4
Homicide and legal intervention	9.7
Diabetes mellitus	9.2
Other causes	107.0
All causes	556.4

A great cause for optimism in the United States has been the decreasing trend of heart disease mortality over the last 30 years. After increasing since 1900 (when satisfactory records were first kept), in 1950 the age-adjusted death rate from diseases of the heart began to decline. It fell from 307.6 deaths per 100,000 population in 1950 to 190.8 in 1982. (The manifest increase in observable cases was due, of course, to the rising proportion of people living to older age levels.)

The exact causes of this trend are not clear, but it is likely that both improvements in medical care and modifications in living habits (diet, smoking, exercise, etc.) have had impacts. This experience has given great impetus to a movement for greater emphasis on prevention and health promotion and for encouragement of healthful life-styles in the U.S. health-care system.

The United States tabulates data regularly on morbidity from all causes of the general population; this is based on periodic household interviews of a nationwide sample of the civilian and noninstitutionalized population. Of the various measures used, the broadest is the number of "restricted activity days" per person per year. (This indicator identifies any disorder in a household member.) In 1981, there were found to be 18.5 restricted activity days per person per year in the United States. The differences by family income were striking:

Family Income per Year	Restricted Activity Days per Person per Year
Less than $7,000	32.1
$7,000–$9,999	23.5
$10,000–$14,999	18.1
$15,000–$24,999	16.2
$25,000 or more	13.6

One reflection on the dynamics of the U.S. health-care system can be seen in contacts with physicians and in inpatient hospital days per person per year in families of different incomes. In 1981, these relationships were as follows:

Family Income per Year	Physician Contacts	Hospital Days
Less than $7,000	5.6	1.32
$7,000–$9,999	4.9	1.16
$10,000–$14.999	4.5	1.06
$15,000–$24,999	4.5	0.84
$25,000 or more	4.4	0.77

Thus, those in the lower income groups—in accordance with their higher rate of morbidity as shown above—have contacts with doctors slightly more often than those in the higher income groups. Nevertheless, for reasons probably related to their general conditions of living, they end up receiving higher rates of hospital care. Thirty years ago, data showed the lower income groups to have higher rates of illness, as they have still, but lower rates of contact with both physicians and hospitals than the upper income groups. The health-care system, in other words, appears to have improved in its degree of equity, but not sufficiently to overcome the generally unhealthful effects of an environment of deprivation or poverty.

Organizational Structure

To analyze the U.S. health-care system today, one must begin with an account of its organizational structure. This component stands at the center of the system model (Figure 1) like the trunk of a tree. Subsequently, the four other components that contribute to this organizational structure will be considered, followed by a discussion of how the whole combination of relationships differs from those of other national systems.

The organizational structure of a health-care system is often described in terms of an array of various health programs. The forms and proportionate role of each program differ greatly among national systems. In the United States, five major types of health programs can be found. They may be analyzed as the principal governmental health authority, other agencies of government with health functions, voluntary health agencies, enterprises with health functions, and the private health-care market. The size, shape, and proportions of these programs define the organizational structure of the U.S. health-care system.

Principal Governmental Health Authority

In most countries, there is a central governmental authority that carries major responsibility for the health protection of the population. In some countries, this responsibility is carried along with other major responsibilities, and this is the arrangement in the permissive health-care system of the United States. Until recently, the U.S. government's equivalent to a Ministry of Health was combined with authority for two other major fields in the Department of Health, Education, and Welfare. In 1978 the responsibility for education was withdrawn, but the resulting Department of Health and Human Services remains responsible for the nation's massive programs of social security and public assistance as well as those for most aspects of health. Within this department, there is a vast organizational structure handling the responsibilities of the U.S. federal government in health resource development, health planning and regulation, and other governmental functions within the national health-care system.

It is not necessary to explore the organization and functions of the U.S. Department of Health and Human Services in detail. It suffices to note that most of the department's responsibilities are fulfilled by allocation of money and delegation of authority to numerous other public and private entities throughout the nation. Being a federation of states, the U.S. Constitution grants the states a great deal of autonomy and responsibility in all social affairs, including health. There are relatively few health functions carried out directly from the national level (principally by the U.S. Public Health Service within the Department of Health and Human Services), such as health examination of immigrants, regulation of drugs that move in interstate commerce, special epidemiological investigations, compilation of national health statistics, or medical services to American Indians.

Below the national level, there is a major health agency in each of the 50 states, although sometimes it is combined with authorities for social welfare and other functions. The administrative configuration and scope of functions of the state health agencies are highly variable. The heads of these agencies are ordinarily appointed by an elected governor; they are responsible entirely to the state governor and not at all to the national health authority. Only insofar as particular standards must be met as a condition for receipt of certain national grants must the state accept national direction. Federal grants for hospital construction, for example, require that the state must have a law on licensure of hospitals; wide leeway is allowed, however, in the provisions of such laws. Similarly, below the level of state government, there are units of local government—counties and cities or sometimes special districts—that also have a major health agency, again with considerable autonomy. On certain health matters, the local health department may carry out functions delegated by the state agency, but on most matters it has full authority within the constraints of the general local government.

Other Agencies of Government with Health Functions

Governmental structures are often determined by historical developments. In public health, agencies grew out of recognition of the need to protect people from hazards of the environment and of epidemic diseases, which were seen to endanger the entire population. Social insurance, however, was a movement to protect the economic position of low-paid workers, who could be ruined by the costs of sickness—costs defined as lost earnings as well as charges for medical care. As a result, the place of social insurance in the structure of government usually has been different from that of public health.

In the United States, the first national social insurance program established to finance medical care was administered by the Social Security Administration, not by the Public Health Service—this was the ''Medicare'' insurance program for the aged, enacted in 1965. When the Medicare program was subsequently withdrawn from the Social Security Administration and combined with the public assistance program of ''Medicaid'' for the health care of the poor, it was placed in yet another non-public-health agency, the Health Care Financing Administration. Several other agencies of the federal government in the United States also administer important health programs. The Department of Labor, with its Occupational Safety and Health Administration, has the main responsibility for protecting the health of workers at their places of work. The health and safety of miners, however, is a concern of the Bureau of Mines in the Department of the Interior. Many aspects of the health of agricultural families and farm workers, including control of the diseases of animals, are a concern of the Department of Agriculture. For certain historical reasons, the control of narcotic drugs has long been in the Department of Treasury. The Veterans Administration is an independent federal authority which, among other things, is responsible for the operation of the nation's largest network of public hospitals—those for military veterans, whether or not their disorders are connected with military service. The separate branches of the armed forces, as in nearly all countries, operate their own large subsystems of health services in time of peace as well as war, under the federal Department of Defense. The Department of Justice is responsible for health facilities in a network of federal prisons.

At the state and local levels in the United States, the multiplicity of governmental agencies concerned with health is still greater. The organizational layout is not the same in any two states. In most states, the medical care programs for the poor—defined in various ways—come under departments of social welfare or public assistance. Factory inspection for accident or disease hazards is usually a function of state departments of labor or industry. Worker's compensation programs, which help workers with work-connected injuries or diseases and are responsible for much medical care and rehabilitation, are generally under the control of special commissions or other agencies. Programs of vocational rehabilitation are often with state departments of education, although a major part of their task is medical. Special state authorities are usually concerned with the licensure of doctors, nurses, pharmacists, and other health personnel. Public water supply and sewage disposal systems are the responsibility of separate departments of public works in many states, and in most states there are special authorities established for the control of air and stream pollution. Even the overall planning of health services is often assigned by governors to a special agency other than the state Department of Health.

At the local level, governmental health responsibilities in the United States are equally as dispersed. Local boards and agencies concerned with welfare (of the poor and disabled), with public schools, with garbage disposal, with water and sanitation, with local government hospitals, with first aid in emergencies, with mental health services, with parks and recreation, and with other programs having health aspects function separately from the local Department of Health. Only a handful of America's 3,100 counties have integrated these many health functions into a single local health agency.

Voluntary Agencies

The permissive character of the health-care system in the United States is vividly demonstrated in the enormous multiplicity of voluntary health agencies. Voluntary agencies typically perform services not being rendered by government, pursue certain objectives with special dedication in order to attain them sooner, advance the interests of a certain population group, or occasionally carry out certain tasks at the behest of official bodies. The term "voluntary agency" is applied ordinarily to organizations that do not conduct a business for profit, hence they are designated "voluntary" in character. There are hundreds of voluntary agencies in the United States which raise funds and carry out programs for fighting certain diseases—cancer, tuberculosis, mental illness, and so on. Other such agencies focus on the health of certain population groups—children, American Indians, war veterans, and so on. Still other voluntary agencies are concerned with certain types of health service, such as visiting nurse care, hospitalization, or blood donations. The voluntary agency may be devoted exclusively to health purposes, or health services may be incidental to certain larger purposes, as in the case of church groups or religious missions.

Most numerous in the United States are the disease-specific voluntary agencies that mobilize the interest and financial contributions of millions of citizens. The American Cancer Society is illustrative. As cancer has become the second highest cause of death, large numbers of people have become deeply concerned about solving the riddle of this complex disease and helping its victims. Although initiated in a few large cities, a national organization was soon formed with branches in every state. Below the state level, there are city or county chapters. Funds are raised from individual donors locally, and a percentage of these is passed along to the national headquarters. A large share of the national funds is used to support cancer-related research projects. Funds kept at the local level are sometimes usd to support ''cancer detection clinics'' or to provide compassionate services to terminal cancer patients. The local, state, and national units of disease-specific voluntary agencies in the United States number in the tens of thousands. In the long run, the initiative taken by voluntary health agencies has often stimulated governmental bodies to do similar work.

Nongovernmental associations of professional health personnel must be counted as another type of voluntary agency. Their funds are raised by membership dues, rather than donations, and their activities are focused largely on advancing the interests of their members. This often includes programs of continuing education and other strategies intended to elevate professional standards. In addition, organizations like the American Medical Association or the American Hospital Association devote substantial effort to opposing legislative proposals that they regard as threatening the independence or economic position of their membership.

Enterprises with Health Functions

Enterprises are relevant to the structure of health-care systems in two ways: first, insofar as a specific company provides direct health services to its employees, and second, when an enterprise is engaged in the commercial provision of health service or is carrying out some other function in a health-care system.

In the United States, in-plant health services are generally of very limited scope, except in large establishments with more than 500 workers. In smaller factories, services are usually limited to first aid by an industrial nurse or perhaps only a medicine chest available to the workers. Large plants or mines may maintain a staff of physicians and nurses who perform periodic and preplacement examinations, treat any intercurrent illness whether job connected or not, and promote education for healthful living. Enterprises in isolated locations, such as railroad junctions or lumber mills, may sometimes operate comprehensive medical care programs for workers. Industrial firms, of course, are obligated by law to protect workers from accidents and occupational diseases, although enforcement is often lax.

Enterprises involved in the health sector as their main commercial objective play an especially large part in the U.S. health-care system. In addition to pharmaceutical companies, there are manufacturers of X-ray and laboratory equipment, surgical instruments and supplies, orthopedic appliances, eyeglasses, hearing aids, dental prostheses, and so on. Relevant to insurance for the costs of medical care (discussed below under economic support), hundreds of companies are engaged in the sale of a vast range of insurance policies financing various "packages" of hospital, medical, and related services. Also, a rising proportion of U.S. general hospitals are coming under the control of for-profit firms, which owned or controlled some 1 percent of general acute care beds in the early 1980s. Nursing homes for the aged and chronically ill have long been predominantly proprietary, with 85 percent of their beds in units operated for profit.

The Private Market

From the vantage point of health-care provision, the U.S. health-care system is overwhelmingly dominated by the private sector. The great majority of physicians and other service providers are private entrepreneurs, although the early 1980s have seen increasing pressures toward group affiliation and even corporatization. Ambulatory medical care (both general and specialist), dental care, pharmacy services, medical and surgical services in hospitals, optical services, and fitting of prosthetic appliances are all furnished predominantly by private practitioners. Personal preventive services may be provided by governmental or other organized entities, but a substantial share of these is delivered by private providers as well. It is especially noteworthy that, even when the financial support for health services has been collectivized, as in the various public or voluntary health insurance programs or in the tax-supported Medicaid program for the poor, the provision of services remains substantially a process in the private market. This is true not only for care in the doctor's private office but also in a hospitalized case, in which the service is rendered to a private patient, and third-party insurers pay essentially a private fee.

Over the last several decades, U.S. physicians have increasingly joined together in groups of different sizes for technical, economic, or professional reasons. Close to half of the American physicians outside of institutions now practice in groups of three or more, working with nurses and numerous allied personnel. The solo practitioner is gradually disappearing. The vast majority of these group-practice doctors, nevertheless, function as private practitioners even though they share their incomes in some way. The provision of dental care is similarly delivered in a private market setting for the vast bulk of services rendered. The same applies to the dispensing of drugs and other services.

The hospital care of short-term patients, on the other hand, is provided principally by nonprofit or governmental facilities (although as noted this, too, is changing). Insofar as certain physicians work full-time in hospitals as residents in training or as full-time specialists in certain fields, mainly pathology and radiology, they may be salaried employees and not in private practice. This pattern has also been growing, but the lion's share of medical or surgical services to patients in American hospitals is still provided by private practitioners.

Production of Resources

The operation of health programs in the organizational structure of every national system of health care depends on the availability of many resources. In the main, these consist of health manpower, health facilities, various commodities (including drugs), and knowledge. All four types of resources must be produced, deployed, and used.

Health Manpower

Perhaps the oldest form of health personnel is the physician. In the United States, there are 135 medical colleges. About half of these institutions are sponsored by state governments as part of state public universities, and half are under the auspices of private universities. All of the schools, however, have received substantial financial support from the federal government for many years. Entry to U.S. medical schools usually requires a university bachelor's degree (requiring four years of study), and medical schooling requires another four years, making eight academic years. Virtually all 50 states require also an internship in a hospital for at least one year, and the vast majority of interns proceed to further training for qualification as specialists. Some 85 percent of active U.S. physicians currently have such specialty credentials.

U.S. medical students must pay high tuitions, although these tend to be higher in the private than in the public schools. For a small percentage of students, there are fellowships and loan programs which may help to meet the costs of tuition and living expenses. For a very small fraction of students, federal or state public subsidy programs finance the entire costs of medical schooling on the condition that the graduate serves in a designated area of doctor shortage (usually rural) for a period equivalent to the years of subsidy.

The optimal supply of physicians required to meet the health needs of a country has long been a subject of discussion and debate. In a period of economic difficulties, such as during the worldwide depression of 1929–1939, there was widespread opinion about a "surplus" of doctors. Then, when economic conditions are favorable and social insurance facilitates financial access to medical care, physicians become very busy and a "shortage" is perceived. Thus, in the permissive U.S. health-care system, there were about 150 doctors per 100,000 population in 1900–1910. This ratio then declined or remained stationary until World War II. By the end of the war, in 1945, a serious shortage was felt, and both federal and state governments gave grants for strengthening the medical schools, both public and private. By 1980, there were more than 200 active physicians per 100,000 and the supply was continuing to increase. In the early 1980s, it was again widely believed that too many doctors were being produced (although not everyone shared this view).

In the affluent United States, there were 433 registered nurses per 100,000 in 1976, plus 227 vocational nurses per 100,000. Until about 1965, the vast majority of these young women were prepared in hospital-based nursing schools requiring three years of training. Then a different educational pattern, which had started earlier, gained momentum—the preparation of professional nurses through two years of academic study in community colleges. By 1980, the vast majority of registered nurses in the United States were being trained through these academic courses lasting two years, acquiring practical experience after they became employed. As in several other professions in this country, nursing leadership sought continuous upgrading, and university-based programs also developed, turning out nurses with a bachelor's degree. Although the majority of registered nurses work in hospitals (61 percent in 1977), 39 percent work in nursing homes for the chronically ill, in public health agencies, in schools, in industrial clinics, in nursing education, in private medical or dental offices, in private duty positions, and in other settings.

The numbers and functions of dental personnel in various health-care systems is an interesting reflection of service policies. In the permissive system of the United States, there are 52 dentists per 100,000 population. There are numerous dental hygienists and dental assistants, but their functions are restricted essentially to preventive work or to assisting the dentists at the chairside. Publicly financed clinics for dental care are scarce.

Health Facilities

The total hospital bed supply in 1977 was 6.3 beds per 1,000 population, of which 5.0 beds per 1,000 were in general hospitals. Although the United States has a smaller supply of general hospital beds per 1,000 than several other countries with cooperative health-care systems, the U.S. rate of admissions to general hospitals in 1977 was quite high—167.2 per 1,000 persons per year—and the average length of stay was quite short.

In the United States, as of 1981, only 27 percent of the general short-stay hospital beds were in institutions owned by governmental agencies. Among the 73 percent of general hospital beds that are privately sponsored, 65 percent are under the auspices of nonprofit bodies (both religious and nonsectarian), and 8 percent are proprietary (for profit). In the late 1970s and the 1980s, however, a growing proportion of hospitals came under the control of for-profit corporations. This increasing "corporatization" or commercialization of American health services has been a source of mounting concern among many medical leaders.

There are two principal types of institutions (other than the private physician's office) that diagnose and treat patients not requiring bed care. These are hospital outpatient clinics and freestanding health centers. Outpatient departments (OPDs) are important in the United States largely as a setting for consultation with specialists and for ambulatory care to poor and/or uninsured patients. Beyond the OPD, a major organized resource for the provision of ambulatory care is the health center.

In the entrepreneurial setting of the United States, health centers were first established in the 1920s as facilities for coordinated provision of preventive services—often by separate governmental agencies for promotion of maternal and child health, for the control of tuberculosis, for hygienic education, and so on. They later came to house official public health agencies. Attempts to extend their scope to provision of medical treatment of the poor were successfully resisted by private physicians, on the ground that this would constitute improper invasion of the sphere of private medicine. Not until the 1960s was the role of the health center in the United States broadened to include general ambulatory medical care for selected population groups. Very poor families in urban slums were the main beneficiaries, but special units—often called simply clinics—were established for migratory farm workers, for residents of blighted Appalachian areas, for low-income children and youth, for American Indians, and for others. Special government subsidies supported these health centers under federal laws.

The health centers just described limit their services essentially to primary health care, including both its preventive and therapeutic aspects. Another important type of freestanding facility in the United States is the private group practice clinic, in which a number of doctors, usually of different specialties, join together as a team to provide a broad range of ambulatory services. In 1975 there were about 8,500 of these private units, far more than the approximately 1,000 health centers supported by governmental grants. Other facilities for organized ambulatory care are focused on industrial workers (supported by management) and on school children (supported usually by educational authorities), but these are devoted essentially to prevention and case detection. Public health agencies, of course, also sponsor clinics for venereal disease control (including treatment), for dental care of children, and so on, and in recent years some of these clinics have broadened their scope to general primary care.

Health Commodities

A third essential type of health resource in any health-care system is a wide variety of equipment for the diagnosis and treatment of disease, supplies for prevention as well as treatment, prosthetic appliances including eyeglasses and hearing aids, dental prostheses, and, perhaps most important, drugs.

Drugs in the economically developed countries are, with few exceptions, produced by pharmaceutical companies and then distributed to the population through large numbers of pharmacies or general health-care facilities (hospitals and health centers). In the permissive health-care system of the United States, the pharmaceutical industry contains hundreds of firms, although about twenty major companies sell most of the products. Newly discovered or invented drugs are protected by patents (which endure for seventeen years) so that they are sold under "brand names," which may command high prices. After a patent expires, the drug's nonpatented or "generic name" may be used to identify the product sold by any manufacturer.

With many companies engaged in drug manufacturing, there is a great deal of advertising to win the preference of physicians. There may be, for example, scores or hundreds of different drugs to combat insomnia and induce sleep, often with very little difference among them—sometimes no difference except their names and perhaps their color or packaging. It has been estimated that more than 25 percent of the price paid by the pharmacist for drugs is attributable to the manufacturer's advertising costs. On top of this, the patient must pay the middleman costs of the pharmacist and sometimes a wholesale distributor. Moreover, since pharmacies must each respond to the prescription orders of numerous doctors, they keep on hand sizable stocks of diverse products, which is very costly. To avoid this problem, many hospitals prepare a drug formulary, which lists only a few hundred drugs that are regularly available in the hospital pharmacy.

The enormous multiplicity of drug preparations in a permissive free enterprise setting has created a number of problems. Beyond substantial expenditures of advertising and pharmacy inventories, there have been several occasions in which firms have been found guilty of collusion to fix prices. Further, with the freedom of hundreds of pharmaceutical companies to manufacture drugs and, formerly, the freedom to make grandiose claims about their benefits, there were bound to be abuses that led sometimes to serious tragedies. As a result, the U.S. government has been stimulated to enact a sequence of "pure food and drug control" laws and regulations, which have greatly restricted the freedom of drug manufacturers.

There has also been virtually complete freedom to establish pharmacies in the United States. As a result, there are about 51,000 drugstores, or one for every 4,500 population—a ratio greatly in excess of need. (Most drugstores have several pharmacists.) To survive economically, the average drugstore must sell many products other than drugs. This may offer certain conveniences for people, but it means that much of the pharmacist's education is wasted, and other functions that might be performed by pharmacies, such as health education or certain routine screening tests, are not done.

Health Knowledge

In the U.S. health-care system, research on countless medical problems is done at every medical school (about 135 institutions) and at many other university departments or schools related to the health sciences. The topics to be investigated have customarily been determined by each scientist, according to his personal interests. In the early decades of the twentieth century, philanthropic bodies like the Rockefeller Foundation gave grants to universities for medical research and conducted such research itself (at Rockefeller Institute). The federal government operated a relatively small Hygienic Laboratory for investigating selected problems of communicable disease. Most biomedical research, however, was done by medical faculty members, often in university-affiliated hospitals.

Since about 1940, these research policies have been changed in order to encourage research on problems of special public interest, and the federal government has provided an increasing volume of research grants in selected fields. At the same time, national research institutes have been established for governmental work in these fields. The National Cancer Institute, for example, conducts research on a wide range of problems relevant to cancer and also makes hundreds of grants each year to private investigators.

Aside from government-funded research, conducted mainly (but not solely) by universities, pharmaceutical companies conduct a substantial amount of research on drugs and their effects on disease. These companies also give grants to medical scientists and clinicians, who are asked to investigate new products. Clinical research (i.e., on patients) must be carried out under strictly prescribed conditions to protect the welfare of all "human subjects." With respect to sociomedical (as distinguished from biomedical) research, many governmental grants go to nonacademic firms devoted to health-care management or administration.

Sources of Economic Support

Most of the discussion of the organizational structure of health programs has explicitly or implicitly made reference to the sources of economic support. Governmental health programs are suported mainly by tax revenues, and voluntary agencies are supported mainly by charitable donations. Private market providers of health care, on the other hand, may be supported by complex combinations of payments by private families, tax revenues from one branch of government, social insurance from another branch, voluntary insurance, and still other sources. This section will assess the different kinds of economic support found in the U.S. health-care system.

Quantitative data on the various sources of economic support for its health-care system are relatively abundant in the United States. These have been gathered both by household surveys and by soliciting information directly from major sources, such as voluntary insurance programs and government agencies.

In 1983, the U.S. population spent directly or indirectly about $355.4 billion on the health-care system. This included expenditures for all components of the system discussed in this chapter, except the education of health manpower (in the U.S. "national accounts," these expenditures are included as part of the education sector). It included both recurrent and capital expenditures that year; recurrent costs, of course, were far greater than capital. This large outlay amounted to 10.8 percent of the gross national product (GNP), a percentage that has been rising steadily for the last half-century.

The sources of these large health expenditures reflect a great deal about the sociopolitical characteristics of the U.S. health-care system. The great bulk of them are for health services, accounting in 1981 for 95.3 percent of the total (the balance of 4.7 percent was for medical research and construction of health facilities). Their distribution in 1980 was as follows:

Source	Percent
Personal individuals and families	32.4
Charitable donations	1.0
Management of enterprises	0.3
Voluntary health insurance	26.6
All private	(60.3)
Social insurance	14.4
Federal government revenues	14.2
State and local government revenues	11.0
All public	(39.6)
All sources	100.0

In very broad terms, it is evident that approximately 60 percent of all U.S. health service expenditures comes from private sources (or the private sector), and 40 percent comes from all public or public sector sources. These relationships epitomize the permissiveness of the U.S. health-care system and help to explain many aspects of its delivery patterns, to be discussed below. As the cost of care has risen, however, the trend has been toward a diminishing role for private household spending and an enlarging role for the major collective mechanisms: voluntary insurance, social insurance, and government revenues.

The seven sources of economic support listed above are actually very crude. For example, the "personal individuals and family" source refers to out-of-pocket expenditures, including repayment of personal loans, but does not include personal payment of insurance premiums. A large share of out-of-pocket expenditures goes to payment for ambulatory medical and dental care, and for drugs, which are not very well buffered by either voluntary or social insurance. Personal expenditures include the cost-sharing requirements under insurance (e.g., deductible amounts or copayments), as well as the payment of charges not protected by insurance at all.

The very small percentage of funds derived from charitable donations may appear surprising, particularly insofar as it includes money spent by large philanthropic foundations (Rockefeller, Ford, Johnson, etc.) on health projects, as well as the donations of small sums to voluntary health agencies by millions of people. In absolute terms, the voluntary donations from charitable sources for health purposes have risen over the years, but the rise of expenditures from the other sources has been much greater—hence, the small percentage. The same applies basically to expenditures by the management of enterprises for the health protection of workers.

The source of funds identified as voluntary health insurance is composed of hundreds of separate organizations. Commercial insurance companies selling policies for health care number around one thousand, and nonprofit Blue Cross and Blue Shield plans paying for hospital and doctor's care number about 120. Other insurance organizations—variously characterized as "prepaid health plans" or "health maintenance organizations" or by other terms—amount to about another 500 entities. The great majority of people protected by these insurance programs are covered through their employment, and the premiums payable are typically shared between employee and employer—the latter often pays the greater share or even the entire amount. The percentages of persons covered by different types of insurance organizations in the United States in 1982 were approximately as follows:

Commercial insurance companies	50
Blue Cross and Blue Shield	35
Prepaid health plans	15
All types of insurance	100

Social insurance in the U.S. health-care system has three major components. One is the mandatory hospital insurance for the aged and disabled beneficiaries of the social security program. Second is the nonmandatory but governmental insurance for doctor's care and certain other medical services for the same population of elderly persons. Together these two are known as Medicare, which is administered by the federal government with the assistance of about 150 private "fiscal intermediaries" who make the direct payments to hospitals, doctors, and others. Much smaller in their total expenditures are the 50 state programs of "worker's compensation" for occupational injuries or illnesses; each of these is different, but a common feature is the payment of insurance premiums by employers. The expenditures relevant here are those made for medical purposes, and not for wage replacements during disability.

Government revenues, as a source of health expenditures, include taxation levied at several political levels. The breakdown in 1980 was roughly 56 percent from federal government sources, and 44 percent from state and local government sources. The major health function, on which both federal and state revenues are spent, is for the medical care of the poor, principally through Medicaid. Federal taxation revenues are derived mainly from individual and corporate income taxes. State revenues come mainly from income and sales taxes. Local government revenues are derived mainly from taxes on property (real estate). The long-term trends have been toward an increase in the federal share of governmental health expenditures, although in recent years (under the Reagan administration) this trend has changed.

The health purposes for which the funds from these several sources are spent are varied. Hospital care, for example, is supported predominantly by voluntary insurance and by social insurance; drugs and dental care are supported predominantly by individuals and families; public health activities (largely preventive) are supported predominantly by government revenues. Physician's care is supported by significant shares from all major sources of funding. The total matrix of economic sources and health purposes in the U.S. health-care system is extremely complex, but the distribution of overall expenditures for different health purposes (from all economic sources) in 1980 was as follows:

Health Purpose	**Percent of Expenditure**
Hospital care (all types)	40.3
Skilled nursing home care	8.4
Physician's care (ambulatory and inpatient)	18.9
Dental care	6.4
Drugs and supplies	7.8
Other personal health care	6.3
Health-care insurance administration	4.2
Public health services	3.0
Medical research	2.2
Health facility construction	2.5
All purposes	100.0

Trends in the above percentages have been toward devotion of increasing shares of the total expenditures to care in hospitals and nursing homes. As a share of GNP, the total expenditures for health purposes have also tended to rise.

Management of Health-Care Systems

Just as financing is essential for the support of health-care systems, so is management. System management in this context is regarded as including four major activities: planning, administration, regulation, and evaluation. Each of these activities is closely related to the others. Problems of terminology, furthermore, may result in a certain action being regarded as deliberate planning in one system, normal administration in a second system, and official regulation in a third. It will be clearest, therefore, to consider all four of these aspects of management together, as they are practiced in the health-care system of the United States.

In the permissive United States, all four aspects of managment stress local responsibility and private sponsorship. The role of government, in general, is kept to a minimum. In the United States, planning for health or any other purposes was so long identified with Soviet communism that it did not appear in any national health legislation until the end of World War II. In 1946, the national Hospital Survey and Construction Act (Hill-Burton) required that federal grants to the states for hospital construction be conditional on the preparation by the state of the "master plan," in which each hospital would theoretically have a designated role in a regionalized system. Not until 1967 did health planning go beyond this, to consider other resources and services, through a program of federal grants to some 200 local "comprehensive health planning" agencies. These bodies were mainly advisory and, in 1974, legislation was enacted to give local health planning agencies greater powers, particularly with respect to hospital construction. Very significantly, however, these local agencies were almost entirely nongovernmental, and very few of them had connections with local departments of health.

The U.S. comprehensive health planning law of 1967 was passed as a sequel to the first national social insurance program for medical care of the aged (Medicare) and the largest public medical care program for the poor (Medicaid). It would seem significant that the need for general health planning was not appreciated until a substantial amount of health money was to pass through government channels. With such public visibility of health expenditures, there was political concern that the funds be wisely spent.

In a sense, any deliberate governmental or nongovernmental action in which resources are to be allocated in some systematic way (outside the mechanisms of the free market) constitutes planning. In this sense, health planning in the United States and elsewhere can be traced to the establishment of the first hospital or the organization of the first department of public health. As customarily used, however, health planning applies to the actions of an agency that functions over and above the health resources and health organizations themselves, exerting an influence on their course of action. In this sense, health planning in the United States has been very weak indeed. Insofar as it has had any noticeable influence, it has been confined to the construction of hospitals, and the decisions have been made by agencies that are both local and nongovernmental. Insofar as the national government has played a part, it has been to issue "guidelines," not regulations or official standards.

General health administration in the United States, like health planning, is characterized by decentralization and voluntarism. This goes beyond the constitutional requirements of state sovereignty. In the Medicare program, for example, the law might have authorized payments to health-care providers through branch offices of the federal government; instead, payments are made to (and relationships maintained with) providers by numerous fiscal intermediaries, which are not only local bodies but in every instance nongovernmental. Likewise, many federally authorized and financed health programs are implemented by grants to local agencies, below the level of the 50 state governments. There are about 3,1000 county governments and a much larger number of municipal governments, to which such health grants may be made, but a major share of them are voluntary nongovernmental bodies. This applies, for example, to grants for mental health services and grants for various types of community health centers. It applies to federal grants for hospital construction or renovation as well.

To underscore the emphasis on local and nongovernmental decision making, almost all federally supported health programs must be governed or advised by a board of local citizens. Sometimes law requires that a majority of the governing board must be "consumers," rather than "providers" of health care. When some health program standard is issued at the state level, at the local level the standard may typically be applied with great leeway. The policies on the education of doctors and other health personnel are essentially up to each educational institution. Within the structure of state governments, the distribution of authority for health matters is so diverse that no two of the states are exactly alike. Likewise, within local governments, there is nearly always a "department of health," but the exact scope of activities carried out is hardly ever the same in two such departments of the same state or another state. Because of the multiplicity of health agencies at the local and state levels, coordinating councils of various sorts abound—sometimes for health as a whole and sometimes in special fields, such as care of the aged or the promotion of mental health.

Insofar as health administration may be characterized by its "style," it is mainly participatory rather than autocratic in the United States. Both in the private and the public sectors, rewards and advancement go to the supervisor who seeks everyone's opinion before reaching a decision. Meetings are held on every possible occasion to permit maximum discussion of problems. Though some of this democratic style of administration may be more apparent than real, there is no question about the theoretical preferences. National tradition in the United States opposes bureaucracy and glorifies efficiency and informality. In health program administration, this tends to mean delegation of great authority from higher to lower levels, and relatively limited accountability through reporting back to the top. Yet, information systems on health services rendered in a program are relatively well developed—to a great extent because such information serves as a basis for financial support.

Regulation in the U.S. health-care system, somewhat paradoxically, is highly developed. To some extent, because of the easygoing form of administration, problems and abuses have developed; in response, regulations have been imposed to prevent further abuses. This is seen in the licensure of physicians which, prior to about 1870, was extremely loose and permissive; scores of poor-quality medical schools graduated physicians of very limited competence. As a result, the state governments developed their own examinations over and above the academic examinations. Somewhat similar has been the development of a regulatory legislation on drugs. In the nineteenth century, hundreds of uncontrolled pharmaceutical companies made extravagant and unjustified claims about their products. New drugs were put on the market without proper testing of their safety (not to mention their efficacy), resulting in tragic deaths of patients. In response, drug control legislation, first enacted in 1906, has become progressively more rigorous.

With respect to specialization in medicine, regulation in the United States was initiated entirely outside of government. Starting with ophthalmology in 1916, "specialty board certification" was developed in one specialized medical or surgical discipline after another. Soon all the specialty boards came under the general jurisdiction of the nongovernmental American Medical Association—more than 50 fields, counting main specialties and subspecialties. Specific regimes of postgraduate training are required in each field, culminating in examinations. Although entirely private in its management, specialty board certification is recognized fully by government for purposes of reimbursement or eligibility to participate in certain public programs. Regarding basic medical licensure by the states, it is significant that the first action to simplify procedures, through a nationally uniform examination, was also taken by a nongovernmental body, the National Board of Medical Examiners.

Regulation by nongovernmental bodies has shown similar development in other fields. In the U.S. "open staff" hospital before 1920, each doctor was theoretically his own master, free to do almost anything he wished. As a consequence, some extremely poor medical and surgical work was done. In reaction, the hospital medical staffs, themselves, set up by-laws to govern what would be permitted within the hospital. In 1917, the American College of Surgeons, a private society, formulated standards for granting its approval of a hospital's policies (especially the medical staff procedures), and, in 1952, the nongovernmental Joint Commission on Accreditation of Hospitals was organized. Similarly, professional associations established codes of ethics. Health insurance organizations set their own rules and regulations. These were all outside the sphere of government, but their control over individual behavior could be just as great. Often such nongovernmental initiative has been taken deliberately to forestall government regulation. Sometimes a regulatory strategy may itself be abused, as in the case of professional ethics, which have been invoked to inhibit innovations in health-care delivery.

Finally, the judicial system provides a certain type of regulation in the U.S. health-care system. The patient who believes that a physician or hospital has brought him harm may bring suit in a court of law. The outcomes of such lawsuits are unpredictable (especially since they are usually tried by juries, and lawyers may be very skillful in their pleading), so that the great majority of cases are settled out of court. Whether settled or tried in court, lawsuits involve such a costly process that nearly all practicing physicians carry ''malpractice insurance,'' which has become increasingly expensive. Regardless of the merits of most malpractice claims, they have served to induce physicians and hospitals to discipline themselves—another form of self-regulatory response to the whole permissive character of the U.S. health-care system.

Evaluation has also become highly developed in the U.S. health-care system for reasons somewhat similar to those involving regulation. So much freedom has characterized the delivery of health services, and their costs have risen so rapidly, that many people were bound to raise questions about the quality and value of those services. When services became increasingly financed by government or by large groups of people, rather than by individuals, the questions became more insistent. As a response, various methods of evaluation have been developed in the U.S. health services. ''Medical audits'' have been promoted in hospitals, based on reviews of patient records in relation to explicit or implicit quality criteria. Under the national Medicare and Medicaid laws, there have been requirements for ''professional standard reviews'' in every community. Most voluntary health insurance organizations have also developed surveillance procedures to detect cases of improper or unjustified medical service. The line between quality control and cost control is not sharp, but it is clear that the U.S. health-care system has generated many forms of evaluation in pursuit of both objectives.

Delivery of Health Services

The several major components of health-care systems culminate in the encounter between a provider and a recipient of health service. To distinguish this more personal process from the other components of the system, it is customarily called the ''delivery of health services.'' These services may be analyzed as primary, secondary, and tertiary, plus a fourth category, in which all levels of service are directed toward selected populations or selected disorders.

Primary Health Service

Primary health services include a wide range of preventive measures plus first-encounter medical care of the patient with a health-care provider—usually a doctor in the industrialized countries. Preventive measures may be environmental (e.g., water purification), educational, or personal, but here only personal prevention is considered. Common forms of personal preventive measures are immunizations, surveillance of expectant mothers and babies, and adult examinations for detection of chronic diseases.

In the United States, primary health service is delivered predominantly by private physicians in their private offices. Increasing proportions of doctors, however, are joining together in small medical groups or group practices (three or more doctors working together and sharing their income in some way), particularly doctors in various specialties. In 1980, nevertheless, the majority were still in individual practice. The patient ordinarily pays for this service out of pocket; even though most of the population has some health insurance protection, it usually does not pay for ambulatory primary care. In fact, even if there is third-party payment for ambulatory services, as under Medicare, preventive services are specifically excluded. Hence, most immunizations are given by private pediatricians, most prenatal examinations by private obstetricians, and most general medical check-ups by private internists.

There are organized public health clinics for these personal preventive services, but they serve only from 15 to 20 percent of the population, mainly the poor. Children are sometimes immunized in schools, and industrial workers may get routine medical examinations in larger plants. Multiple screening tests may be done at workplaces or elsewhere, and the patient with any positive finding is typically referred to a private physician.

The treatment aspects of primary health service are also most often rendered in private medical offices, typically those of specialists, since general practitioners or family practice specialists constitute only a small fraction of the doctors. Patients of low income, however, frequently seek primary medical care in the outpatient departments of hospitals, most often in the emergency room. Scheduled clinics in various specialties are held only in a small proportion of hospitals, usually in large cities. Since about 1965, various types of community health centers have been established in poverty sections of large cities and in some rural areas. At these units, a wide range of primary services is offered by salaried doctors and allied staffs, although only a small fraction of the overall ambulatory care encounters occur in these settings.

Secondary and Tertiary Health Services

Secondary and tertiary health services are highly developed in the United States, reflecting its permissive health-care system. Until relatively recent times, any community or group that could raise the money to build a hospital was free to do so and to furnish the facility with whatever sophisticated diagnostic or treatment equipment it could afford. The same freedom applied to physicians who could specialize in whatever field they could find postgraduate training, so that more than 85 percent of physicians became specialists. An approach to regionalization of hospital facilities was made in 1946, with the Hospital Survey and Construction Act, and again in 1966, with the Act for Regional Medical Programs on Heart Disease, Cancer and Stroke, but the regionalization concept remains largely a theoretical idea. In reality, almost any patient is free to consult any high-powered specialist for a minor problem (provided he or his insurance can pay the cost), and almost any doctor is free to hospitalize his private patient for diagnosis and treatment that could just as well be given in the office of a general practitioner.

The concept of a pyramidal framework of health service, in which the patient is seen by primary care personnel before access to secondary or tertiary care, is implemented in certain health maintenance organizations (HMOs) in the United States. HMOs, however, cover only about 12 percent of the population. The freewheeling pattern noted above characterizes health-care delivery in the average community. Patients have direct access to specialists in private practice, and only a minority of the average specialist's patients come on referral from another doctor. In general hospitals, medical staff organization is typically "open," so that applications for staff affiliation by most qualified physicians are approved. A general hospital of 100 beds in a city might have 100 physicians and surgeons on its medical staff, although only 10 or 20 of them might have patients hospitalized at any one time. Each doctor is responsible for his own patients, seeking consultation from another staff member only when he deems it appropriate. Because of this great permissiveness and the hazards of improper care, medical staffs in most American hospitals have established numerous self-disciplinary committees—on surgery, drug therapy, length of stay of patients, record-keeping, and so on—to monitor each other.

Traditionally, both hospitals and attending physicians have been reimbursed for inpatient care on a fee basis. Although most physicians are still paid on a fee-for-service basis, a slowly increasing proportion of hospital doctors have become based in the hospital full-time and paid by salary. This has long applied to pathologists and radiologists, but it is becoming more frequent for internists, surgeons, and other specialists who serve as the full-time heads of clinical departments, as heads of outpatient services, continuing medical education, or medical rehabilitation, and in other fields. There are also some HMO hospitals, with entirely full-time salaried medical staffs, similar to those in governmental general hospitals, like the network of the Veterans Administration. Furthermore, government legislation in the early 1980s has begun to shift the method of paying for hospital services from retrospective charges to prospective rates based on the diagnostic category (the diagnosis-related group, or DRG) of each case. In spite of these trends, as of the early 1980s, the open staff general hospital was the norm in America, with only mental hospitals, some special government general hospitals, and institutions attached to medical schools having a full-time salaried "closed staff" of physicians as the usual pattern.

Finally, the large urban public hospital, limited essentially to serving the poor, is an important component of the pattern of delivery for secondary and tertiary care. It is a hangover of the late nineteenth and early twentieth centuries, when programs such as Medicaid were not available to finance the care of the poor in the customary community hospital. With such financial support programs in the mainstream hospital system, these special public hospitals now serve principally low-income patients not eligible for Medicaid or other third-party support. Because of rising costs of hospital maintenance and the restrictions in local revenues (on which most of these hospitals depend), public hospitals for the poor face increasingly chronic financial difficulties.

Care of Special Populations and Disorders

In all types of health-care systems, there are special programs—encompassing primary, secondary, and tertiary care—for the care of certain population groups, and for the control of certain disorders. For various historical and political reasons, as well as for economy and efficiency, special forms of delivery of health care have been developed for these populations and disorders.

In the U.S. health-care system, where private buying and selling of health service is the norm, it is noteworthy that military personnel are served by a highly structured and comprehensive health-care program, financed entirely by government funds. The army, navy, air force, and marines each has its own network of health facilities—hospitals, clinics, and field posts. All personnel are public employees, salaried according to their military ranks (without relation to the specific services they render). The same basic structure prevails in times of war or peace. Health promotion and illness prevention are emphasized and integrated with the delivery of treatment services. Even after retirement, high-ranking officers continue to be entitled to these comprehensive services, without personal costs. If service of a highly specialized type is needed, but available only at a distant place, the patient will be transported there promptly; if this resource is private, the bill is paid by the military establishment.

After military service, the U.S. veteran becomes entitled to a remarkably broad range of medical care. If a disorder is connected with military service, its care is a responsibility of the federal Veterans Administration for life. For any other disorder suffered by the veteran, hospital care is provided through a nationwide network of Veterans Administration facilities, which are usually affiliated with medical schools to ensure high quality, so long as the veteran states it would cause him financial hardship to obtain the care privately. Normally, about 75 percent of Veterans Administration hospital beds are occupied by veterans with conditions unrelated to military service. The United States is unique in supporting so broad a scope of health services for veterans—a fact doubtless related to the lack of a national health insurance program for the general population.

A similarly comprehensive range of services is provided to American Indians through special facilities on or near Indian reservations. Originally, these public services were managed by the Bureau of Indian Affairs in the Department of Interior, but in the 1950s they were transferred for administration by the U.S. Public Health Service.

Other programs for health care of special populations in the United States include those for railroad workers, for employees of special projects such as the Tennessee Valley Authority, or for migratory farm workers. Merchant seamen are another population for whom a special network of federal hospitals has long been operated at major port cities. Special programs for industrial workers and school children have been noted already, and in colleges and universities the scope of health services for students is typically comprehensive. In contrast to customary U.S. patterns of health-care delivery, through private medical and allied practitioners, services in all these programs are provided by salaried personnel working in organized frameworks.

Among disorders, for which special subsystems of health-care delivery are organized in the United States, mental illness is probably the most important. A large share of ambulatory psychiatric care is, indeed, provided by individual psychiatrists in the mainstream of private medical practice, but a substantial amount of such care is furnished to low-income patients through thousands of special mental health clinics, under public or voluntary auspices. These clinics typically are staffed by teams of psychiatrists, psychologists, social workers, nurses, and others—all working on a salary basis. Hospitalization for mental illness occurs predominantly in special mental hospitals, financed and operated by state governments (although general hospitals have been increasingly admitting short-term patients with psychiatric diagnoses). Tuberculosis, before its steep decline in incidence and prevalence, also warranted a special network of clinics and hospitals (sanatoriums) for its detection and care.

Looking Ahead

The highly permissive and pluralistic character of the U.S. health-care system suggests the character of its major problems. There is a broad consensus that health-care costs have risen excessively and much too rapidly. The free market in medical care has been so uncontrolled, even for services paid for by governmental insurance, that prices have spiraled to much higher levels than the general consumer price index. The Medicare program for medical care for the aged, for example, permits the doctor (by not "accepting assignment") to charge the patient any fee he wishes. Hospital charges have become particularly high as hospital technology has increased, hospital personnel per patient have multiplied, and salaries have risen.

With the escalation of costs, access of the lower income groups to needed care has become more difficult. Government programs to finance care for the poor, like Medicaid, have been cut back both at the federal and state levels. Even in the social insurance Medicare program, copayments required from the patient have increased so that the elderly have had to pay an increasing out-of-pocket share of the cost of their care. The political environment established by the Reagan administration in the 1980s has promoted reduction in public expenditures for all human services and much greater reliance on private sector financing.

A special aspect of the current political ideology has been a striking privatization of the health-care industry. Voluntary nonprofit hospitals, which serve better-off patients, have been acquired by commercial hospital chains. Voluntary and even public hospitals have been turned over to management by private corporations, in the expectation that this will enhance efficiency and productivity. Up to this writing, evidence of such effects has not been demonstrated, and some studies have shown higher costs associated with commercialization of hospital services.

To stem the tide of rising medical and hospital costs, major reliance has been on promoting competition among providers. The new ''preferred provider organization'' (PPO), for example, is a mechanism by which groups of doctors and/or hospitals agree to serve certain public or private beneficiaries at competitively lower prices. For some years, the prepaid HMO has shown the economies achievable by modification of physician incentives, especially with regard to hospital use, and now a number of variations on the HMO theme are being explored. Although competition is politically favored in preference to regulation, the very largest innovation in public medical care policy has been essentially regulatory. This has been the introduction of prospective payment to hospitals according to the DRG of each patient under Medicare, and, in some states for all insurance payers, rather than by charges retrospectively for each unit of service.

While the pressure of rising costs has been responsible for many of the changes being seen in the U.S. health-care system, long-term forces with broader objectives than cost containment continue to have an impact. The movement for social financing of health care, to ensure its availability to everyone, continues. Legislation for national health insurance lost the priority position it held in the 1970s, but there can be no doubt that it will move forward again. Hawaii enacted mandatory state health insurance in 1975, and other states may follow suit, along the lines that led to national legislation in Canada. Much depends, however, on which political party holds national power.

The enthusiastic promotion of prevention and sound lifestyle, which has occupied center stage in recent years, is likely to continue. It is unlikely that this policy will result in a lower need for medical care, however. As men and women live longer, due to the prevention or postponement of both communicable and noncommunicable diseases, they live on to the age when cancer or other disorders strike. Moreover, they live on with hypertension, diabetes, glaucoma, arthritis, cardiovascular problems, and other disorders that are not cured but are controlled by good medical care. Maintenance of the quality of life in the company of chronic disease is quite possible, but it has its costs.

Continuing specialization and technological advancements render the solo medical practitioner increasingly obsolete. Despite the ideology of individual freedom for health-care professionals, the grouping of doctors, nurses, technicians, and others in teams—under either public or private auspices—can be expected to continue. The increasing organization of health-care delivery suggests that fee-for-service payments will be replaced by various social mechanisms of financing and that all personnel, including doctors, will eventually be paid salaries based on their qualifications, responsibilities, and their hours of work. The perverse incentives of fees-per-medical act will be replaced by incentives to win the respect of one's peers.

All this means more deliberate planning of the U.S. health-care system, more rational regulation to promote quality and avert abuse, and strategies to help ensure that each person receives the health services he or she requires. The World Health Organization goal of Health for All by the year 2000 should certainly be attainable in the United States. The heterogeneity and pluralism of the U.S. health culture will not vanish, but organization and coordination are capable of achieving harmonious performance and equity in the future.

References

Cambridge Research Institute. 1976. *Trends Affecting the U.S. Health Care System*. Washington, D.C.: Government Printing Office.

Davis, Karen. 1975. National Health Insurance—Benefits, Costs, and Consequences. Washington, D.C.: Brookings Institution.

Donabedian, Avedis, Solomon J. Axelrod, and Leon Wyszewianski. 1980. *Medical Care Chartbook*. Ann Arbor, Mich.: Health Administration Press.

Freyman, J. G. 1974. *The American Health Care System: Its Genesis and Trajectory*. Baltimore, Md.: Williams and Wilkins.

Goodman, L. J. and A. R. Mason. 1978. *Physician Distribution and Licensure in the United States*. Chicago: American Medical Association.

Gray, B. H., ed. 1983. *The New Health Care for Profit: Doctors and Hospitals in a Competitive Environment*. Washington, D.C.: National Academy Press.

Health Insurance Association of America. 1983. *Source Book of Health Insurance Data 1982–1983*. Washington, D.C.: The Association.

Jonas, Steven, ed. 1981. *Health Care Delivery in the United States*. Second ed. New York: Springer Publishing.

Kane, Robert L. et al., eds. 1976. *The Health Gap—Medical Services and the Poor*. New York: Springer Publishing.

Kovner, A. R. and D. Neuhauser, eds. 1986. *Health Services Management—Readings and Commentary*. Third ed. Ann Arbor, Mich.: Health Administration Press.

Lave, Judith R. and Lester B. Lave. 1974. *The Hospital Construction Act: An Evaluation of the Hill-Burton Program, 1942–1973*. Washington, D.C.: American Enterprise Institute.

Levey, Samuel and N. P. Loomba. 1973. *Health Care Administration: A Managerial Perspective*. Philadelphia: J. B. Lippincott.

Levin, Arthur, ed. 1980. *Regulating Health Care*. New York: Academy of Political Science.

Marmor, T. R. 1973. *The Politics of Medicare*. Chicago: Aldine Publishing.

Roemer, Milton I. 1978. *Special Medicine: The Advance of Organized Health Services in America*. New York: Springer Publishing.

———. 1981. *Ambulatory Health Services in America: Past, Present, and Future*. Rockville, Md.: Aspen Corporation.

Roemer, Ruth, C. Kramer, and J. E. Frink. 1975. *Planning Urban Health Services—from Jungle to System*. New York: Springer Publishing.

Roemer, Ruth and George McKray, eds. 1980. *Legal Aspects of Health Policy: Issues and Trends*. Westport, Conn.: Greenwood Press.

Saward, E. W., ed. 1976. *Regionalization of Personal Health Services*. Revised ed. New York: Prodist.

Shonick, William. 1976. *Elements of Planning for Area-Wide Personal Health Services*. St. Louis, Mo.: C. V. Mosby.

Sidel, Victor W. and Ruth Sidel. 1983. *A Healthy State: An International Perspective on the Crisis in United States Medical Care*. New York: Pantheon Books.

Silverman, Milton and P. R. Lee. 1974. *Pills, Profits, and Politics*. Berkeley, Calif.: University of California Press.

Somers, Anne R. 1971. *Health Care in Transition—Directions for the Future*. Chicago: Hospital Research and Education Trust.

Starr, Paul. 1982. *The Social Transformation of American Medicine*. New York: Basic Books.

Stern, Bernhard J. 1946. *Medical Services by Government: Local, State, and Federal*. New York: Commonwealth Fund.

Stevens, Rosemary. 1971. *American Medicine and the Public Interest*. New Haven, Conn.: Yale University Press.

U.S. Public Health Service. 1979. *Health Status of Minorities and Low Income Groups*. Washington, D.C. (DHEW Pub. HRA 79–625).

———. 1979. *Healthy People: The Surgeon General's Report on Health Promotion and Disease Prevention*. Washington, D.C. (DHEW PHS Pub. No. 79–55071).

———. 1984. *Health: United States, 1984*. Washington, D.C.: National Center for Health Statistics (DHHS Pub. No. PHS 85–1232).

Zubkoff, Michael, ed. 1976. *Health: A Victim or Cause of Inflation?* New York: Prodist.

BIBLIOGRAPHY

General Resource Materials

Organization for Economic and Community Development. *Measuring Health Care 1960–1983: Expenditures, Costs, and Performance*. Paris: OECD, 1985.

UNESCO. *Statistical Yearbook*. Paris: UNESCO, various years.

United Nations Department of International Economic and Social Affairs. *Demographic Yearbook*. New York: UNDIESA, various years.

———. *Population and Vital Statistics Report*. New York: UNDIESA, various years.

The World Bank. *World Development Report*. New York: Oxford University Press, various years.

World Health Organization. *Primary Health Care: Report of the International Conference on Primary Health Care, Alma-Ata, USSR, 6–12 September 1978. Geneva: WHO, 1978.*

———. *World Health Statistics Annual*. WHO: Geneva, 1986.

———. *Health Services in Europe*. Regional Office for Europe, third ed. Copenhagen: 1981.

Comparative Studies and Monographs

Abel-Smith, B. *Cost Containment in Health Care: The Experience of 12 European Countries (1977–1983)*. Brussels: Commission of the European Communities, 1984.

———. *Value for Money in Health Services*. London: Heinemann, 1976.

Banta, H. D and K. B. Kemp, eds. *The Management of Health Care Technology in Nine Countries*. New York: Springer Publishing Company, 1982.

Blanpain, J., L. Delesie, and H. Nys. *National Health Insurance and Health Resources: The European Experience*. Cambridge, Mass.: Harvard University Press, 1978.

Bridgman, R. *Hospital Utilization: An International Study*. Oxford: Oxford University Press, 1979.

Culyer, A. J., ed. *Health and Health Indicators*. Oxford: Martin Robertson, 1983.

de Kervasdoue, J., J. Kimberly, and V. Rodwin, eds. *The End of an Illusion: The Future of Health Policy in Western Industrialized Nations*. Berkeley, Calif.: University of California Press, 1984.

Douglas-Wilson, I. and G. McLachlan, eds. *Health Services Prospects: An International Survey*. London: Nuffield Provincial Hospital Trust, 1974.

Elling, R. H. *Cross-National Study of Health Systems: Political Economies and Health Care*. New Brunswick, N.J.: Transaction Books, 1980.

Fry, J. and W. Farndale. *International Medical Care: A Comparison and Evaluation of Medical Care Throughout the World*. Wallingford, Pa.: Washington Square East, 1972.

Glaser, W. A. *Health Insurance Bargaining*. New York: Gardner Press, 1978.

———. *Paying the Doctor: Systems of Remuneration and Their Effects*. Baltimore, Md.: Johns Hopkins Press, 1970.

Ingman, S. R. and A. E. Thomas, eds. *Topias and Utopias in Health: Policy Studies*. Chicago: Aldine Publishing, 1975.

Kaser, M. *Health Care in the Soviet Union and Eastern Europe*. London: Croom Helm, 1976.

Kohn, R. and K. White, eds. *Health Care: An International Study*. London: Oxford University Press, 1976.

Leichter, H. M. *A Comparison Approach to Policy Analysis: Health Care Policy in Four Nations*. Cambridge: Cambridge University Press, 1979.

McLachlan, G. and A. Maynard. *The Public/Private Mix for Health*. London: Nuffield Provincial Hospital Trust, 1982.

Maxwell, R. *Health and Wealth*. Lexington, Mass.: Lexington Books, 1981.

Maynard, A. *Health Care in the European Community*. London: Croom Helm, 1975.

Mizrahi, A., Sandier, A., and S. Sandier. *Medical Care, Morbidity and Costs*. Oxford: Pergamon Press France, 1983.

OECD. *Financing and Delivering Health Care: A Comparative Analysis of OECD Countries*. Paris: OECD, 1987.

Raffel, Marshall, ed. *Comparative Health Systems*. State Park, Pa.: Pennsylvania State University Press, 1984.

Roemer, M. *Comparative National Policies on Health Care*. New York: Marcel Dekker, 1977.

———. *Health Care Systems in World Perspective*. Ann Arbor, Mich.: Health Administration Press, 1976.

Roemer, M. I. and R. Roemer. *Health Care Systems and Comparative Manpower Policies*. Los Angeles: University of California Press, 1981.

Sokolowska, M. et al., eds. *Health, Medicine, Society: Proceedings of the International Conference on the Sociology of Medicine, Warsaw (Jablonna) August 20–25, 1973*. Dordrecht, the Netherlands and Boston: D. Reidel, 1976.

INDEX

ABOUT THE EDITOR AND CONTRIBUTORS

SHLOMO BARNOON, Ph.D., is Senior Lecturer and Director of the Division of Health Economics and Administration, Health Sciences Center, Ben Gurion University, Beersheba, Israel.

FRITZ BESKE, M.D., is Director of the Institute for Health Systems Research, Kiel, FRG.

PAUL O. CHUKE, M.D., formerly Professor of Medicine at the University of Nigeria, is Program Manager for General Health Protection and Promotion in the Regional Office for Africa of the World Health Association.

M. RAHMI DIRICAN, M.D., D.P.H., is Professor of Public Health in the Department of Public Health, Uludag University Medical School, Bursa, Turkey.

ADRIENNE EPSTEIN, R.N., M.P.H., is Director of Nursing at a neighborhood health center in Boston, Massachusetts, USA.

PAUL EPSTEIN, M.D., M.P.H., is a family practice physician at The Cambridge Hospital, Cambridge, Massachusetts, and an Instructor of Medicine at Harvard Medical School, Cambridge, Massachusetts, USA.

MARK G. FIELD, Ph.D., is Professor of Sociology at Boston University, and a Fellow in the Russian Research Center as well as a Lecturer in the Department of Health Policy and Management, School of Public Health, at Harvard, Boston, and Cambridge, Massachusetts, USA.

IVÁN FORGÁCS, M.D., is Director of the Institute of Social Medicine in the Postgraduate School of Medicine, Budapest, Hungary.

JÜRGEN GROSSER, M.D., is Prorektor for Medicine at the Bereich Medizin (Charité) Der Humboldt-Universität zu Berlin, Berlin, GDR.

STEPHEN HARRISON, Ph.D., is Lecturer in Health Services Organization in the Department of Social Policy and Health Services Studies at the University of Leeds, England.

DIANA JELLEY, M.D., is a family practice physician in northern England.

MARLOW KWITKO, M.D., M.P.H., formerly Secretary of Medical Services of the Ministry of Social Security, now works as Special Associate of the Secretary of Health in the state of Santa Catarina in Florianópolis, Brazil.

MAREK LUBICZ, Ph.D., is Assistant Professor at the Institute for Organization and Management of the Technical Institute of Wroclaw, Poland.

EVA JANE McHAN, Ph.D., is Assistant Professor in the Department of Community Medicine, College of Medicine, King Saud University, Riyadh, Saudi Arabia.

JEREMIAH NORRIS is Program Officer for the Pritech Project at Management Sciences for Health, in Washington, D.C., USA.

JOSEPH S. PLISKIN is Professor in the Department of Industrial and Management Engineering and Deputy Rector at Ben Gurion University, Beersheba, Israel.

JULIUS B. RICHMOND, M.D., a former Surgeon General of the United States, is Director of the Division of Health Policy Research and Education at Harvard University, Boston, Massachusetts, USA.

ELEUTÉRIO RODRIGUEZ NETO, M.D., is Director of the Public Health Center of the University of Brasilía and Technical Assistant of the Gabinete Civil da Presidencia da Republica in the Ministry of Health, Brasilía, Brazil.

MILTON I. ROEMER, M.D., is Professor of Health Services at the University of California, Los Angeles, California, USA.

ADRIAN A. DE ROO, Ph.D., is Professor in the Department of Health Care Organization in the Faculty of Medicine of Erasmus University, Rotterdam, Netherlands.

RICHARD B. SALTMAN, Ph.D., is Associate Professor in The Program in Health Policy and Management of the Division of Public Health, University of Massachusetts at Amherst, USA.

ANDRÉS A. SANTAS, M.D., was Professor of Surgery, Dean of the School of Public Health, and Rector of the University of Buenos Aires, Argentina.

PEDRO, J. SATURNO, M.D., M.P.H., is Subdirector for Health Planning and Human Resources in the Ministry of Health, Madrid, Spain.

WILLIAM E. STESLICKE, Ph.D., is Associate Professor in the College of Public Health of the Univeristy of South Florida, Tampa, USA.

ABRAAM SONIS, M.D., D.P.H., is Director of the School of Public Health at the University of Buenos Aires, and Advisor to the Minister of Public Health.

W. CEZARY WLODARCZYK, Ph.D., is Head of the Organization and Management Section, Institute of Occupational Medicine and Senior Lecturer in Health Management at the Medical Academy, Lodz, Poland.

FRANCISCO J. YEPES LUJAN, M.D., M.P.H., directs a Child Health Program in the Ministry of Health, Bogotá, Colombia.

JOHN G. YOUNGMAN, M.S.S.C., M.P.H., is Deputy Medical Superintendent of the Royal Brisbane Hospital, Herston, Queensland, Australia.